Rasayana

Traditional Herbal Medicines for Modern Times

Each volume in this series provides academia, health sciences and the herbal medicines industry with in-depth coverage of the herbal remedies for infectious diseases, certain medical conditions or the plant medicines of a particular country.

Edited by Dr Roland Hardman

Volume 1
Shengmai San, edited by Kam-Ming Ko

Volume 2
Rasayana, by H.S. Puri

Rasayana

Ayurvedic herbs for longevity and rejuvenation

H.S. Puri

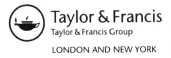
Taylor & Francis
Taylor & Francis Group

LONDON AND NEW YORK

First published 2003
by Taylor & Francis
11 New Fetter Lane, London EC4P 4EE

Simultaneously published in the USA and Canada
by Taylor & Francis Inc,
29 West 35th Street, New York, NY 10001

Taylor & Francis is an imprint of the Taylor & Francis Group

Typeset in 11/13pt Garamond 3 by Graphicraft Limited, Hong Kong
Printed and bound in Great Britain by
TJ International Ltd, Padstow, Cornwall

Every effort has been made to ensure that the advice and information in
this book is true and accurate at the time of going to press. However,
neither the publisher nor the authors can accept any legal responsibility or
liability for any errors or omissions that may be made. In the case of drug
administration, any medical procedure or the use of technical equipment
mentioned within this book, you are strongly advised to consult the
manufacturer's guidelines.

British Library Cataloguing in Publication Data
A catalogue record for this book is available from the British Library

Library of Congress Cataloging in Publication Data
A catalog record has been requested

ISBN 0-415-28489-9

Contents

Foreword   viii
Preface to the series   xii
Preface   xv

 1 Introduction   1

 2 What are *Rasayana*?   4

 3 *Tridosha*   10

 4 *Rasayana* preparations   13

 5 Aak (*Calotropis* spp.)   16

 6 Akrakara (*Anacyclus pyrethrum*)   20

 7 Amalaki (*Phyllanthus emblica*)   22

 8 Anantmul (*Hemidesmus indicus*)   43

 9 Ashwagandha (*Withania somnifera*)   46

10 Badam (*Prunus amygdalus*)   59

11 Bala (*Sida* spp.)   64

12 Banslochan   71

13 Bhalatak (*Semecarpus anacardium*)   74

14 Bhringraj (*Eclipta prostrata*)   80

15 Bhuiamla (*Phyllanthus* spp.)   86

16 Brahmi (*Bacopa monnieri*)   94

17 Chitrak (*Plumbago zeylanica*)   98

18 Chuara (*Phoenix dactylifera*)   102

19 Draksha (*Vitis vinifera*)   105

20 Gaduchi (*Tinospora cordifolia*)   107

21 Gokshru (*Tribulus terrestris*)   116

22 Guggal (*Commiphora wightii*)   124

23 Haritaki (*Terminalia chebula*)   135

24 Hing (*Ferula foetida*)   141

25 Jaiphal and Javitri (*Myristica fragrans*)   144

26 Kabab Chini (*Piper cubeba*)   147

27 Kalmegh (*Andrographis paniculata*)   151

28 Kawanch (*Mucuna pruriens*)   157

29 Keshar (*Crocus sativus*)   164

30 Kikar (*Acacia nilotica*)   170

31 Kuchla (*Strychnos nux vomica*)   175

32 Kulanjan (*Alpinia galanga*)   180

33 Kutaki (*Picrorhiza kurrooa*)   184

34 Kuth (*Saussurea Spp.*)   190

35 Malakangani (*Celastrus paniculatus*)   196

36 Mandukparni (*Centella asiatica*)   200

37 Mundi (*Sphaeranthus indicus*)   209

38 Musli (*Curculigo orchioides*)   212

39 Neem (*Azadirachta indica*)   215

40 Peepali (*Piper longum*)   219

41 Punernava (*Boerhavia diffusa*)   227

42 Pushkarmul (*Inula racemosa*)   233

43 Salai Guggal (*Boswellia serrata*)   237

44 Salep (*Orchis latifolia*)   242

45 Semal Musli (*Bombax ceiba*)   247

46 Shankhpushpi (*Convolvulus pluricaulis*)   250

47 Shatawari (*Asparagus racemosus*)   255

48 Som Ras (*Amanita muscaria*)   262

49 Sonth (*Zingiber officinale*)   265

50 Talamkhana (*Hygrophila spinosa*)   270

51 Tulsi (*Ocimum tenuiflorum*)   272

52 Vacha (*Acorus calamus*)   281

53 Vata Vriksh (*Ficus* spp.)   289

54 Vatsnabh (*Aconitum* spp.)   295

55 Vibhitaki (*Terminalia bellirica*)   299

56 Vidari Kand (*Pueraria tuberosa*)   303

57 Vidhara (*Argyreia speciosa*)   309

58 Some *Rasayana* formulations   312

Index   337

Foreword

Ayurveda, the Ancient Science of Hindus and Indians, dates back about 7000 years. It has eight branches, one of which is *Rasayana Tantra*. The word *rasayana* literally means the path that *rasa* takes (rasa: the primordial tissue or plasma; ayana: path) (*Charaka*). It is also considered as the science which restores youth, alleviates suffering (diseases) and bestows longevity (*Sushruta*). It is believed in Ayurveda, that the qualities of the *rasa-dhatu* influence the health of other *dhatus* (tissues) of the body. Hence, any medicine that improves the quality of *rasa* are called as *rasayanas*, resulting in the strengthening or promoting of the qualities and health of all tissues of the body. These *rasayana* plants are said to possess the following properties:

— Prevent ageing
— Re-establish youth
— Strengthen life
— Strengthen brain and mind
— Prevent disease
— Promote healthy longevity

Rasayana Tantra appears to have been practiced as an independent clinical discipline primarily as a positive health medicine. With the passage of time this important branch of knowledge has ceased to be in practice (except the knowledge and use of a few herbs) in its appropriate form. Comprehensive efforts are needed to revive this useful discipline for the welfare of humanity at large.

The ability to adapt to a given habitat is a distinctive feature of all living organisms. Any type of demand (external or internal) in this habitat elicits either a specific or non-specific response (Selye,1983). This non-specific response to any demand has been defined as *stress* and the demand as *stressor* by Hans Selye. As per his description there are three stages of response to any given situation of stress, which together constitute the *general adaptation syndrome* (GAS) (Selye,1946), the stages being a) alarm reaction b) resistance and c) exhaustion. Thus, the ability to develop resistance and to maintain it is crucial for coping with a variety of stressors encountered in human life. The desire to control the coping mechanisms has led to the origin of the *science of adaptation*. The branch of Ayurveda which deals with the *science of adaptation* is called *Rasayana Tantra*. Ayurveda may not coin the term *adaptogen*, but those practices, or substances / herbs / medicines which help a person cope with his day to day stresses are known in Ayurveda as *Rasayanas*. Modern research has proved that herbs listed as *Rasayanas* possess *adaptogenic properties* as well (Dahanukar, 1986.).

All of the above imply that they improve and increase the resistance of the body. The scientific studies carried out on most of the *rasayana* herbs showed that these plants non-specifically activated the reticuloendothelial system (RES) and other components of the immune system as well (Dahanukar, 1986). Knowing that the central nervous system, endocrine system and the immune system participate in intense cross-talk (Ader *et al.*, 1990; Glaser and Kiecolt-Glaser, 1994), it was easy to hypothesize that by acting on the immune system these *rasayanas* could exert broad-based effects by initiating a massive cascade of events involving various neurotransmitters, hormones and amines of the stress response cycle.

With the emerging science of ecogenetics, it is becoming evident that genetic predisposition can alter responses to the external environment. However, at present most of the data is on diseases, which manifest in genetically predisposed persons on exposure to the external stressors. Can *rasayanas* (or adaptogens or immunomodulators) influence genetic control and favour the maintenance of homeostasis in stressful situations? The research on *Amruta* (*Tinospora cordifolia*) opens up a new vision in this direction, as early experiments have shown that it increases the bone marrow proliferative fractions leading to leucocytosis. A slight increase in dose reverses this process and inducing *apoptosis*, and this apparent paradox was believed to be because of its effect on c-myc, a gene that causes both proliferation as well as induces apoptosis depending on the environment. These are some of the recent advances seen in the field of *rasayana drugs*. Looking at it it appears that rasayana herbs act as:

— an adaptogen
— an immunostimulant
— an immunomodulater
— pro-host probiotic
— anti-mutagenic

But Ayurveda has much more in it to be included under *rasayana therapy*. Looking at only a few herbs will be doing an injustice to the holistic approach of Ayurveda, hence a brief description of *Rasayana Tantra* may be necessary here.

According to Ayurvedic concept *rasayana therapy* simultaneously affects the body and the mind and bring about physical and psychic improvement. This therapy prevents the effects of early ageing, develops intelligence and increases the body-resistance against diseases.

Rasayana means vitalizing / rejuvenating. In the words of *Charaka* with a *rasayana*, *one obtains longevity, regains youth, vitality and vigour, gets a sharp memory, intellect and freedom from diseases, gets a lustrous complexion and the strength of a horse.* Sushruta is more specific, describing a *rasayana* as one which, *is anti-ageing, increases life-span, promotes intelligence and memory and increases resistance to disease.*

Any drug, diet or conduct that leads to the replenishment of the *dhatus* and enlivens the body and mind is *rasayana*. *Rasayana* not only rejuvenates the body and mind, it also prevents disease. There are a number of drugs/materials described which possess the qualities of maintaining health, prolonging life and warding off diseases. They are all grouped as *rasayana* in Ayurveda. A close look at the concept of *rasayana* of Ayurveda and various research findings on *rasayana* suggests that *rasayana therapy/ drug* may have its effect on our *ojas, immunity, resistance*, etc. Hence the following points related to the concept of *resistance, immunity* as described in Ayurveda may be useful:

1. The qualitative, quantitative and functional balance of the body-elements maintains strength which, in general, causes resistance to diseases. *Raktam* (Blood) has

been attached much importance because it's normal condition reflects good health and general resistance power.

2.   Ayurveda has described a separate substance named *ojas* which has been said to be the essence of all the *dhatus* and is considered to be an excellent body element. Therefore, the excellence of the body in totality is *ojas*. It reflects the excellent performance of the man as a whole. Therefore, resistance power of the body depends on the quality and quantity of *ojas*.

3.   Bala (strength or power) has been classified as *sahaja* (natural, hereditary), *kalakrita* (variable as per age and season) and *yuktikrita* (acquired by good diet, drug and exercise etc.). This is why some families have a specific resistance to specific diseases; some diseases are born in a specific age and season and generally speaking those, who are well built, fall less ill.

4.   Again the *bala* (resistance) has been divided into *vyadhi pratibandhakatwa* and *vyadhi bala virodhitwa* bala. The former is the specific resistance against a specific disease so that those diseases will never afflict the man. Today, vaccines substitute this type of resistance. The latter does not stop the onset of the disease but can only minimise its severity. In another context it has been said that the overweight or emaciated, those of weak build, who have a deficient diet and who are mentally weak, are more susceptible to disease (Ch.Su.28/7).

There are various ways of classifying *rasayana therapy* in Ayurveda. They are basically either based on the method of administering the *rasayana* therapy, such as *kutipravesika* (indoor) or *vataatapika* (outdoor); or based on the effect. *Kaamya* (invigorating and vitalizing), *medhya* (promoting intellectual factors), *achara* (address psycho-somatic activities), *naimittika* (used to promote resistance against disease following illness) and *vrishya* (virilifying or sex-stimulant). Also remember that *Rasayana Tantra* is one of the eight branches (Asthanga Ayurveda) of Ayurveda. And, before administering *rasayana* the individual needs to undergo the *shodana/panchakarma* (purification therapy) process. *Kaya-kalpa* is nothing but another name for *rasayana*.

The importance of Ayurveda in countries outside of India continues to increase. In order to meet the demand in the United Kingdom for qualified personnel, there has been established, for the first time in the UK, a first degree course in the subject at Thames Valley University. It is a three-year degree course with the opportunity afterwards for continuing the course in India for a fourth year at Kottakal (or Manipal University). This degree course is run in conjunction with the world's first Charitable Ayurvedic Hospital outside of India and Sri Lanka which is based in London.

In the light of the extreme importance of *rasayana* in Ayurvedic therapy it is appropriate that Dr Harsharnjit Puri's book on *rasanaya* is being published by Taylor & Francis. I congratulate him on producing this excellent reference book with detailed explanations on the activity of each drug.

However, as a persistent defender of the intellectual property and patent rights of Ayurvedic doctors and Indian Ayurveda, I hope that this book will be read by those with a spirit of learning and not as a commercial tool for attempts to synthesize these medicines or for using them as herbs in non-Ayurvedic traditions.

Gopi Warrier
Chairman
Ayurvedic Charitable Hospital
British Ayurvedic Medical Council

References

Ader R, Felten D and Cohen M (1990). Interactions between the brain and the immune system, Ann. Rev. Pharmacol. Toxicol. (pp. 30, 561–602.)

Dahanukar, S A (1986). Study of influence of plant products on Adaptive Processes, PhD thesis, Dept of Pharmacology and therapeutics, University of Mumbai, Mumbai.

Dahanukar, S A, Nirmala M Thette, Nirmala N Rege (1999). Immunomodulatory Agents from plants, ed. By M Wagner, Birkhausen Verlag Basel / Switzerland, pp. 289–323.

Glaser R and Kiecolt, Glaser J (1994). Handbook of human stress and Immunity, Academic Press, San Diego.

Selye H (1946). General adaptation syndrome and diseases of adaptation. J Clin Endocrinol. 6, pp. 117–230

Selye H (1983). The stress concept: past, present, and future, In, Stress Research, Issues for the Eighties, ed. By C L Cooper, (pp.1–21) John Wiley & Sons, New York.

Preface to the series

Global warming and global travel are among the factors resulting in the spread of such infectious diseases as malaria, tuberculosis, hepatitis B and HIV. All these are not well controlled by the present drug regimes. Antibiotics too are failing because of bacterial resistance. Formerly less well known tropical diseases are reaching new shores. A whole range of illnesses, for example cancer, occur worldwide. Advances in molecular biology, including methods of *in vitro* testing for a required medical activity give new opportunities to draw judiciously upon the use and research of traditional herbal remedies from around the world. The re-examining of the herbal medicines must be done in a multidisciplinary manner.

Since 1997 twenty volumes have been published in the Book Series **Medicinal and Aromatic Plants – Industrial Profiles**. The series continues. It is characterised by a single plant genus per volume. With the same Series Editor, this new series **Traditional Herbal Medicines for Modern Times**, covers multi genera per volume. It accommodates for example, the Traditional Chinese Medicines (TCM), the Japanese Kampo versions of this and the Ayurvedic formulations of India. Collections of plants are also brought together because they have been re-evaluated for the treatment of specific diseases, such as malaria, tuberculosis, cancer, diabetes, etc. Yet other collections are of the most recent investigations of the endemic medicinal plants of a particular country, e.g. of India, South Africa, Mexico, Brazil (with its vast flora), or of Malaysia with its rainforests said to be the oldest in the world, etc.

Each volume reports on the latest developments and discusses key topics relevant to interdisciplinary health science research by ethnobiologists, taxonomists, conservationists, agronomists, chemists, pharmacologists, clinicians and toxicologists. The Series is relevant to all these scientists and will enable them to guide business, government agencies and commerce in the complexities of these matters. The background to the subject is outlined below.

Over many centuries, the safety and limitations of herbal medicines have been established by their empirical use by the *healers* who also took a holistic approach. The *healers* are aware of the infrequent adverse affects and know how to correct these when they occur. Consequently and ideally, the pre-clinical and clinical studies of a herbal medicine need to be carried out with the full cooperation of the traditional healer. The plant composition of the medicine, the stage of the development of the plant material, when it is to be collected from the wild or when from cultivation, its post-harvest treatment, the preparation of the medicine, the dosage and frequency and much other essential information is required. A consideration of the intellectual property rights and appropriate models of benefit sharing may also be necessary.

Wherever the medicine is being prepared, the first requirement is a well documented reference collection of dried plant material. Such collections are encouraged by organisations like the World Health Organisation and the United Nations Industrial Development Organisation. The Royal Botanic Gardens at Kew in the UK is building up its collection of traditional Chinese dried plant material relevant to its purchase and use by those who sell or prescribe TCM in the UK.

In any country, the control of the quality of plant raw material, of its efficacy and of its safety in use, are essential. The work requires sophisticated laboratory equipment and highly trained personnel. This kind of *control* cannot be applied to the locally produced herbal medicines in the rural areas of many countries, on which millions of people depend. Local traditional knowledge of the *healers* has to suffice.

Conservation and protection of plant habitats is required and breeding for biological diversity is important. Gene systems are being studied for medicinal exploitation. There can never by too many seed conservation *banks* to conserve genetic diversity. Unfortunately such banks are usually dominated by agricultural and horticultural crops with little space for medicinal plants. Developments such as random amplified polymorphic DNA enable the genetic variability of a species to be checked. This can be helpful in deciding whether specimens of close genetic similarity warrant storage.

From ancient times, a great deal of information concerning diagnosis and the use of traditional herbal medicines has been documented in the scripts of China, India and elsewhere. Today, modern formulations of these medicines exist in the form of e.g. powders, granules, capsules and tablets. They are prepared in various institutions e.g. government hospitals in China and Korea, and by companies such as Tsumura Co. of Japan with good quality control. Similarly, products are produced by many other companies in India, the USA and elsewhere with a varying degree of quality control. In the USA, the dietary supplement and Health Education Act of 1994 recognised the class of physiotherapeutic agents derived from medicinal and aromatic plants. Furthermore, under public pressure, the US Congress set up an Office of Alternative Medicine and this office in 1994 assisted the filing of several Investigational New Drug (IND) applications, required for clinical trials of some Chinese herbal preparations. The significance of these applications was that each Chinese preparation involved several plants and yet was handled as a *single* IND. A demonstration of the contribution to efficacy, of *each* ingredient of *each* plant, was not required. This was a major step forward towards more sensible regulations with regard to phytomedicines.

Something of the subject of western herbal medicines is now being taught again to medical students in Germany and Canada. Throughout Europe, the USA, Australia and other countries pharmacy and health-related schools are increasingly offering training in phytotherapy.

TCM clinics are now common outside of China. An Ayurvedic Hospital now exists in London and a degree course in Ayurveda is also available here.

The term *integrated medicine* is now being used which selectively combines traditional herbal medicine with *modern medicine*. In Germany there is now a hospital in which TCM is integrated with western medicine. Such co-medication has become common in China, Japan, India, and North America by those educated in both systems. Benefits claimed include improved efficacy, reduction in toxicity and the period of medication, as well as a reduction in the cost of the treatment. New terms such as adjunct therapy, supportive therapy, and supplementary medicine now appear as a consequence of such co-medication. Either medicine may be described as an adjunct to the other depending on the communicator's view.

Great caution is necessary when traditional herbal medicines are used by those doctors not trained in their use and likewise when modern medicines are used by traditional herbal doctors. Possible dangers from drug interactions need to be stressed.

I find exceedingly helpful the CAB abstracts *Review of Aromatic and Medicinal Plants*, editor Debbie J. Cousins of CABI Publishing, Wallingford, Oxon, 0X10 8DE, UK. Email; cabi@cabi.org

Many thanks are due to the staff of Taylor & Francis who have made this series possible and especially to the volume editors and their chapter contributors for the authoritative information.

Dr Roland Hardman
January 2002

Preface

Ayurveda – the science of life, has been divided into eight disciplines. Whereas the first six disciplines can be easily related to similar topics of modern medical science, the last two *Rasayana* and *Vajikarna*, are unique in themselves and until recently were least understood. Initially *Rasayana* was equated with tonics, elixirs and alteratives, which helped rejuvenation of all systems in the body and hence longevity. *Vajikarna*, also spelled *Bajikarna* – which means to impart (sexual) power of the horse, and also translates as the science of procreation, were considered aphrodisiacs.

This overemphasis on herbs as elixirs and for sexual purposes is not unique to Ayurveda; the study of other oriental *materia medica* reveals more or less the same story. Recent developments have also shown that the concept of sexual deficiencies, real or imaginary, is widespread all over the world in different populations, as has became evident from the success of a preparation for erectile dysfunction (impotence) in males.

Whereas in modern times the emphasis is on sexual pleasure, in ancient India the preparations were required for reproduction to replenish the depleted population. Manpower was required, not only for day-to-day agricultural and industrial activities but also for wars to defend the existing territory and to acquire more land from nature and from other communities. With little knowledge in the prevention and cure of diseases, the death rate was very high, both from natural and unnatural causes. It necessitated the search for herbs, which would not only help in reproduction but also in prolonging life by keeping the body healthy and disease free.

The herbs used for the above purposes had diverse physiological actions on the body, such as sexual stimulant, tranquilizer, liver protection, diuretic, bronchiodilator, etc. When subjected to detailed pharmacological activity in the last century, in most cases these herbs had a mild pharmacological effect on the body and it was said that herbs used as *Rasayana* and *Vajikarna* helped the body due to their placebo effect.

After India's independence in 1947, more attention was paid to research on Indian medicinal plants, particularly those used in Ayurveda, but for about half a century much of the information on these herbs remained confined to India, as most of these research findings were published in Indian journals, which had only local circulation and were not even abstracted by multinational publishers. The international journals at that time were not interested in the publication of the routine type of research work, or the Ayurvedic polyherbal, polymineral preparations, processed in the traditional way, where nothing was known about the exact chemical nature of the active constituents with certainty. Mostly the articles on Indian medicines submitted to these journals were returned back to the author with the remark *local interest only*.

Studies on ginseng, *Panax ginseng*, was a trendsetter for research on herbs, considered as a tonic. Ginseng did not have a strong pharmacological activity but it showed diverse beneficial effects on the human body. In the meantime, in the Soviet Union (the present Russia and other Republics), a new group of herbs, called adaptogens, were discovered. It was observed that by the use of these herbs, the body adapts itself to adverse environmental conditions. These herbs were found to combat stress, kept infections away by their immunomodulating activity and thus helped to promote a long life of good quality.

Recent research has shown that many Ayurvedic herbs used as *Rasayana* act as adaptogens. In this book, an effort has been made to refer to all the lesser known articles on these herbs, so that the interested reader may obtain detailed information about them. In addition to these, some other herbs, which in Indian folklore are considered to have *Rasayana* type activities, have also been included, with the hope that further research on them may discover some new therapeutic active substance.

In the introductory chapters of the book the concept of *Rasayana*, and an allied subject *Tridosha* is explained, along with the methods used for preparing various Ayurvedic products. The main part of the text is concerned with the herbs used as *Rasayana*: each chapter is devoted to a single herb. In the Contents, the Indian names of these herbs are followed by their botanical names in parentheses. In the text, English names are also mentioned; botanical and Indian names are italicized. While describing various formulations, to avoid confusion, instead of botanical binomial nomenclature, mostly generic names of the plants are given. Where more than one part of the herb is used, the plant part is given along with the name of the herb. In the cases where a particular herb is processed, specific information about this has been provided. When describing a herb, Ayurvedic name, botanical name, brief description, distribution of the plant and illustration is followed by its uses in folklore and Ayurveda. Brief information on pharmacology and therapeutic studies have also been provided if recent research confirms the common claims for the herb. An account of some important polyherbal, polymineral formulations used as *Rasayana* and *Vajikarna*, are also given.

When Dr R. Hardman, the series editor, mentioned the new series, *Traditional Herbal Medicine for the Modern Times*, I suggested he include a book on *Rasayana*. In the earlier part of my career, I had surveyed the literature and conducted some research on the plants used in both *Rasayana* and *Vajikarna*. The present book, which describes herbs, is the first part of the study on *Rasayana*. In the second part, information will been given about the role that *Rasayana* plays in our daily life, along with a description of animal products, gems and minerals. I am grateful to Dr Hardman for the guidance and help while preparing the manuscript for the book. During my stay at Herb Pharm Inc., Williams (Or. USA), Mr Ed Smith was kind enough to provide me with a computer and other facilities during the preparation of the manuscript. Thanks are also due to Dr Naresh, of the Institute of Microbial Technology, Chandigarh (India), for library help and occasional discussion, Mr V.K. Sawhney for typing some sections and Mr Naresh Bagga, for the line drawings of the plants.

My son Avon Puri, my wife Harminder Puri, Thorin Halverson, Ashneet Puri and Vikram Malhotra also helped me during the preparation of the manuscript for this book.

H.S. Puri

1 Introduction

Disease (dis-ease), is the disturbance of *ease* i.e. comfort, freedom from constraint, annoyance, awkwardness, pain or trouble both bodily and mental. Since time immemorial, man has tried to lead a disease free life. In one of the oldest repositories of human knowledge, *vedas* of Aryans (*veda* means to know, knowledge), the plants with medicinal virtues have been identified as *oushidhis* which are to be distinguished from *ahara* the edible plants. After *vedas*, further developments in various spheres of human life gave rise to Indian medicine called Ayurveda (*Ayuh* – life, *veda* – science). Dhanwantri, said to be the father of Indian medicine, lived in 7th century BC., as compared to Hippocrates who lived in 5th century BC. After Dhanwantri, the system of Ayurveda developed further, and peaked at the time of *Charak Sanhita* and *Sushrut Sanhita*, the treatises on medicine and surgery written about 1000 BC to 1000 AD. *Charak Sanhita* is said to be a compilation of proceedings of a symposium held in the Himalayas, to discuss the cure of various diseases which had originated at that time due to urbanization. For this purpose, the ancient scholar divided Ayurveda into the following eight disciplines:

1   Internal medicine
2   Ophthalmology and otorhinolaryngology
3   Surgery
4   Toxicology
5   Psychiatry
6   Paediatrics
7   *Rasayana*, which in broad terms means rejuvenator
8   *Vajikarna*, the literal meaning is to have the sex power of a horse, but is often considered as fertility inducer or procreator.

As the present studies show, it is difficult to distinguish between *Rasayana* and *Vajikarna*. The sexual system is fully dependent on the proper function of mind and body, so a good *Vajikarna* has to be a good *Rasayana*. Initially *Rasayana* preparations were herbal and were prescribed as dietary supplements. Some were administered under controlled conditions, whereas the *Vajikarna* included poisons, minerals, animal products and narcotics like *Cannabis* and opium.

Further developments in Ayurveda took place with the incorporation of herbs discovered in other countries and by contacts with medical scholars from other parts of the world. These developments lead to the incorporation of more and more substances, particularly minerals in Ayurvedic *materia medica*. By the time of *Bhavparkasha* in the fifteenth century AD, Ayurveda had become a composite science, covering all aspects of human activities, even including recipes on nutritive foods.

Initially, Ayurveda developed as the medical science of the Aryans settled mainly in the Indo-Gangetic region, but later, findings of physicians from other parts of India were also incorporated into it. In east and south India, Ayurveda developed with the same basic principles but with a focus on local flora, and on physiotherapy. Progress in gemology and metallurgy had its effect on medicine also. For boosting the effects of herbal preparations, a large number of minerals, particularly mercury, with a miraculous power against microbes, became an integral part of Ayurvedic treatments (for details see chapter on Some *Rasayana* Formulations).

During all these stages, Ayurveda covered all aspects of human life. The aim was not only to make a man healthy but happy too. It did not deal with man and medicine only, but with a way of life, which included social, moral, and religious education, based on very intricate philosophies of Indian sages. These learned men postulated many theories. They gave their views about the origin of the universe, the composition of matter, and the actions and interactions in our environment, which disturb the systems of our bodies and gives rise to many diseases and discomforts. Ayurveda combined philosophy with science, so the life processes, which cannot be understood by wisdom (*budhi*) have been explained on the basis of reasoning (*yukti*). These philosophical thoughts are too complex for the present purposes and only the salient features, in a simplified manner, are given in the following chapters.

It was postulated that human health is related to constitution of body, age, sex, geographical region, race, ancestry, and resistance power or immunity. Good health is something more than the absence of diseases or infirmity. It is a state of complete mental, physical and social well being. As per Ayurvedic theories, the approach to health is holistic, with less emphasis on symptomatic relief. Treatment does not mean healing the affected part or a particular system, but the whole body. The treatment aims at correcting the site of origin of disease, the channels of accumulation and the site of manifestation of body poisons. For example, when there is a breathing problem, in the conventional system antispasmodics and bronchodilators are prescribed but in Ayurveda polyherbal preparations are given, in which some of the ingredients may have an antispasmodic effect but some others act on the stomach and intestine, from where the disease might have originated. This diagnosis is based on *tridosha*, the three biological factors in the human systems, around which Ayurvedic physiology, pathology and therapeutics revolve. In broad terms *tridosha* represents metabolic disturbances, and various treatments are given to keep the three *doshas* in order. Balancing of the *doshas* is required for a good old age and also for the day-to-day activities of modern life. It has been stressed that medicaments, particularly *Rasayana*, work only if the conditions within the body are conducive for their effect. During treatment, due importance has also been given to the mind, which is a powerful agent in causation and cure of diseases. Emotions, anger and pride are also treated as diseases. These affect the health, happiness and longevity of an individual.

Recent studies also confirm these observations. According to a leading Indian cardiologist (Dr H.S. Wasir) negative emotions like greed, ego, anger and too much materialistic attachment lead to high blood pressure, aggravation of angina and heart attack. Positive emotions have a beneficial effect on heart function and prevent an upsurge in blood pressure. Music, meditation, and yogic excesses help in settling the mind. A good way of life is also conducive to good health. *Aachar* – good conduct, *Vichar*

– good thoughts, *Vyahar* – good interpersonal dealing, and *Ahar* – good food habits, help. Both malnutrition and over-nutrition adversely affect our health and longevity. Over-nutrition is excessive intake of calories, saturated fats of animal origin, sugar and lack of complex carbohydrates from tubers. The diseases affecting longevity are hypertension, brain stroke, cancer, diabetes, obesity, cirrhosis and other hepatic disorders, alcoholism, cardiomyopathy, and AIDS etc. The ancient Indian physicians were aware of these, and most of the herbs prescribed as *Rasayana* treated one or more of the above diseases.

2 What are *Rasayana?*

The agents which cure body and mental diseases, delay old age, increase mental power, generating power, vital energy, eyesight, impart intelligence, memory, aid proper digestion and clear complexion are *Rasayana* (Shastri, 1979). These nourish the whole body by strengthening the primordial tissue *Rasa*, the essence of all food we take, and which the body can assimilate. If this essence is well distributed in all systems, the body remains healthy. By their physico-chemical action *Rasayana* purify and promote *dhatus* (tissue). They augment the body's disease resistance capacity, as well as the ability for restorative reaction and counteract all the deleterious effects including that of ageing.

The *Rasayana* keep tissues, enzymes, membranes and tranquility of the mind in their normal functioning conditions through anabolic processes. They help if the tissues have become inactive, are to be revitalized and their composition changed. They achieve this by increasing *bala*, the physiological and immunological strength of the body. They are good for all people, at all stages, at all times but they do not prevent ageing and do not assure immortality.

Rasayana may be compared to alteratives, which work as *blood cleansers* by their diuretic and antihepatotoxic action. Alteratives also restore the proper functions of the body and increase health and vitality (Hoffmann, 1998). They alter the body's metabolism in various ways so that the tissue can best deal with the range of function from nutrition to elimination. Some of these herbs eliminate waste from the body through kidney, liver, lung or skin, while others work by stimulating digestive functions and still others act as antimicrobial agents. Some *Rasayana* also help in the disposal of waste *ama*. *Agni* is the biological fire burning inside the body, which acts on food so that energy is generated by digestion. If waste is not excreted from the body properly and *ama* is deposited in the tissues, it may disturb various systems. The herbs are given to strengthen the tissue to counteract all the ill effects of *ama*.

In Ayurveda, human life has been divided into four spans according to growth and development:

1 From birth to the age of 20, all tissues of the body grow.
2 20–40 years of age, tissues continue to grow.
3 40–60 years is the age of stagnation. If an individual has a balanced diet, cheerful life, adequate nourishment, and is free of worries and anxiety, the person can maintain good health. At this stage the mental activities expand, and power of judgment increases.

4   After the age of 60, in spite of good quality of life, senescence starts. Metabolism of the tissues decreases, waste is not excreted properly, and the bone joints become dry and fixed.

The body can be rejuvenated at stages 3 and 4 and during senescence by *Rasayana*. These can be used as a dietary supplement, but in the case of chronic diseases, old age, etc. where *kaya kalp* (rejuvenation) is required, a special treatment, called *Rasayana* therapy, is provided under the supervision of medical experts.

RASAYANA THERAPY

Before the start of actual therapy, the internal and external organs of the body are cleansed and the system is made more receptive to assimilation of medication. It has been stressed that *Rasayana* administered without these treatments is like seed sown on barren land, from where no good results can be expected. This pretreatment is given only to those persons who have enough strength to bear it.

Pretreatment for *Rasayana* therapy

Samshodhna (*Diet restriction*)

One week before the start of therapy, the person should resort to a simple diet consisting of only steamed vegetables and fresh fruits. He should not be given sugar, alcohol or animal products. Milk and honey are allowed.

Purvakarma (*Preparatory treatment*)

Involves massage with warm oil, and application of heat on the body by a massage therapist. The massage should be so vigorous that a large amount of latent heat of the body is generated. For this purpose sesame oil is generally used but sometimes some other medicated oils, which are supposed to have better properties, are applied.

Panchkarma (*Cleansing of internal organs of the body*)

Virechna	purging to clean the small intestine
Basti	to clean the large intestine
Vamna	emetics to clean the stomach
Naysya	nasal drops to clear the respiratory passage
Raktaoksha	bloodletting by leeches may be done to those patients who have excess of blood in their body. Nowadays blood is donated to the blood bank. It is optional.

Administration of herbs

After *panchkarma* the patient is admitted into a hut (*kuti prveshika*) for the administration of *Rasayana* preparations. The hut should be in a pollution-free area, well ventilated, facing north, and painted with slaked lime to make it germ-free.

The preparations required during *Rasayana* therapy vary, at the discretion of the health provider. Generally the patient is given a restricted diet, along with only that quantity of medication which the patient can easily digest. The medicine should be fully utilized by the body and not passed into faeces undigested. The medicine should not create any digestive disturbance, such as indigestion, hyperacidity or constipation. If any of these conditions persist for some time, a laxative or a colon cleanser should be given.

Herbs such as garlic, *neem, amalaki*, etc. were commonly used for this therapy but now polyherbal preparations with animal products such as musk, amber, coral, pearl, gems, minerals, and metals are prescribed. Some of the formulations may consist of red sulphide of mercury, prepared in the presence of gold, along with processed poisonous herbs like aconite, nux vomica, etc. The preparation is given to the patient in the early hours of the morning (within three hours of sunrise). During administration of mercurial compounds, the patient should have a pure vegetarian diet. He should not remain thirsty or hungry. He should avoid excessive sleep, swimming, talking, anger, sadness, desire, excessive happiness, bathing, worry, irritation, depression, sex, and fragrances. He should lead a simple, pious, and religious life.

After *kuti prevesh*, the patient should start steadily with a diet of rice water, followed by rice gruel, rice and split beans, rice with beans, and finally he may be given a normal diet with a teaspoonful of *ghee* (butter oil). The patient should remain in a relaxed condition, and should have a whole body massage daily with warm sesame oil. This treatment is said to make the arteries softer and smoother, the constitution of the blood changes, clots are dissolved, and new cells are formed.

RASAYANA AND VAJIKARNA

Vajikarna are Ayurvedic aphrodisiacs, and may be used in place of *Rasayana*. There is no clear-cut distinction between the two, and these may be substituted for each other. In general *Vajikarna* are used for the production and purification of *shukra* (this term is used for vital fluid, and also for sperm and spermatic fluid). The vital fluid is considered the essence of all functions of the body, which result in fame, beauty, strength and power. It is the result of all metabolic activities of the human body. If any system of the body is disturbed, the formation of vital fluid does not take place, but in a person who is healthy, energetic, active, has good digestion, sleep, active life, nutritive diet, regulated routine, a good household atmosphere, affectionate wife, and who consumes milk, *ghee*, citrus fruits and stays away from excessive amorous activities, the vital fluid does not get depleted and hence these persons do not require any medication (aphrodisiac).

Some recent research on *Rasayana* and *Vajikarna*

Puri (1970a, b, 1971, 1972) gave an account of the herbs used in various *Rasayana* and *Vajikarna* preparations. The other studies carried out on these aspects are as follows:

For mental diseases

Udupa (1973) was the first to study the effects of herbs used as *Rasayana* on psycho-somatic stress. Singh and Murthy (1989) treated patients with epilepsy syndrome with various *Rasayana* preparations for one year. Seventy-five per cent of patients had less severe fits. Dwivedi and Singh (1992) prescribed *Medhya Rasayana* (the herbs said to be a brain tonic), for convulsive disorders. The treatment showed significant improvement in terms of frequency, duration and severity of seizures. Pandey and Pandey (1995) used *Rasayana* because of their sedative and tranquillizing property for the treatment of psychological and psychosomatic disorders. These preparations reduced anxiety, apprehension, and kept the mind calm and cool.

As adaptogens and immunomodulators

Srivastava *et al.* (1990) tried *Rasalyana* preparations on people/persons exposed to high altitudes. These herbs also helped in generalized weakness (Jayaram *et al.* 1993). Praveen Kumar *et al.* (1994) noted that the oral administration of *Rasayana* preparations protected mice from cyclophosphamide-induced leukopaenia. In this case white blood cell count increased and there was an increase in bone marrow cellularity. The herbs were found useful in chemotherapy-induced myelosuppression.

Wagner (1994), after a detailed study, concluded that *Rasayana* preparations, which act both as herbal immunostimulants and adaptogens, regulate the immunological and endocrine systems, with relative low doses, without damaging the autoregulative functions of the organisms. These induced a general increase in non-specific resistance against infectious and non-infectious stresses. Mulgund and Uchil (1994) noted that herbal formulations used as *Rasayana* were powerful immunostimulants. All the groups treated with these herbal extracts showed a significant increase in macrophage function, indicating their role in protection against stress. The rise in plasma cortisol following stress was inhibited. Srivastava (1995) studied the effects of Ayurvedic adaptogens on psycho-physiological performance of volunteers, up to three months at an altitude of 4800–6000 m. These herbs improved the physical performance and sensitivity index of oxygen availability.

In another experiment, Shetty (1995) studied the *Rasayana* effect of a herbal preparation consisting of six herbs, by prescribing it 3 g daily for 6 months. Extensive clinical, biochemical, psychological, and anthropometric assessment, with direct or indirect bearing on the ageing process, was done initially and at the end of six months. Analysis of clinical parameters indicated that with the preparation, the diastolic blood pressure came down within normal limits. Menon *et al.* (1996) observed that *Brahma Rasayana* with more than twenty ingredients, inhibited methylcholanthrene (200μg) induced sarcoma development. The preparation inhibited carcinogenesis by 80 per cent and enhanced mouse life. Praveen Kumar *et al.* (1996) carried out further studies on the oral administration of four *Rasayana* preparations. These significantly increased total leucocyte count and bone marrow cellularity. These had natural killer cell activity and antibody dependent cellular toxicity in mice exposed to gamma radiation. The effect of *Rasayana* preparation could be due to increased stem cell proliferation and also on free radical-induced injury produced by radiation.

In a review article Dahanukar and Thatte (1997) mentioned that *Rasayana* protected animals from infections, shortened recovery time, and lowered mortality rates.

They made antibiotics more effective at lower doses. *Rasayana* worked by enhancing leucocytosis and by neutrophil destruction. Important immune functions such as phagocytosis, intracellular killing and macrophage activity also increased in treated animals.

As an anti-inflammatory agent

Pathak *et al.* (1992) treated osteoarthritis patients, first subjecting them to physiotherapy, for example heating the body systems with massage to cause perspiration, followed by administration of a polyherbal *Rasayana* preparation containing *Ashwagandha, Guggulu*, etc., with positive results.

References

Dahanukar, S.A., Thatte, U.M. (1997) Current status of Ayurveda in Phytomedicine. *Phytomedicine,* 4, 359–368.

Dwivedi, K.K., Singh, R.H. (1992) A clinical study of Medhya Rasayana therapy in the management of convulsive disorders. *Journal of Research in Ayurveda and Siddha*, 13, 97–106.

Hoffmann, D., *The Herbal Handbook*. Healing Arts Press, Rochester, Vermont 1998.

Jayaram, S., Walwaikar, P.P., Rajadhyaksha, S.S. (1993) Evaluation of efficacy of a preparation containing combination of Indian medicinal plants in patients of generalised weakness. *Indian Drugs*, 30, 498–500.

Kumar, P., Kuttan, R.V., Kuttan, G. (1994) Chemoprotective action of Rasayana against cyclophosphamide toxicity. *Tumori*, 80, 306–308.

Kumar, P., Kuttan, R.V., Kuttan, G. (1996) Radioprotective effects of Rasayanas. *International Symposium on Radiomodifiers in Human Health*. Manipal, India. 28–31 December 1995 (Uma Devi, P., Bisht, K.S., eds) *Indian Journal of Experimental Biology*, (1996) 34, 846–850.

Menon, L.G., Kuttan, R., Kuttan, G. (1966) Inhibition of chemical-induced carcinogenesis by Rasayana – an indigenous herbal preparation. *Journal of Experimental and Clinical Cancer Research*, 15, 241–243.

Mulgund, S.P., Uchil, D.A. Comparative immunomodulatory and antistress effect of plant extracts. *Update Ayurveda – 94*, Bombay, 24–26th February 1994.

Pandey, K.K.K., Pandey, S.B. (1995) Sedative and tranquilising properties of Medhya drugs – a pharmacodynamic concept. *Aryavaidyan*, 84, 198–200.

Pathak, B., Dwivedi, K.K., Shukla, K.P. (1992) Clinical evaluation of Snehan, Swedana and an ayurvedic compound drug in sandhivata vis-a-vis osteoarthritis. *Journal of Research and Education in Indian Medicine*, 11, 27–34.

Puri, H.S. (1970a) Indian medicinal plants used in elixirs and tonics. *Quarterly Journal of Crude Drug Research*, 10, 1555–1566.

Puri, H.S. (1970b) Chavanprasha – an ancient Indian preparation for respiratory diseases. *Indian Drugs*, 7, 15–16.

Puri, H.S. (1971) Vegetable aphrodisiacs of India. *Quarterly Journal of Crude Drug Research*, 11, 1742–1748.

Puri, H.S. (1972) Aphrodisiacs in India. *Indian Drugs*, 9, 11–14.

Shastri, K. *Rastrangni* by Sharma, Sadanand, (translation of Sanskrit text into Hindi). Motilal Banarsi Das, Delhi, India 1979.

Shetty, B.R. Studies on the Rasayana effect of an Ayurvedic compound drug in apparently normal aged persons. *Seminar on Research in Ayurveda and Siddha, CCRAS*. New Delhi, 20–22nd March 1995.

Singh, R.H., Murthy, A.R.V. (1989) Medhya Rasayana therapy in the management of apsmara *vis-à-vis* epilepsies. *Journal of Research and Education in Indian Medicine*, 8, 13–16.

Srivastava, K.K. (1995) Adaptogens in the high mountains, *Indian Journal of Natural Products*, 11, 13–19.

Srivastava, K.K., Grover, S.K., Ramachandran, U.R. (1990) Membrane integrity changes at high terrestrial altitudes. *Probe*, 29, 112–117.

Udupa, K.N. (1973) Psychosomatic stress and Rasayana. *Journal of Research in Indian Medicine*, 8, 1–2.

Wagner, H. (1994) Therapy and prevention with immunomodulatory and adaptogenic plant drugs. *Update – Ayurveda-94*, Bombay, 24–26 February 1994.

3 *Tridosha*

The origin of disease in the body, as per Ayurveda, is due to metabolic disturbances in the various systems. The aim of the *Rasayana* is to correct this system by balancing various *ras* (extracts which are manifested by a particular taste). Whatever we eat, it has one or more of the six *ras* (tastes): sweet, acidic, salty, bitter, astringent and pungent.

Sweet *ras*

It is mainly in carbohydrates (starch- and sugar-containing substances). It nourishes *sapt dhatus* (seven tissue systems in the body), i.e. chyme, blood, liver, flesh, bones, bone marrow and semen. It is good for five senses, i.e. eye, ear, nose, tongue and skin. In excess it causes laziness, obesity, diabetes, and high blood pressure, etc.

Acidic *ras*

It is mainly present in acidic fruits, except in *amalaki* (*Emblica officinalis*), yogurt, and fermented preparations. This *ras* stimulates saliva, increases the power of digestion, imparts strength to the body, and keeps the sense organs in order. In excess it causes hyperacidity and loss of sexual power.

Salty *ras*

It is mainly present in minerals. It makes food tasty and digestible. Excess of salt causes thirst, heat, softness of muscles, premature greying of hair, wrinkles, hair loss and loss of libido.

Bitter *ras*

The main sources are herbs. It cleans the mouth, increases glandular secretion, digests food and strengthens all senses. It has an anti-inflammatory effect. It helps in skin diseases, liver functions and obesity. If bitters are taken in excess they cause inflammation, burning sensation and make a man impotent.

Pungent *ras*

Mainly spices give rise to this *ras*. Spices do not have a good taste of their own but make food tasty. They act as antidote to toxins and kill microbes in the food. They cause diuresis and help in obesity. Excess of pungent *ras*, reduces power, energy, and may cause sedation and hallucination.

Astringent *ras*

It is mainly in tannin-containing unripe fruits, barks and roots. Astringents are not good to taste and cause dryness of the body and constipation. Excess of this *ras* causes loss of virility, paralysis or other diseases of the nervous system.

RELATIONSHIP BETWEEN *RAS* AND *DOSHA*

If a particular *ras* is deficient or in excess, it disturbs the equilibrium or three *dosha* of the body: *vata*, *pitta* and *kapha*. These *doshas* are sometimes equated with three *humours* of Greek: air, bile and phlegm. These control all functions of the human body, i.e. the biomotor force, metabolic activity and the preservative principles. When all these are in balance in the body, they are the *regenerator* but if there is an imbalance in them then they become the *destroyer*. There is an action and interaction between these *ras* and *doshas*. Sweet *ras* suppresses *vata*; sweet, astringent and pungent tastes suppress *pitta*; bitter, astringent and pungent tastes suppress *kapha*; but if bitter, pungent and astringent are in excess then *vata* is corrupted; with acids, salt and bitter in excess *pitta* is corrupted while sweet, acid and salt affect *kapha*. Sweets, acids and salt suppress bad effects of *vata*, astringent, sweet and pungent help in *pitta*, and astringent, bitter and pungent suppresses *kapha*. Thus it is clear that a particular *ras* increases or decreases a particular *dosha*. The balanced diet, which keeps the three *doshas in order*, has no *ras* in excess or in short supply.

In *Charak Sanhita* it has been stated that no self-inflicted disease originates without disturbance of these *doshas*. Out of these three *doshas*, *vata* dominates *pitta*. *Vata* causes the movement of *kapha*, the same way air causes movement of clouds in the sky. If a particular *dosha* is corrupted it affects a particular system but if two *doshas* are involved then the bad effect increases manifold. If both *pitta* and *vata* are corrupted then the effect is like that of high winds on wild fire. This fire can only be controlled by *kapha*, which acts as water. If all the three *doshas* become unstable the result is disastrous.

The three *doshas* are:

Vata

It is equated with *vayu* or *baya* or *bios* of Greek. It is the life or vital force. It differentiates the cells into different structures, creates blood vessels, lymphatic system and nerves. *Vata* in the body becomes corrupted by the use of light, dry, easily digestible food for a long time, by eating highly nutritious substances with little roughage, by eating food in small quantities several times a day for long duration, by consuming excessive cold drinks, excessive work, from stress arising from non-fulfillment of goal, due to worry, grief, panic, fear, excessive sex, sleeping late at night, and by taking a bath for a long time. All these deplete the vital energy from the body in the same way as it is lost during ageing. Indigestion and constipation also have a bad effect on *vata*. They produce gas and may cause arthritis, muscular pain and headache. If *vata* remains stable then all the five senses of the body, body systems and organs remain stable, otherwise it causes many complications leading to chronic diseases, and untimely death.

Pitta

It generates and preserves body heat. It manifests itself in various forms in different biochemical activities mainly concerning digestion and assimilation of food. It brings about metabolic activity. It is equated with heat or fire. *Pitta* is situated between the duodenum and stomach. It digests food by separating *ras*, chyme, urine, faeces, and liberates energy for the body. *Pitta* works in close association with liver and spleen to produce blood. The bad effects of *pitta* are due to regular use of hot, spicy, fried, sour, and salty food, by eating food late in the evening just before sleeping, by remaining thirsty for a long time, by exposure to heat and sun for a long time, by remaining irritable and angry. Excess of *pitta* causes excess body heat, which results in hyperacidity, haemorrhage, loss of calcium or urinary diseases like incontinence and burning micturition. It may cause headaches, which result in restlessness, irritation and noise phobia. If *pitta* flares up cold, soft, sweet, bitter and astringent substances should be used but fried, salty, spicy, acidic, non-vegetarian food, alcohol, tobacco, hard work and sunshine should be avoided.

Kapha

It has a cooling and preservative property, and it acts like the water jacket of the internal combustion engine. It provides the humidity required by the various systems of the body particularly, bile, mucous membranes, gastric juices, pancreatic juices and other systems. A person who has a good diet and good way of living remains free from the bad effects of *kapha*. It helps the growth of the body by anabolic activities, develops strength and vigour in laziness, obesity and thinness of body, and stimulates the mind, enabling courage, tolerance, and selflessness, whilst discouraging greed and lust. It imparts knowledge to do the good things by intelligence.

Kapha becomes corrupted by sweet, sour, fatty, and highly nutritious foods which are hard to digest. It causes diseases which are cold in nature such as the common cold, cough, bronchial troubles, loss of appetite, insomnia, and laziness. It increases mucus, saliva, perspiration, and causes loss of virility. To control *kapha* avoid strong, cold, humid wind, excess sleep, sex, greediness and lust.

4 *Rasayana* preparations

The simplest mode of administering a herb is to take it as it is, to pound it or to use its juice after filtration. These are the least processed forms and all constituents of the herb are made available to the body. However fresh herbs are often not readily available throughout the year. Some fresh herbs not only taste bad but are even nauseating. The best alternative to fresh herbs is to use properly dried herbs in powder form (*churn*). Usually the *churn* are mixed with salt or sugar to make them more palatable. These powders are usually administered with a fluid medium, because in a dry form they are difficult to swallow or sometimes may even choke the respiratory passage. For *Rasayana* powders, the common medium for administration is boiled lukewarm cow's milk, sweetened with sugar, honey, cow's *ghee* or a mixture of both milk and *ghee*. (*Ghee* is prepared by heating the butter to remove the fat-insoluble, proteinaceous and other matters and water, so that only fatty acids and the constituents soluble in fat are left. It is surprising to find that though butter has been a common household item in India since ancient times, it has rarely been used for the administration of Ayurvedic preparations.)

The other methods of administration of powdered herbs are infusion, decoction and distillation. To make an infusion, the herb is immersed in water, usually kept overnight, filtered and used. In decoction the herb is boiled in water until the water is reduced to half or so, filtered through a cheese cloth and heated further until the decoction is reduced to one-fourth. The infusion or decoction may be used in place of juice, if fresh herbs are not available. For distillation, fresh leaves or flowers, dry root or seed are boiled in water in a closed container and the steam that arises is condensed, so that the volatile active constituents of the herb are dispersed in water (*aqua*).

Ghansatva are concentrated, sometimes standardized aqueous extracts of the herbs made from the decoction in the form of a thick paste or dry powder. These are now preferred by the pharmaceutical industry because they reduce the bulk of the herbs, and can be easily incorporated into capsules or pills, are easy to formulate, have a longer shelf life and the end products have good consumer appeal. Sometimes syrups or alcoholic preparations are made from these extracts.

The herbal products, in general, have an expiry period of one year but if stored in airtight containers they may be used for up to two years, whilst the mineral products may be used indefinitely. The early Ayurvedic physicians were aware that the aqueous decoctions did not extract all the constituents from the herbs, so they developed methods to generate alcohol from the solvent during fermentation, in which ethanol soluble constituents of the herbal mixtures could be dissolved. These preparations are called *Asav* and *Arishta*, to which sweetening agents such as raw sugar, honey and flowers of *Woodfordia floribunda*, etc., which can be fermented easily, are initially added. Due to the alcohol these preparations have a long shelf life, taste good and provide immediate energy and therapeutic agent to the body. *Asava* and *Arishta* differ in their method of preparation. *Arishta* are prepared from the decoctions of the herbs, whereas *Asav* are made from dry powders. In both cases all the herbs are allowed to ferment in airtight earthen pitchers for 40–50 days. Before the fermentation of herbal materials it is ensured that the pots are clean. They are then fumigated with camphor, sandal and *agar* wood (*Aquillaria agallocha*), or with long pepper powder and *ghee*. The water to be used should not be alkaline and should be free of inorganic matter. When the period of fermentation is complete, the solution is filtered and stored in bottles. The fermented end product mainly consists of ethanol, glycerol, lactic acid, acetic acid, besides other products. This can be used for an indefinite period. In a study of *Draksharishta*, it was seen that before fermentation the mixture contained 34.91 per cent sugar, but after fermentation the product had 19.17 per cent sugar, 8.70 per cent, alcohol, 0.24 per cent glycerin, 0.21 per cent lactic acid and 1.38 per cent acetic acid. The pH of the medium changed from 6.40 to 5.00.

Avleha or *lehya* (linctus) are semi-solid preparations prepared from dry powders, decoctions and the pulp of the herbs, along with sugary substances, honey, *ghee* and/or oil. During preparation, sugar is boiled in the extract/decoction of the herbs or water, until thick in consistency. A fine powder of herbs, minerals and spices is then added to warm thick syrup and stirred so that a homogenous mixture is formed, followed by *ghee* or oil when still hot. Honey should be added after cooling the preparation. *Avleha* should be dried to such an extent that there is neither too little nor too much moisture.

The term *Bhasam* literally means ash. In practice, in this case, minerals, gems or hard animal products, after treatment with herbs, are calcined at a very high temperature to form ash and then this ash-like end product is heated and powdered repeatedly. When this process has been repeated 100 times, the *bhasam* is known as *Shatputi* (*shat* is hundred) but after 1,000 times it is known as *Sahastraputi* (*sahastr* is thousand). For each mineral or exoskeleton of animals, different methods are followed. These products do not degrade during storage and can be used indefinitely.

Ghrita or Ghritam are preparations made from oil or *ghee*. These contain fat soluble constituents. *Ghrita* are prepared by heating juice, paste, decoction, infusion, etc. of the herbs in *ghee* and oil until all the water evaporates. The resulting mass is filtered to remove fat insoluble materials. The fat is preserved for use as a medicine. Where vegetable oils alone are used, heating is stopped when froth appears, but when *ghee* is used, heating is stopped when the froth subsides. For internal uses these preparations can be stored for sixteen months after manufacture, but for external use there is no expiry period.

Pak are the preparations made from milk, *ghee*, dry fruits, herbs, minerals and spices. These preparations are mainly used as nutrients or aphrodisiacs. The usual method for their preparation is to boil milk until thick and solid. This condensed milk is fried in *ghee* and sugar powder or thick sugar syrup, herbs, minerals, chopped dry fruits and spices, etc. are added to it when warm. The whole mass is made into chocolate or candy balls of about 25 g each.

Before use poisonous herbs or minerals are subjected to mitigation called *marn* (to kill) or *sodhana* to purify but it is actually a process to reduce the toxicity so as to make them available to the body within safe therapeutic doses.

In this process toxic materials are generally boiled or treated with some herbs or chemicals in fluids such as cow's urine, cow dung solution, water, milk, etc. After treatment the herb/mineral is dried and processed further before use.

In India, cane sugar juice is used for making raw sugar (brownish in colour) and for sugar manufactured by western technology. In addition to these, an indigenous method of refining sugar has been used for a very long time. The end product, called *Mishri*, consists of lumps of transparent, bold crystals. This sugar candy is considered to have a cooling effect and is used in auspicious ceremonies and in Ayurvedic medicaments as a sweetening agent. In the present book, the term sugar candy has been used for *Mishri*, to differentiate it from other forms of sugar.

In Ayurveda five types of salts are recognised. Out of these a man-made preparation called *black salt* is considered a good carminative and is included in many formulations for digestive problems. It is prepared by fusing saltpetre (nitre), *Terminalia chebula*, and common salt. In the presence of organic matter at high temperatures the salt turns into a deep violet amorphous mass.

5   Aak

Calotropis procera (Ait.) R.Br.
C. gigantea (L.) R. Br. ex Ait.
Family: Asclepiadaceae

THE PLANTS AND THEIR DISTRIBUTION

Both *Calotropis* species are common, wild, latex-containing shrubs, growing on waste-land in the arid zones of India. The plants are characterized by thick leathery leaves, with white incrustation. In *C. procera* (Fig. 1A) leaves are 5.5 to 15 cm long and 4 to 8 cm broad, ovate or oblong with acuminate apex. In *C. gigantea* (Fig. 1B) the leaves are 10–20 cm long and 8–10 cm broad, obovate to oblong with a cordate base. Flowers are white or pink in colour. The fruit is a follicle and seed is with pappus.

USES IN FOLKLORE AND AYURVEDA

In Ayurveda, two types of *aak* have been recognised, one with white flower (*C. procera*) and the other with red flower (*C. gigantea*). Root (Fig. 1C), latex, and the flower of both species are used in medicine. These herbs are said to have a strong mercury-like action on the human body, so these plants are often referred to as *vegetable mercury*.

The root bark occurs in irregular short pieces, slightly quilled or curved, externally greyish yellow, soft and spongy, internally yellowish white. The taste is acrid and bitter.

Root bark is alterative, tonic, antispasmodic, expectorant, and in large doses an emetic. It has a *Digitalis*-like effect on the heart. It is used as a substitute of ipecacuanha for inducing vomit. It also helps in dysentery. It increases glandular secretion, especially bile. For syphilis, it is smoked like tobacco. It is used as an antimicrobial agent and is said to be as effective as mercurial preparations. The latex is applied externally for chronic skin diseases such as leprosy and eczema.

Ayurvedic preparation

An aphrodisiac is prepared by pulverising a mixture of 125 dry flowers and 12 g each of clove, nutmeg, mace, and *Anacyclus pyrethrum* root. To use, 500 mg of this preparation is stirred in milk and administered three times a day (Nadkarni, 1954).

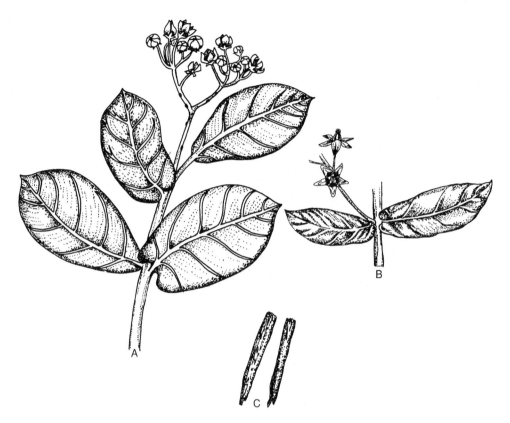

Figure 1 Calotropis procera: **A** branch, **C** dry root, **B** *C. gigantea* branch.

THERAPEUTIC INDICATIONS AND PHARMACOLOGICAL STUDIES

In diarrhoea and dysentery

The root bark powder, within the first day of the treatment of diarrhoea, changed the faecal matter into a semi-solid mass. In dysentery cases, mucus and tenesmus were relieved. The bark was not effective when dysentery was accompanied by blood (Jain *et al.* 1985).

In migraine headaches

In the morning, before sunrise, tender leaves were given in a capsule with water on an empty stomach. After treatment for three days, all patients suffering from migraine headaches got relief (Prasad, 1987).

Hepatoprotective effect

Basu *et al.* (1992) tried chloroform root extract of *C. procera* in experimentally-induced acute and chronic liver injury by carbon tetrachloride.

In inflammations

A single dose of the aqueous suspension of the dried latex was effective to a significant level against the acute inflammatory response (Kumar and Basu, 1994).

In bronchial asthma

Sharma and Sharma (1992) tried powders of both *C. procera* and *C. gigantea* on 75 patients of bronchial asthma, and observed good results. In another experiment, equal quantities of *C. gigantea*, *Piper nigrum* and *P. betle* leaf juice were made into pills of 200 mg each. They were quite effective in the cases of asthma (Thirunavukkarasu, 1995).

Cytotoxic effect (anticancerous property)

On the basis of Ayurvedic principles, out of 500 plants, Smit *et al.* (1995) selected forty four plants, which were supposed to have anticancerous properties. Of these fourteen plants out were investigated for cytotoxicity on human colorectal carcinoma cell line. Extracts of *C. procera* flowers displayed the strongest cytotoxic activity.

Chemical studies

The herb juice is reported to contain calactin, calotropin, calotoxin and uscharidin, all of which are poisonous in nature (Chouhan *et al.* 1992). In latex, a powerful bacteriolytic enzyme, a very toxic glycoside calactin and a non-toxic proteolytic enzyme calotropin have been identified. It is more proteolytic than papain and bromelain (Himalaya Drug Co-Herbal database).

Toxicological studies

The accidental instillation of herb juice of both *C. procera* and *C. gigantea* resulted in local poisoning (Chouhan *et al.* 1992). In higher doses, root bark caused nausea, vomiting and diarrhoea, headache, burning micturition, and leucorrhea. The toxic constituents of latex had a caustic effect on mucous membranes and tender skin. It increased heart beat and respiration, leading to distress and death. Calotropin, a compound in latex, is more toxic than strychnine (Himalaya Drug Co. – Herbal database).

References

Basu, A., Sen, T., Ray, R.N., Nag Chaudhuri, A.K. (1992) Hepatoprotective effects of *Calotropis procera* root extract on experimental liver damage in animals. *Fitoterapia*, 63, 507–514.

Chouhan, B.S., Gupta, I.L.A., Rathore, G.S., Mathur, C.B. (1992) *Calotropis* injury to eye. *Afro Asian Journal of Ophthalmology*, 10, 124–125.

Jain, P.K., Kumar, N. Verma, R. (1985) Clinical trials of Arka Mula Tvaka, bark of *Calotropis procera*, Ait (R.Br.) on Atisar and Pravihika – a preliminary study. *Journal of Research in Ayurveda and Siddha*, 6, 89–91.

Kumar, V.I., Basu, N. (1994) Antiinflammatory activity of the latex of *Calotropis procera*. *Journal of Ethnopharmacology*, 44, 123–125.

Nadkarni, K.M. *Indian Materia Medica*, Vol. I. Popular Prakashan, Bombay, India 1954.

Prasad, G. (1985) Action of *Calotropis procera* on migraine (Family Asclepiadaceae). *Journal of National Integrated Medical Association*, 27, 7–10.

Sharma, P.P., Sharma, J.M. Therapeutic evaluation of *Calotropis* spp. in the management of bronchial asthma: a clinical study. *International Seminar of Traditional Medicine*, Calcutta, 7–9 November 1992.

Smit, H.F., Woerdenbag, H.J., Singh, R.H., Meulenbeld, G.J., Labadie, R.P., Zwaving, J.H. (1995) Ayurvedic herbal drugs with possible cytostatic activity. *Journal of Ethnopharmacology*, 47, 75–84.

Thirunavukkarasu, S. (1995) A clinical evaluation of Siddha herbal drugs for bronchial asthma: Eraippu Noi. *International Seminar on Recent Trends in Pharmaceutical Sciences*, Ootacamund, India. 18–20 February 1995.

6 Akrakara

Anacyclus pyrethrum DC
Syn: *A. pyrethrum* (L.) Lagsca
Family: Asteraceae (Compositae)

The English name of this root is pellitory. In Germany, *A. officinarum*, also known as *A. pyrethrum* or *Pyrethrum germanicum* was used earlier.

THE PLANT AND ITS DISTRIBUTION

The plant does not grow in India, and is imported mainly from Spain, Algeria, Morocco and other Mediterranean countries. It is commonly adulterated with other roots of similar shape. It is a perennial plant, the stems of which in the earlier stages lie prostate on the ground before arising erect. The leaves are smooth, alternate and pinnate with deeply cut segments. Each stem bears one large flower head; the disk flowers are yellow and ray flowers white, tinged with purple beneath.

The root is slightly twisted, cylindrical, tapering brownish to greyish brown in colour, wrinkled, about 0.5 cm thick, with a tuft of grey hairs and bright black spots. The fracture is short and horny. The cut surface is pale white in colour and shows a radiate structure in the centre, with many oleoresin glands in the bark. The root has slight odour, taste is pungent with a tingling sensation.

USES IN FOLKLORE AND AYURVEDA

Earlier, it was used in Europe for relieving toothache and in promoting free flow of saliva in cases of mouth and throat dryness. A gargle of the infusion was prescribed for relaxing mouth muscles and in partial paralysis of the tongue. Patients seeking relief from rheumatic or neuralgic affections of the head and face were advised to chew the root daily for several months. It was supposed to purge the brain (cerebral stimulant) and thus help in epilepsy, gout, sciatica and in lethargy (fibromyalgia).

In India, because of its powerful irritant nature, it is considered a stimulant for the nervous system and is included in the preparations used as a sex stimulant. It is also an ingredient in recipes for paralysis, hemiplegia, chorea and rheumatism.

In Unani system of medicine, a decoction obtained by boiling in 100 ml of water, a mixture of *Anancyclus pyrethrum* 2 g, ginger 1 g, liquorice 2 g is prescribed for 30–45 days in facial palsy.

Ayurvedic preparation

Akrakaradi Vati

Method   Mix fine powders of *akrakara* 1 part, ginger (dry) 1 part, *Piper cubeba* 1 part, saffron 1 part, long pepper 1 part, nutmeg 1 part, clove 1 part, sandalwood 1 part, opium 4 parts, and make pills of 125 g each.

Uses   To delay the time of ejaculation during sexual intercourse.

Chemical studies

The root has resin, inulin, some inorganic compound and an active principle pyrethrin.

7 Amalaki

Phyllanthus emblica L.
Syn: *Emblica officinalis* Gaertn
Family: Euphorbiaceae

THE PLANT AND ITS DISTRIBUTION

The tree grows wild in the deciduous the forests of the Indian subcontinent and along the foothills of the Himalayas. It flowers in March to May and the fruit ripens in the cold season. Leaves are feathery, with small, oblong, pinnately arranged leaflets (Fig. 2A). The fruits are depressed globes (Fig. 2B). The fruit of the wild variety is the smallest, 2–2.5 cm in diameter and 7–10 g in weight. This fruit has more fibres, is astringent and is more acidic in taste. *Amla* is often cultivated and two horticultural varieties *Biju* and *Kalmi* are well known. In *Biju* variety the fruits are fleshy globes, 2.5–3.6 cm in diameter weighing 10–15 g. The *Kalmi* variety has the biggest fruit, which may grow up to 5 cm in size. The fresh fruit is waxy and when ripe its pale yellow colour is often tinged with pink. The dry fruit (Fig. 2C) is smaller in size, sub-hexagonal and wrinkled. The colour varies from greyish black to yellowish brown, depending on the stage of ripening when it is harvested. The dry fruit separates easily into six parts and on applying pressure releases trigonous seed. Sometimes the commercial samples of the fruit are waxy brownish. These are obtained by drying the boiled fruit. By boiling, the contents of the fruits gelatinize, resulting in a waxy pulp.

Morton (1957) has given an account of this tree.

In Ayurveda, the various characteristics of the fruit described are: *Shreephala* – fruit of prosperity, *Shiva* – auspicious, nectar, *Divyadhara* – the basis of divine quality, *Sayastha* – arrests old age, *Dhatri* – mother like, sustains the life, *Vrishya* – invigorating, *Shitphal* – fruit cooling in effect.

USES IN FOLKLORE AND AYURVEDA

According to Ayurveda, *amalaki* is sour but not acidic like other fruits. It is astringent but sweet. On tasting the fruit, it is initially sour, but sometimes with a sweet aftertaste, which becomes more apparent if water is drunk afterwards.

The common uses of the fruit are:

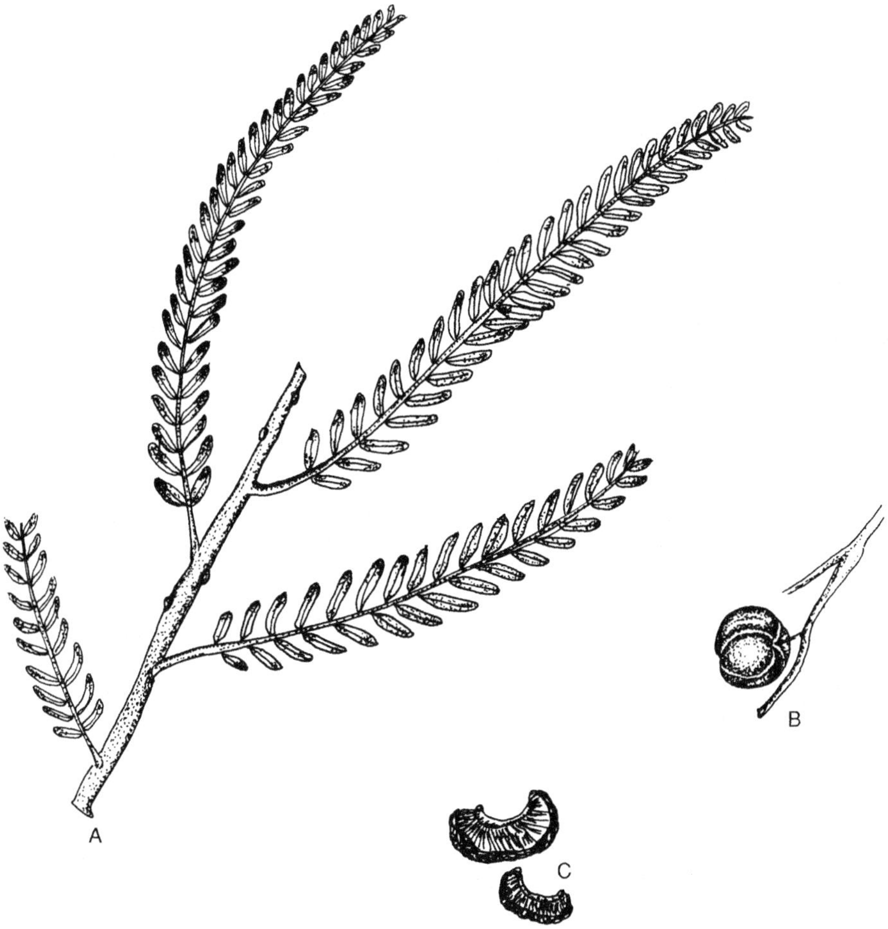

Figure 2 Phyllanthus emblica **A** leaves, **B** fresh fruit, **C** dry fruit.

As a *Rasayana*

Amalaki is considered best among *Rasayana* so called *Acharasayana*. It clears all the three *doshas* present in the human body. A regular use of *amalaki* is presumed to prolong lifespans, up to 120 years for humans. Its use not only increases human life but also improves the quality. It imparts memory, balanced intellect, health, youthfulness, lustrous body and a clear voice. It helps reduce tendencies for headaches, confusion of thought, psychic disorders and memory loss. *Amla*, when administered with *ghee*, honey and oil for one month, is a geriatric tonic for general debility, lack of disease resistance and memory loss. It overcomes the degenerative effects of old age. In winter, when vitality is low, *amla* with *ashwagandha*, *ghee* and honey is restorative and invigorating.

In stomach troubles

A decoction of the fruit is useful in dyspepsia, chronic dysentery and diarrhea. It is cooling and a refrigerant, diuretic and laxative. A sherbet of the fruit made with lemon juice helps acute dysentery, constipation, piles, enlarged liver and dropsy.

As an expectorant

It is a stimulant and expectorant in chronic bronchitis.

In diabetes

It is used for sugar control in diabetes. A tablespoon of the juice with a cup of bitter gourd (*Momordica charantia*) juice, or with equal quantities of powder of seed kernel of *Syzgium cumini*, taken daily for two months stimulates the pancreas and causes insulin secretion.

In eye diseases

The eyes should be washed with a solution of *amla* juice. The juice is administered internally with honey. It is said to restore eyesight and reduce intraocular tension.

As a hair tonic

As a hair tonic, for hair growth and pigmentation, hair is washed with an infusion prepared by soaking *amla* overnight in water. For detergency, soap pod (*Acacia concinna*) and soap nut (*Sapindus mukorossi*) may be added to *amla* before soaking. A hair oil is prepared by boiling a decoction or juice of *amla* in the sesame oil until all water from the mixture evaporates. While preparing this medicated oil, *Centella asiatica*, *Eclipta alba* and some aromatic herbs may be used along with it.

Household preparations

Amla is a household remedy in many parts of India and may be used as follows:

Powder

The fine powder of the fruit is administered as such, or with water or milk.

Decoction

The powder in the form of decoction and may be administered as such, or used as a washing agent as detailed above.

Poultice

The coarse powder is heated with water and applied to wounds or swellings.

Medicated hair oil

As detailed above under hair tonic.

Medicated ghee

The juice or decoction of *amalaki* is boiled along with other herbs in butter oil (*ghee*) until all the water evaporates.

Preserve

The big *Kalami Amla* (horticultural variety) fruit is stored in saline water for a couple of days, washed, pierced with stainless steel needles and stored in a glass pot with alternate layers of sugar and fruit. After a few days the sugar (which turns into syrup) is separated from the fruits, heated until thick and poured back on the fruits. After many days the sugar infiltrates the fruit, which becomes soft and loses much of its astringency and sourness. This preserve is often administered with silver foil for headaches, as a nervous tonic. While making the preserve, precautions are taken to prevent iron objects from touching the *amalaki* fruits as these turn the preserve black.

Compound Ayurvedic preparations

Amla is an ingredient of a large number of Ayurvedic preparations. The important ones, in which *amla* is the main ingredient are: *Amalaki Rasayana, Triphala*, and *Chavanprasha*. Keeping in view the importance and popularity of these products, a detailed account of these is given after the therapeutic and pharmacology studies on *amla*.

THERAPEUTIC INDICATIONS AND PHARMACOLOGICAL STUDIES

Bordi *et al.* (1985) have written a article on the juice of this fruit.

As an anabolic agent

It raised the total protein level and increased the body weight. Clinical research has shown the positive effects of this fruit on the body, which include enhanced cellular regeneration, increased lean body mass, enhanced production and secretion of interferon and corticosteroids. *Amla* preparation caused a significant increase in body weight. Nitrogen balance studies also showed that it has an anabolic effect (Singh and Guru, 1975, Tewari *et al.* 1968).

Antiemetic

This effect was observed by Yaqueenuddin *et al.* (1990).

Antioxidant effect

Experiments conducted at Niwa Institute of Immunology in Japan have shown it to be a potent scavenger of free radicals as it has a high level of superoxide dimutase (SOD) activity (Treadway, 1988). Earlier it was considered that the fruit's antioxidant activity was due to ascorbic acid, but work done by Thresiamma *et al.* (1996) and Ghoshal *et al.* (1996) indicated that it is due to ellagic acid and four hydrolyzable tannins.

As an antidiarrhoeal

The antidiarrhoeal activity is generally attributed to the astringent action of tannins in the fruit on the mucosal proteins, resulting in the formation of a protective layer and thus the arresting of intestinal inflammation.

As an antimicrobial

It has antiviral, antibacterial and antifungal activity. When *Amla* was studied for inhibitory effects on human immunodeficiency virus-1 reverse transcriptase, it exhibited significant activity. Bioassay-guided studies indicated that putranjivain A and four other compounds are potent inhibitory substances (El-Mekkawy, 1995).

Antimutagenic effect

It protected *Salmonella typhimurium* against nitro-o-phenylenediamine-induced mutagensis (Grover and Simran Kaur, 1989).

As an immunomodulator

Amla has been found to enhance natural killer cell activity and antibody-dependent cellular cytotoxicity. It elicited a twofold increase in spleen NK cell activity on third day of tumour inoculation, which became highly significant later on. It increased the lifespan of tumour-bearing rats by 35 per cent. The anti-tumour property is due to cell mediated toxicity (Suresh and Vasudevan, 1994).

As a cytoprotectant

When animals fed with lead and aluminium salts were given aqueous extract of *amla*, histopathological studies revealed that *amla* could prevent the cytotoxicity of metals more successfully than vitamin C (Roy *et al.* 1991). Crude *amla* extract before administration of cesium chloride reduced the clastogenic effect of the compound *in vivo* on mouse bone marrow. It reduced the frequency of chromosomal aberrations (Ghosh *et al.* 1993). Gulati *et al.* (1995) observed that 50 per cent alcohol extract and quercetin isolated from alcohol extract showed significant hepatoprotection against alcohol and paracetamol in rats. Ellagic acid from *amla* afforded protection against radiation-induced toxicity (Thresiamma *et al.* 1996).

As a nutritive tonic

Earlier the therapeutic efficacy of the *amla* was considered to be due to the presence of vitamin C in the fruit (Siddique and Ahmed, 1985). It was observed that one fruit of *amla* contained vitamin C equivalent to nine oranges. Recent studies also confirmed that bioavailability of vitamin C from *amla* fruit is better than that from the synthetic ascorbic acid, probably due to the presence of some accessory factors in the fruit. Roy *et al.* (1987) observed that 10 ml of *Amla* syrup, containing 8.7 mg of vitamin C was as effective as 100 mg of synthetic vitamin C. It is one of the fruits containing chromium and some of the beneficial effects of it may be due to this element (Janjua, 1991). *Amla* preparations showed good effects in generalised weakness (Jayaram *et al.* 1993).

In acne vulgaris

When *Sunder vati* (consisting of *Holarrhena pubescens*, *Emblica officinalis*, *Embelia ribes* and *Zingiber officinale*) was studied in a double blind randomized placebo-controlled clinical evaluation, a significant reduction in lesions was indicated (Pranjpe and Kulkarni, 1995).

In heart problems

The effect of alcoholic extract of *amla* was studied on myocardial necrosis. It increased the cardiac glycogen level significantly with marked changes in serum-free fatty acids levels. Serum glutamic oxaloacetic transminase (SGOT), serum glutamic pyuruvate transminase (SGPT), and serum lactic dehydrogenase (LDH) were significantly less in the group treated with this fruit (Tariq *et al.* 1977).

In hyperacidity

Cases of hyperchlorhydria with burning sensation in the abdomen, cardiac and gastric regions benefited from application of the fruit powder. A decoction prepared by taking 5 g *amla* in 80 ml of water (reduced to 20 ml) was given after main meals to patients. There was significant relief in symptoms after 30 days (Tripathi *et al.* 1992). When water extract of *amla* was administered to patients of hyperhidrosis, excellent results were achieved in 29 of 40 cases (Zachariah, 1984).

In hypercholesterolaemia

In a trial, when 15 g of fresh *amla* was taken daily for four weeks, it reduced cholesterol by 21 per cent. Feeding *amla* to hypercholesterolaemic rabbits for 12 weeks increased lipid mobilization, catabolism and retardation of lipid deposition in the extra hepatic tissues. The lipid level in the aorta increased but it was much less compared with the control (Mand *et al.* 1991). *Amla* reduced serum cholesterol levels significantly and had an antiatherogenic effect. It was confirmed that this effect of *amla* is due to a group of compounds and not vitamin C alone (Thakur and Mandal, 1984). Mathur *et al.* (1996) studied the hypolipidaemic effect of fruit juice in cholesterol-fed rabbits and an antiatherosclerotic effect was observed. It lowered serum cholesterol, triglyceride, phospholipid and LDL value by 82 per cent, 66 per cent, 77 per cent, and 90 per cent respectively. Rabbits treated with *amla* juice excreted more cholesterol and phospholipids, suggesting that the juice changed the mode by which these compounds are absorbed.

In leucorrhoea

A one g dose of equal quantities of *amla* and *guggal* with honey, three times a day was effective in leucorrhoea (Seshagiri Rao *et al.* 1985). *Triphala*, when used, was also effective (Singh and Londhe, 1993).

In ulcers

When the patients of duodenal ulcer and non-ulcer dyspepsia, were administered *amla*, they showed improvements, with a significant drop in acid and pepsin secretion (Varma *et al.* 1977, Chawla *et al.* 1982). Complete radiological recovery was reported in the peptic ulcer patients. *Amla* exhibited prophylactic affect against histamine-induced ulcers in albino rats (Singh and Singh, 1985). Intraperitoneal administration of ellagic acid from *amla*, in a 5 mg/kg dose, markedly reduced the occurrence of gastric lesion and acid secretion-induced stress (Murakami *et al.* 1991). Pakrashi and Bandyopadhyaya (1996–1997) have also studied the effects of *amla* extract on peptic ulcers.

AYURVEDIC PREPARATIONS

1 *Triphala*

This *Rasayana* is made by pulverizing a mixture of dry fruits of *P. emblica*, *Terminalia bellirica* and *T. chebula*. Different opinions exist about the proportion of each fruit in the formulation of *Triphala*. The various views are as follows:

1   One part each of the three fruits, by weight.
2   One part *T. chebula*, two parts *T. bellirica* and three parts *P. emblica*, by weight.
3   One part *T. chebula*, two parts *T. bellirica* and four parts *P. emblica*, by weight.
4   One fruit of *T. chebula*, two of *T. bellirica* and four fruits of *P. emblica*, by number. (This does not appear appropriate as the weight of individual fruit on the same tree varies and the resultant product based on the number of fruits cannot be of uniform quality).

Uses in Ayurveda

Triphala is one of the most widely used Ayurvedic preparations and a household name in India. It is a fine combination of three *Rasayana* fruits, which interact and potentiate each other. As with the Ayurvedic concept, it destroys *kapha* and *pitta*. It is a laxative, digestive, carminative, good for eyes and gives relief in diabetes, leprosy and in chronic fevers. The other major uses of *Triphala* are:

For arthritis

Boil 10 g *Triphala* in 200 ml of water until reduced to one-fourth and add one teaspoon of honey to this decoction. Drink this decoction twice daily, in the morning and evening. It is an anti-inflammatory agent and induces sleep.

As a blood purifier

For healthy skin and in diabetes, take 3 g *Triphala*, 3 g turmeric, and 6 g sugar. Drink this mixture with water for 60 days.

For chronic headaches

Take 30 g of *Triphala* and 10 g each of *Swertia* spp., turmeric, *Azadirachta indica* bark and *Tinospora* spp. Make a fine homogenous mixture. Take 10 g of this powder and boil it in 800 ml of water until reduced to 200 ml, strain and drink along with 10 g of *Commiphora wightii* gum.

In convalescence

Mix equal quantities of fine powders of *Triphala*, *Withania somnifera*, *Glycyrrhiza glabra* and *Asparagus racemosus*. The dose is 3 g with honey, before meals for 30–40 days.

For improving eyesight and coughs

Make an infusion of 10 g *Triphala* in 400 ml of water and keep overnight. In the morning filter the infusion and wash the eyes with it (it may cause irritation to eyes). Internally, take 10 g *Triphala* with one teaspoon of *ghee*.

For obesity

Regularly drink two teaspoons of honey with one teaspoon of *Triphala* and a glass of cold water.

For oral hygiene

As a tooth powder for dental cavities, spongy, bleeding gums and malodour, etc., make a fine powder by mixing *Triphala*, *Acacia* bark and *Butea* gum 50 g each, ginger and black pepper 10 g each, dehydrated alum (alum is heated to remove water until it swells), common salt, turmeric, *Cyperus scariosus*, *Embelia ribes*, *Azadirachta* leaves and *Quercus* gall (20 g each). Pass the powder through a sieve of 100 mesh or so, so that there are no coarse or gritty particles. Massage this powder on the gum, not on the teeth. Let the powder remain there for about 20 minutes. If there is an excess of saliva in the mouth, it should be spat out but water for gargling should not be used during the duration of treatment. The mouth may be rinsed afterwards.

(Note: this powder contains quite a number of astringent substances, some of them very rich in tannins, so the mouth may become very dry after its use in some cases.)

For premature grey hairs

Drink a mixture of two teaspoons of honey, half a teaspoon *ghee* and one teaspoon of *Triphala* first thing in the morning, when stomach is empty.

For stomach troubles

For indigestion A mixture of fine powders of *Triphala* 10 g, black salt 1 g, divided into three doses, is used three times a day.

As a laxative Boil 20 g *Triphala* in 400 ml of water until reduced to 100 ml. Add 10–20 ml of castor oil and drink before retiring. It is a very good colon cleanser.

For flatulence Mix fine powders of *Triphala* 15 g, raw sugar 10 g, ginger 5 g, and take a dose of 5 g twice daily.

For loose motions with mucus a) Take 3 g *Triphala* with honey or b) a mixture of equal parts of *Triphala*, *Cyperus scariosus*, *Aconitum heterophyllum*. Dose 3 g twice daily. Avoid fried, spicy and hard-to-digest food items. (Note: *A. heterophyllum* is a non-poisonous aconite, bitter in taste. It does not contain the toxic aconitine group of alkaloids and is safe even for infants, to whom it is often prescribed as an antidote to poisons.)

Compound preparations of Triphala

Sooksham Triphala

Ingredients: *T. bellirica*, *T. chebula*, *P. emblica* 66.7 g each and *Kajjali* 10 g (made by triturating mercury 5 g, and sulphur 5 g). *Sooksham Triphala* is used for the same purposes as *Triphala* but *Kajjali* is said to enhance its effect.

Mahatriphaladi Ghrit

Method *Triphala* powder 500 g, and 500 ml juice of each of *Eclipta*, *Adhatoda vasica*, *P. emblica*, *Fumaria indica*, *Tinospora*, goat milk 500 ml, *ghee* 500 g. Separately take 15 g each of long pepper, sugar, black grapes, blue lotus flowers, *Triphala*, liquorice, *Withania*, *Tinospora*, and *Solanum surattensis* (*S. xanthocarpum*).
   Boil *Triphala* (500 g) in 4 litres of water until reduced to half a litre. Filter it and add to it 15 g powder of each of nine herbs. Mix this decoction in *ghee* followed by juices and milk. Heat the whole mass until all the water evaporates and only fatty matter is left.

Dose 5–10 g (1–2 teaspoons) twice daily with milk, sweetened with sugar.

Indications Cleans the eye, restores eyesight, prevents formation of cataract and saves eyes from all types of diseases. It is alleged that regular use of this compound for 5–6 months can improve eyesight to such an extent that glasses may not be required.

Phalghrit

Method Take ten g each of liquorice, *T. bellirica*, *T. chebula*, *P. emblica*, *Saussurea lappa*, turmeric, *Berberis* spp., *Picrorhiza kurroa*, *Embelia ribes*, *Piper longum*, *Cyperus scariosus*, *Citrullus colocynthis* root, *Withania somnifera*, *Acorus calamus*, *Hemidesmus indicus*, *Cryptolepis buchanani*, *Callicarpa macrophylla*, fennel, asafoetida (fried), *Alpinia galanga*, *Santalum album*, *Pterocarpus santalinus*, jasmine flower, lotus flowers, bamboo manna (silica), celery, *Baliospermum montanum* and sugar along with 600 g *ghee*, 250 ml cow's milk and 250 ml water.

Make a paste from the coarse powders of all the herbs with water and *ghee*, add milk and the remaining water. Heat until all the water evaporates. Strain the fatty matter through muslin cloth and preserve.

Dose 5–10 g in the morning.

Indications: It exerts beneficial effects on the sexual system of both males and females. It is particularly useful in infertility and threatened miscarriage. Couples desirous of a child should start this medication months before conception and the expectant mother should continue this during pregnancy. This treatment facilitates normal delivery and a healthy child.

Therapeutic indications and pharmacological studies on Triphala preparations

Anthelmintic activity

Gaind *et al.* (1964) noted this activity.

As an anti-oxidant

Vani *et al.* (1997) observed radical scavenging properties in *Triphala* extract. It was effective in preventing superoxide-induced haemolysis of red blood cells. The extract also prevented lipid peroxidation in rat liver mitochondria.

Anti-inflammatory, analgesic and antipyretic property

Ghosh *et al.* (1989) observed these activities in *Triphala*. Doiphode (1993) prescribed *Sooksham Triphala* to 73 patients suffering from fevers, headaches, body aches and coughs. Out of these 49 patients showed signs of improvement.

As an antidiabetic

Triphala (90 mg/kg orally) had a significant hypoglycaemic activity in fasting rats (Ghosh *et al.*, 1990).

In obesity

For weight loss, Pranjape *et al.* (1990) prescribed 250 mg *Triphala guggal*, three times daily with lukewarm water before meals for three months. Kulkarni (1995a, b, c) used *Sooksham Triphala* in obesity and observed a significant weight loss with reductions in skin-fold thickness, hip and waist circumference, serum cholesterol and triglyceride levels. It was moderately useful in lipoma.

In leucorrhoea

Triphala decoction yielded good results, when given to the patients with symptoms of leucorrhoea (Singh and Londhe, 1993).

2 Amalaki Rasayana I

Method Cut transversely into two pieces, one big and one small, the stem of mature *Butea* tree. From one side of the bigger stem piece, scoop out wood to form a container-like structure. With the smaller piece make a lid. Fill the container with fresh green *amla* fruit and seal it with the lid. The whole assembly is covered on the outside with the coarse cloth and plastered with wet clay about 2.5 cm thick. Heat the container in slow burning cow dung cakes, remove it from the fire after 2–3 hours and take out the cooked fruits. Macerate these fruits by hand to remove the stones and fibres from the pulp. To this pulp add equal quantities of *ghee* and one and a half times as much honey to form a paste.

Dose Before administering this preparation, *Panchkarma* is required and the patient is confined to a hut for one month. Water and food should not be used, only giving cow's milk 2–3 times a day. The initial dose of this *Rasayana* is 50 g, which may be increased up to 200 g, depending on the digestive power of the patient.

Indications The above treatment is said to rejuvenate all body systems with increased mental power, resistance and immunity. It is alleged to transform old men into young, with new hair and teeth, and induce physical power like that of an elephant.

3 Amalaki Rasayana II

It is a simpler form of the above *Amalaki Rasayana*. It is prepared by blanching the fresh fruit for five minutes in boiling water. When soft, stones and fibres are removed and the pulp of the fruit is dried in the sun. *Add amla juice* to this pulp, macerate and dry. This process is repeated daily for 21 days. On the 22nd day store the completely dry powder in an airtight container.

Dose: 2 g in the morning on an empty stomach with honey or with cold milk and honey. Do not use hot milk with honey.

Amalaki Rasayana imparts positive nitrogen balance to the body. It is digestive, laxative and diuretic (Singh and Guru, 1975).

4 Chavanprasha

It is also spelt as *Cyavanaprasa, Chyavanprasha*.

According to a legend in Rigveda, the sage *Chavan* got the formulation of this supreme *Rasayana* for rejuvenation and longevity from the twin divine physicians

Ashwini Kumars and by using the formulation *Chavan* became young again. For the benefit of mankind he widely disseminated the knowledge about this preparation. People in ancient India called it *Chavanprasha Avleh* (*prasha* means diet, and *avleh* is linctus), so its meaning is "the dietary linctus as revealed by *Chavan*".

Due to the aggressive publicity of the commercial section, *Chavanprasha* has become so popular in India that it accounts for one-third of the total sales of all Ayurvedic products. It has been introduced in the western world with great success.

According to Ayurveda, as a dietary supplement it strengthens the organs under the ribs. It is very effective in the convalescence of weak individuals, children and old people suffering from coughs, colds, urinogenital problems and in all disturbances of *vata, pitta* and *virya* (vital fluid). It makes the body strong and lustrous, sharpens the memory, contributing to a happy mind. The dose is 10–15 g in the morning and before retiring in the evening. The dose can be increased or decreased as per the digestive power of the patient.

Formulation of Chavanprasha

The formulation of *Chavanprasha* consists of two groups of herbs, *Ashtvarga* (eight herbs) and *Dashmul* (ten roots), in addition to many other ingredients.

Ashtavarga

The plants of the *Ashtvarga* group became rare or extinct about 500 years ago. The renowned author Bhavamisra (c1500–1600AD) suggested substitutes in his book *Bhavaprakasa Nighantu*, as referenced by Chunekar and Pandey (1969). Bhavamisra said, "What to say to common men is that as the herbs of *Ashtvarga* are not available to kings even so the learned physicians should substitute the herbs of *Ashtvarga* by the other herbs of the same physiological activity." Bhavamisra suggested the following substitutes for various members of *Ashtavarga*:

For *Meda, Mahameda:*	*Asparagus racemosus*
For *Jeevak* and *Rishbhak:*	*Pueraria tuberosa*
For *Kakoli* and *Ksheer Kakaoli:*	*Withania somnifera*
For *Ridhi* and *Vridhi:*	*Dioscorea bulbifera*, or *Tacca aspera* tubers.

Some other Ayurvedic experts did not agree with these substitutes and they suggested the following herbs:

In place of *Jivak:*	*Tinospora* spp. or *Centaurea behen*
In place of *Rishbhak:*	*Orchis* spp., or bamboo manna, or *Salvia haematode*
In place of *Meda:*	*Orchis mascula*
In place of *Mahameda:*	*Paederia foetida, Asparagus adscendens*
In place of *Kakoli:*	*Curculigo orchioides*

In place of *Ksheer Kakaoli*:	*Chlorophytum arundinaceum* or the other members of white *Musli*
In place of *Riddhi*:	*Sida spp.* herb or seed
In place of *Vridhi*:	*Orchis latifolia* or *Sida rhomboidea*

Recent research workers, after extensive ethnobotanical surveys of the Himalayas, from where *Ashtavarga* was probably collected, have identified the various members as follows:

Ridhi Vridhi:	*Habenaria interemedia* D. Don
Jivak:	*Microstylis* spp.
Rishbhak:	*Microstylis wallichii* Lindl.
Kakoli:	*Fritellaria oxypetala* Royle
Kshirkakaoli:	*Lilium polyphyllum*
Meda, Mahameda:	*Polygonatum verticillatum* Moench.

Dashmul

These ten plants are further divided into two groups: *laghu* (herb) and *Vrihta* (tree shrub).

Laghu   This consists of *Desmodium gangeticum*, *Uraria picta*, *Solanum indicum*, *S. xanthocarpum*, and *Tribulus terrestris*. These herbs grow mainly in the wild areas and are handcrafted, which is tedious and uneconomical, so it is common practice to use the whole herb with an admixture of adjoining flora in place of genuine herb roots.

Vrihat   This includes *Oroxylum indicum*, *Aegle marmelos*, *Gmelina arboreum*, *Clerodendrum phlomoides*, and *Stereospermum suvaleons*. The Ayurvedic texts mention the use of these plants' root bark but in these cases stem bark is used instead.

Recent studies on *Dashmula* by Gupta *et al.* (1983, 1984) have shown that its decoction produced aspirin-like antipyretic and anti-inflammatory effects. It reduced the spontaneous motor activity. It potentiated the pentobarbitone hypnosis and antagonized the amphetamine-induced hyperactivity. It also exhibited tranquilizing, sedative activity. The above research justified the use of *Dashmula* in pains, backache, gout, sciatica, pyrexia, inflammation and oedema.

Composition of Chavanprasha

The composition of this product varies from place to place and from person to person. The various manufacturers, on the basis of their experience, substitute the herbs with some other herbs/materials or fortify the preparation with minerals, animal products, etc. The number of formulations is so large that enumeration of the majority of these will be beyond this book's scope. For present purposes, as an example, a comparative study of various ingredients in *Charak Sanhita*, Puri (1970), Alam (1977), Ayurvedic Pharmacopoeia (personal communication) and by a commercial house, Baidyanath (personal communication), is given in Table I.

It is commonly advocated that fresh *amalaki* fruit should be used for the preparation of *Chavanprasha* but Alam *et al.* (1977), on the basis of chemical analysis of the end product, recommended the use of dry fruit also. These authors observed that the product manufactured by cooking at a low heat for a longer duration is of better quality than the product manufactured at a higher temperature. Earlier it was thought that therapeutic efficacy of *Chavanprasha* is due to vitamin C, but Alam *et al.* (1977) could detect only 19 mg/100 g ascorbic acid from the product prepared at low temperatures from dry fruit and 17 mg/100 g from that of the fresh fruit. The product obtained using a high temperature had 2.14 mg/100 g and the commercial samples 8.30 to 12.67 mg/100 g vitamin C. Shishoo *et al.* (1997) determined the vitamin C contents of *amalaki* and *Chavanprasha* by sensitive 0-phenylenediamine fluorometric methods. The pericarp of a large variety of *amla* contained 2.915 mg/g, the smaller variety 3.775 mg/g, the freeze-dried powder 23.24 mg/g and the room-temperature dried powder 21.04 mg/g of vitamin C. None of the three market samples of *Chavanprasha* investigated contained any vitamin C, which probably gets destroyed during processing.

Method of preparation   Boil 1,000 *amalaki* fruits in a vessel containing 16 litres of water. Crush 90 g of each of the herbs mentioned in Table I (except bamboo manna and spices (cardamom, long pepper, cinnamon leaves, cinnamon, *Mesua ferrea*)) and tie them loosely in a cloth to form a bag-like structure. Boil this bag in the vessel containing *amla* fruits and 16 litres of water until the water is reduced to one-fourth. When cool, the bag is taken out of water and discarded, while the *amalaki* fruit are kept for making pulp. From the cooked fruits, seeds and fibrous materials are separated by passing them through bamboo sieves or through thick filter cloth. The pulp is fried in *ghee* and oil until dehydrated. A decoction of the herbs obtained above is added to this fried paste and boiling is continued. When the mixture is like a thick slurry, 4.50 kg sugar is mixed and heating is continued until a jam-like consistency is obtained. The product is allowed to cool and 500 g honey, 352 g of fine bamboo manna powder, 175 g of finely powdered long pepper and all spices are added to the end product.

A mechanical way of preparing *Chavanprash* is to crush blanched *amalaki* fruit to form a paste. This paste is passed through a stainless steel sieve to remove non-digestible portions such as fibres, the seed coat, etc. The paste is then heated with a decoction of herbs. Pectin tests (as with jam) can be performed by treating the finished product with alcohol or by dropping paste in a glass of water. Bearing in mind the modern trend of using less fat, it has been shown that *Chavanprasha* made without frying the pulp in oil or *ghee* does not deteriorate for many years if properly cooked. Honey can be omitted in this preparation and sugar can be reduced. For diabetics invert sugar may be used instead of cane sugar.

Alam *et al.* (1977) analysed various samples of *Chavanprasha*. The samples contained 22.29 to 27.70 per cent reducing sugars, 6.16–6.21 per cent non-reducing sugars and 3.62–4.13 per cent total fats. The genuine sample had 14.04–18.32 per cent reducing sugars, 1.24–12.66 per cent non-reducing sugars and 2.19–7.67 per cent fats. A commercial sample contained 68.9 per cent total sugars and 8.33 per cent fats.

Dose   10–15 g in the morning and before retiring in the evening. If digestion is impaired by its use and food intake is reduced, then decrease the dose as per the digestive power of an individual.

Contraindications   Polyurea, acidic urine, constipation, flatulence, diarrhoea, and nocturnal spermatic emission.

Precaution   Chavanprasha is often made more palatable by adding more sugar and honey than that prescribed in ancient texts. Most of the commercial preparations contain up to 570 g of sugar and 60 g honey in one kilogram of preparation, without any warning for diabetics or individuals who are overweight or have high levels of cholesterol.

Chavanprasha *Special*

Chavanprasha is often fortified with gold and silver foil, saffron, musk (this is now mainly synthetic), red sulphide of mercury, stag horn or other ingredients which are supposed to have an invigorating effect. One such formulation is as follows:

Ingredients   2 kg *Chavanprasha avleh*, 25 mg processed gold, 10 g processed tin, 2 g saffron, 10 g stag horn ash, 10 g mica (processed 100 times), 2 g silver foils, 5 g *Makardhawaj* (red sulphide of mercury).

Method   Start with trituration of saffron, followed by other inorganic materials, one by one, until the whole mass is homogenous. Mix this mass in *Chavanprasha*. If the preparation is too thick and proper mixing is not possible add honey to lower the viscosity.
   Dose 5–10 g.

Uses   It increases the aphrodisiac effect of *Chavanprasha* many times and stimulates all the body systems. It should only be used in winter or in cold areas. It is said to have a very strong heating effect on the body and so should not be used in hot areas or during hot weather.

Therapeutic studies on Chavanprasha

It has an anabolic effect so is recommended for catabolic diseases like chronic infection, mainly pulmonary. Ojha *et al.* (1973) observed an increase in body weight and a 24-hour retention of urinary and faecal nitrogen in experimental animals fed on it. In other studies Varma *et al.* (1973) concluded that *Chavanprasha* toned up cardiovascular and respiratory systems and improved metabolism, particularly protein metabolism, and decreased urinary nitrogen and creatine levels. It affected the positive nitrogen balance. There were increases in serum protein levels, correcting the albumin–globulin ratio. The secretion of urinary muco-polysaccharides and hydroxy-proline decreased which suggested decreased connective tissue breakdown (this occurs at a higher rate in old people). The decrease in acetylcholine and histamine suggested improved adrenocortical function. It toned testicular activity with a significant increase in urinary testosterone. It improved respiratory stress, induced improved stress tolerance by correcting levels of neurohumours. Ojha *et al.* (1975) used *Chavanprasha* as an adjunct in the treatment of pulmonary tuberculosis; the clinical features were chronic lung infection and malnutrition. It showed results comparable to those of anabolic steroids, vitamins and protein supplements, with significant increases in body weight, without any side effects. When administered with antitubercular drugs there was not only amelioration of symptoms but a relative quick therapeutic response.

Savrikar and Bhangle (1984) carried out clinical studies with this preparation, while Tersia *et al.* (1982) noted that *Chavanprasha* was effective in increasing the body weight and haemoglobin levels considerably. Jose and Kuttan (1995) observed that aqueous extract inhibited oxygen free radicals. It had an effect on potent inhibitors of lipid peroxide formation and acted as a scavenger of hydroxyl and superoxide radicals *in vitro*. Mehrotra *et al.* (1995) noted adaptogenic and antifungal properties in it.

Chemical studies

The fruit is very rich in vitamin C. The tannins of the fruit consist of gallic acid and ellagic acid, which prevent the decomposition of vitamin C in both the raw form as well as in the finished product (Brahamchari and Gupi, 1958). In another study, analysis of the fruits collected in winter showed the following results: vitamin C 921 mg/100 ml in juice, 720/100 mg in pulp, calcium 0.05 per cent phosphorus 0.02 per cent, iron 1.2 mg and nicotinic acid 0.2 mg.

Table 1 Comparative study of different formulations of *Chavanprasha*

Ayurvedic name	Botanical name	Part used	Charak Smhita	Puri (1970)	Alam (1977)	Ayurvedic Pharmaco poeia	Commercial (Baidynath)*
Abhya (Haritaki)	Terminalia chebula	fruit	+	–	+	+	+
Adusa (Vasa)	Adhatoda vasica	leaves root	+	+	+	+	
Agaru	Aquillaria agallocha	wood	+	+	+	+	+
Aganimantha	Premna integrifolia Clerodendrum phlomoides	root bark	+	+	+	+	
Amalaki	Phyllanthus emblica	fruit	+	+	+	+	+
Amrita (Gaduchi)	Tinospora cordifolia	stem	+	+	+	+	+
Ashtvarga	(no specific herbs)						+

Table I continued

Ayurvedic name	Botanical name	Part used	Charak Smhita	Puri (1970)	Alam (1977)	Ayurvedic Pharmacopoeia	Commercial (Baidynath)*
Bala	Sida cordifolia	herb			+	+	
		seed					+
		root	+	+			+
Banslochan	(Bamboo concretion)		+	+		+	+
Bhuiamalaki	Phyllanthus amarus	herb	+		+	+	+
Bilva	Aegle marmelos	bark	+	+	+	+	+
Brhati	Solanum indicum	herb	+		+	+	+
Chandan (white)	Santalum album	wood			+	+	+
Chandan (red)	Ptercarpus santalinus	wood	+	+			
Dashmula	(no specific herbs)						+
Draksha	Vitis vinifera	fruit	+	+	+	+	+
Ela (small)	Elettaria cardamomum	fruit	+	+	+	+	+
Ela (big)	Amomum subulatum	fruit	+				
Gambhari (Kasmiri)	Gamelina arborea	root	+	+	+		
		bark				+	+
Ghee	Butter fat		+	+	+	+	+
Gokshru (small)	Tribulus terrestris	root	+	+	+	+	+
Gokshru (big)	Pedalium murex	fruit					+
Jivak	Ipomea digitata	root			+		+
Jivanti	Leptadenia reticulata	root	+		+	+	
Kaknasa	1. Marytenia diandra	root	+				+
	2. Lee aquata			+			
	3. Pentatrapsis microphylla					+	
Kakoli	1. Withania somnifera	root	+		+		
	2. Lilium polyphyllum					+	
Kakrasinghi	Rhus succedanea	galls	+	+			
Kantkari	Solanum surattense	herb	+		+	+	+
		root		+			
Kesar	Crocus sativus	style					+
Madhu	Honey		+	+	+	+	+
Mashparni	Teramnus labialis	herb	+	+	+	+	+
Meda	1. Asparagus racemosus	root			+		
	2. Habeneria intermedia			+			
	3. Polygonatum verticillatum					+	
Musta	Cyperus rotundus	root	+		+	+	

Table I continued

Ayurvedic name	Botanical name	Part used	Charak Smhita	Puri (1970)	Alam (1977)	Ayurvedic Pharmaco poeia	Commercial (Baidynath)*
Nagkesar	Mesua ferrea	stamen	+	+	+	+	+
Patala	Stereospermum	root	+				
	tetragonum	bark		+	+	+	+
	Syn.						
	S. suaveolens						
Patha	Cissampelos pariera	leaves	+				+
Patra (twak) (Dalchini)	Cinnamomum zeylanicum	bark	+	+	+	+	+
Pippali	Piper longum	fruit	+	+	+	+	+
Prishanparni	Uraria picta	herb	+	+			
	Syn. (U.lagopoides)	root			+	+	
Punernava	Boerhaavia difusa	root	+	+	+	+	+
Pushkara mul	1. Inula racemosa	root		+	+	+	
	2. Saussurea lappa		+				
Riddhi	1. Curculigo orchiodes	root	+				
	2. Habeneria intermedia			+		+	
	3. Dioscorea bulbifera				+		
Rishbhak	1. Microstyllis wallichi	root	+				
	2. Pueraria tuberosa				+		
Shalparni	Desmodium gangeticum	herb		+			
		root	+		+	+	
Sathi	1. Curcuma zedoria	root	+	+	+		
	2. Hedychium spicatum					+	
Shakar (Misri)**	Sugar		+	+	+	+	+
Sringi	Melaphis chinensis	leaves			+	+	
Shoynka	Oroxylum indicum	bark	+		+	+	
Tejpat	Cinnamomum spp	leaves	+	+	+	+	+
Til oil	Sesame oil		+	+	+	+	+
Utpala	Nymphea stellata	flower rhizome	+		+	+	+
Vanmung	Phaseolus aconitifolius or P. trilobus	root	+	+			
Vidarikand	Pueraria tuberosa	root		+	+	+	

* In addition to these, processed mica, ash of stag horn and red sulphide of mercury is also added.
** It is a sugar refined in Ayurvedic way.

The original formulation in the ancient texts recommended higher quantities of *Amalaki* fruit but the end product if prepared with this quantity is unpalatable, so the subsequent formulations contained lesser quantity of *Amla* and more of sugar.

References

Alam Muzaffer Varadrajan, T.V., Dayala Venkatakrishna, D. (1977) Some studies on Cyavanaprasa preparation and standardisation. *Journal of Research in Indian Medicine, Yoga and Homeopathy*, 12, 64–71.

Bordia, A., Verma, S.K., Mehta, I.K. Andreais, A.M.R. (1985) Comparative effects of amla juice: review. *Indian Drugs*, 23, 72.

Brahmachari, H.D., Gupi, V.S. (1958) Role of tannins in stabilising the ascorbic acid content of the fruit. *Indian Journal of Applied Chemistry*, 21, 173–174.

Chawla, Y.K., Dubey, P. Singh, R., Nandy, S., Tondon, B.N. (1987) Treatment of dyspepsia with amalaki (*Emblica officinalis*) with an Ayurvedic drug. *Vagbhata*, 5, 24–26.

Chunekar, K.C., Pandey, G.S. *Bhavprakash Nighantu* (in Hindi). Chokhamba Vidya Bhawan, Varansi, India 1969.

Doiphode, V.V. (1993) Suksham Triphala in general practice. *Deerghayu International*, 3, 21–23.

El-Mekkawy, S., Meselhy, M.R., Kusumoto, I.T., Kadota, S., Hattori, M., Namba, T. (1995) Inhibitory effects of Egyptian folk medicines on human immunodeficiency virus (HIV) reverse transcriptase. *Chemical and Pharmaceutical Bulletin*, 43, 641–648.

Gaind, K.N., Mital, H.C., Khanna, S.R. (1964) Anthelimintic activity of triphala. *Indian Journal of Pharmacy*. 26, 106–107.

Ghosal, S., Tripathi, V.K., Chauhan, S. (1996) Active constituents of *Emblica officinalis*: Part I: The chemistry and antioxidative effects of two new hydrolysable tannins, emblicanin A and B. *Indian Journal of Chemistry*, section B. *Organic including Medicinal*, 35, 941–948.

Ghosh, A., Sharma, A., Talukder, G. (1993) Comparison of the protection afforded by a crude extract of *Phyllanthus emblica* fruit and an equivalent amount of synthetic ascorbic acid against the cytotoxic effect of calcium chloride in mice. *International Journal of Pharmacognosy*, 31, 116–120.

Ghosh, D., Thejomoorthy, P., Veluchamy, G. (1989) Antiinflammatory, antiarthritic and analgesic activities of Triphala. *Journal of Research in Ayurveda and Siddha*, 10, 168–174.

Ghosh, D., Uma, R., Thejomoorthy, P. Veluchamy, G. (1990) Hypoglycaemic and toxicity studies of Triphala: a Sidha drug. *Journal of Research in Ayurveda and Siddha*, 11, 78–89.

Grover, I.S., Simran Kaur (1989) Effect of *Emblica officinalis* Gaertn (Indian Gooseberry) fruit extract on sodium azide and nitro-o-pheylenediamine-induced mutagensis in *Salmonella typhniureum*. *Indian Journal of Experimental Biology*, 27, 207–209.

Gulati, R.K., Agarwal, S., Agrawal, S.S. (1995) Hepatoprotective studies on *Phyllanthus emblica* Linn. and quercetin. *Indian Journal of Experimental Biology*, 33, 261–268.

Gupta, R.A., Singh, B.N., Singh, R.N. (1983) Pharmacological studies on *Dasamula kvatha*. Part I. *Journal of Research in Ayurveda and Siddha*, 4, 73–84.

Gupta, R.A., Singh, B.N., Singh, R.N. (1984) Pharmacological studies on *Dasamula kvatha*. Part II. *Journal of Research in Ayurveda and Siddha*, 5, 38–40.

Janjua, K.M. (1991) Role of minor minerals on human health. Diabetic control with chromium containing herbs. Part IV. *Hamdard Medicus*, 34, 104–106.

Jayaram, S., Walwaikar, P.P., Rajyadhyaksha, S.S. (1993) Evaluation of efficacy of a preparation containing combination of Indian medicinal plants in patients of generalised weakness. *Indian Drugs*, 30, 498–500.

Jose, I.K., Kutan, R. (1995) Inhibition of oxygen free radicals by *Emblica officinalis* extract and Chavanprasha. *Amala Research Bulletin*, 15, 46–52.

Kulkarni, P.H. (1995a) Clinical assessment of effect of Sookshma Triphala in Lipoma, in Kulkarni, P.H., ed., *Ayurveda Research Papers II*, pp. 66–71, *vide* MAPA 9605-2700.

Kulkarni, P.H. (1995b) Clinical assessment of effect of Sookshma Triphala in Lipoma. *Biorhythm*, 72–77, *vide* MAPA 9605-2713.

Kulkarni, P.H. (1995c) *Clinical study of effect of Sukshma (subtle) Triphala Guggulu (TG 3X)*, in P.H. Kulkarni, ed., *Ayurveda Research Papers* II, pp. 50–59, *vide* MAPA 9605-2716.

Mand, J.K., Soni, G.L., Gupta, P.P., Singh, R. (1991) Effect of Amla (*Emblica officinalis*) on the development of atherosclerosis in hypercholesterolemic rabbits. *Journal of Research and Education in Indian Medicine*, 10, 1–7.

Mathur, R., Sharma, A., Dixit, V.P., Verma, M. (1996) Hypolipidaemic effect of fruit juice of *Emblica officinalis* in cholesterol fed rabbits. *Journal of Ethnopharmacology*, 50, 61–68.

Mehrotra, S., Rawat, A.K.S., Singh, H.K., Shome, U. (1995) Standardisation of popular Ayurvedic adaptogenic preparation *Chavanprash* and ethnobotany of its ingredients. *Ethnobotany*, 7, 1–15.

Morton, J.F. (1957) Emblic (Phyllanthus emblica) rich but neglected source of vitamin C. *Economic Botany*, 31, 223–264.

Murakami, S., Isobe, Y., Kijima, H., Nagai, H., Muramatu, M., Otomo, S. (1991) Inhibition of gastric H+, K+-ATPase and acid secretion by ellagic acid. *Planta Medica*, 57, 305–308.

Ojha, J.K., Bajpai, H.S., Sharma, P.V., Khanna, M.N., Shukla, P.K., Sharma, T.N. (1973) Chavanprasha as an anabolic agent: experimental study (preliminary work). *Journal of Research in Indian Medicine*, 8, 11–19.

Ojha, J.K., Khanna, M.N., Bajpai, H.S., Sharma, P.V., Sharma, T.N. (1975) A clinical study of Chavanprasha as an adjunct in the treatment of pulmonary tuberculosis. *Journal of Research in Indian Medicine*, 10, 1–4.

Pakrashi, A., Bandyopadhyaya, S. (1996–97) Effect of *Phyllanthus emblica* extract on peptic ulcer. *Phytomedicine*, 3(supp.), 66.

Puri, H.S. (1970) Chavanprasha: an ancient Indian preparation for respiratory diseases. *Indian Drugs*, 7, 15–16.

Pranjpe, P., Kulkarni, P.H. (1995) Comparative efficacy of four Ayurvedic formulations in the treatment of acne vulgaris: a double blind randomised placebo controlled clinical evaluation. *Journal of Ethnopharmacology*, 49, 127–132.

Paranjpe, P., Patki, P., Patwardhan, B. (1990) Ayurvedic treatment of obesity. A randomized double-blind placebo-controlled clinical trial. *Journal of Ethnopharmacology*. 29, 1–11.

Roy, A.K., Dhir, H., Sharma, A., Talukder, G. (1991) *Phyllanthus emblica* fruit extract and ascorbic acid modify hepatotoxic and renotoxic effects of metals in mice. *International Journal of Pharmacognosy*, 29, 117–126.

Roy, S., Khan, S.U., Siddiqui, H.H., Arora, R.B. (1987) Bioavailability of ascorbic acid in children as a method of standardisation of amla and vitamin C rich herbal extracts. (AH-II) *Hamdard Medicus*, 30, 229–238.

Savrikar, S.S., Bhangle, P.K. (1984) Clinical study of Chavanprasha Avaleh. *Nagarjun*, 27, 117–119.

Seshagiri, Rao, Kusumkumari, K., Netaji, B., Subhakta, P.K.J.P. (1985) A pilot study of Svet pradra (Leucorrhoea) with Amalaki Guggul. *Journal of Research in Ayurveda and Siddha*, 6, 213.

Shishoo, C.J., Shah, S.A., Rathod, I.S., Patel, S.G. (1997) Determination of vitamin C content of *Phyllanthus emblica* and Chyavanprash. *Indian Journal of Pharmaceutical Sciences*, 59, 268–270.

Siddique, T.O., Ahmed, J. (1985) Vitamin C contents of Indian Medicinal plants: a literature review. *Indian Drugs*, 23, 72.

Singh, I.P., Guru, L.V. (1975) The effect of Amalaki rasayana on experimental rats with special reference to their nitrogen balance. *Journal of Research in Indian Medicine*, 10, 141–146.

Singh, K.P., Singh, R.H. (1985) Recent advances in the management of amalpitta Parinam sula (non-ulcer dyspepsia and peptic ulcer dyspepsia). *Journal of Resesarch in Ayurveda and Siddha*, 6, 32.

Singh, R.K., Londhe, C.S. (1993) Use of Triphala Kwath in Swet Pradera (leucorrhoea). *Deerghayu International*, 9, 15–17.

Suresh, K., Vasudevan, D.M. (1994) Augmentation of murine natural killer cell and antibody dependent cellular cytotoxicity activities by *Phyllanthus emblica*, a new immunomodulator. *Journal of Ethnopharmacology*, 44, 55–60.

Tariq, M., Hussain, S.J., Asif, M., Jahan, M. (1977) Protective effect of fruit extracts of *Emblica officinalis* Gaertn and Terminalia belerica Roxb., in experimental myocardial necrosis in rats. *Indian Journal of Experimental Biology*, 15, 485–486.

Tersia, T.L., Sridhar, B.N., Pillai, B.K.R. (1982) Effect of Chyavanaprasha on malnutrition. *Journal of Research in Ayurveda and Siddha.* 3, 119–123.

Tewari, A., Sen, S.P., Guru, L.V. (1968) The effect of Amalaki (*Phyllanthus emblica*) rasayana on biologic systems. *Journal of Research in Indian Medicine*, 2, 189.

Thakur, C.P., Mandal, K. (1984) Effect of *Emblica officinalis* on cholesterol-induced atherosclerosis in rabbits. *Indian Journal of Medical Research*, 79, 142–146.

Thresiamma, K.C., George, J., Kuttan, R. (1996) Protective effect of curcumin, ellagic acid and bixin on radiation-induced toxicity. *Indian Journal of Experimental Biology*, 34, 845–847.

Treadway, Linda (1988) Amla, traditional food and medicine. *Herbalgram*, 31, 26–27.

Tripathi, P.C., Shaw, B.P., Mishra, R.K., Mishra, P.K. (1992) The role of amalaki in the management of amlapitta. *Indian Medicine*, 42, 11.

Vani, T., Rajani, M., Srakar, S., Shishoo, C.J. (1997) Antioxidant properties of the Ayurvedic formulation Triphala and its constituents. *International Journal of Pharmacy*, 35, 313–317.

Varma, M.D., Singh, R.H., Udupa, K.N. (1973) Biological, endocrine and metabolic studies on the effect of rasayana on aged persons. *Journal of Research in Indian Medicine, Yoga and Homeopathy*, 8, 1–9.

Varma, M.D., Singh, R.H, Gupta, J.P., Udupa, K.N. (1977) Amalaki rasayana in the treatment of chronic peptic ulcer. *Journal of Research in Indian Medicine, Yoga and Homoeopathy*, 12, 1–9.

Yaqueenuddin, Quereshi, I., Mirza, M., Yaqeen, Z. (1990) Pharmacological evaluation of the antiemetic action of *Emblica officinalis* Gaertn. *Pakistan Journal of Scientific and Industrial Research*, 33, 268–269.

Zachariah, G. (1984) *Emblica officinalis*: A remedy for hyperhidrosis. *Antiseptic*, 81, 312–315.

8 Anantmul

Hemidesmus indicus R. Br
Family: Asclepiadaceae

THE PLANT AND ITS DISTRIBUTION

It is also known as Indian Sarsaparilla. It should be distinguished from American Sarsaparilla, *Smilax aristolochaefolia* Mill and Jamaican Sarsaparilla, *Smilax ornata* Hook f.

It is a latex containing creeper (Fig. 3A) with opposing leaves that are 5–10 cm long with white streaks. Flowers are in bunches, greenish from outside but violet from inside. Follicles are 10 to 15 cm long. It grows in the sub-tropical forests of east and south India. The root of *anantmul* is 1–2 cm thick, blackish brown and wrinkled on the outside. The central woody portion is quite distinct (Fig. 3B). It has a pleasant camphoraceous smell and a mild bitter, astringent taste. The active ingredients are contained in the bark.

In Ayurveda, there is a confusion about the botanical identification of another herb *sariva*. Some authors think that *H. indicus* is white *sariva* (Karnick, 1977).

USES IN FOLKLORE AND AYURVEDA

As per Ayurveda, it is cooling, sweet, anabolic, heavy, oily, bitter, aromatic laxative, sudorific and a blood purifier. It stimulates the flow of bile and is antidote to *tridosha* and body toxins. It helps in leucoderma, malodour from the body and bronchial problems, leucorrhoea, gastroenteritis, inflammation, physical weakness, fatigue, weight loss, threatened miscarriage and kidney stones. It cures skin diseases and ulcerations, especially those of syphilitic origin. The other major uses of this herb are:

Diuretic effect

The decoction of root increases urine output by three to four times. When used with *Tinospora* spp. this herb's effect is enhanced further.

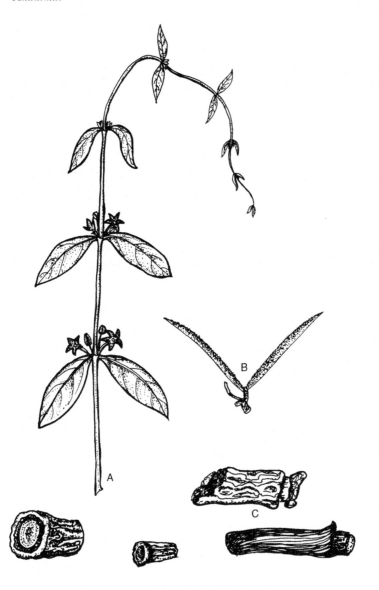

Figure 3 Hemidesmus indicus **A** branch, **B** follicles, **C** dry root pieces.

In urino-genital problems

With *Tinospora* and cumin, it relieves inflammation of urethra and burning micturition. The decoction of 3 g powder of the herb helps with prostate problems.

In sexually transmitted diseases

With *Tinopspra* spp., it is a valuable remedy for third and fourth stages of syphilis and its numerous manifestations. It may be used as follows:

1   Give a decoction made from equal parts of *Citrullus colocynthis* root, *anantmul*, *Ichnocarpus*, *Hedyotis auriculata*, to the patient as per the drinking capacity along with long pepper and *Commiphora wightii* powder.
2   Pulverize 5 parts of *anantmul*, 4 parts of *Vetiveria*, 5 parts of *Cyperus scariosus*, 6 parts of *Picrorhiza* and 4 parts of ginger. Prescribe a dose of 5–10 g of this preparation.

For infants and children

Hot infusion of the root with milk and sugar is a tonic for children with chronic coughs and diarrhoea.

As a laxative

Make a paste of 25 g each of *anantmul*, *Pavonia odorata*, *Cyperus rotundus*, ginger and *Picrorhiza*. Prescribe 10 g of this paste, twice daily with warm water.

THERAPEUTIC INDICATIONS AND PHARMACOLOGICAL STUDIES

It suppressed both the cell mediated and humoral component of the immune system (Atal *et al.* 1986).

The glycosides had an anti-tumour property (Deepak *et al.* 1997).

Chemical studies

The following compounds have been reported; coumarins, volatile oil, crystalline principle hemidesmine (Nadakarni, 1954), two sterols–hemidesterol and hemidesmol (Chunekar and Pandey, 1969) and pregnane glycoside (Deepak *et al.* 1997). The major component of the essential oil has been identified as p-methoxy salicylic aldehyde.

References

Atal, C.K., Sharma, M.L., Kaul, A., Khajuria, A. (1986) Immunomodulating agents of plant origin. *Journal of Ethnopharmacology*, 18, 133–141.
Chunekar K.C., Pandey, G.S. *Bhavprakash Nighantu* (in Hindi) Chowkhamba Vidya Bhawan, Varanasi, India 1969.
Deepak, D., Srivastava, S., Khare, A. (1997) Pregnane glycoside from *Hemidesmus indicus. Phytochemistry*, 44, 145–151.
Karnick, C.R. (1977) Ethnobotanical, pharmacognostical and cultivation studies of *Hemidesmus indicus* R. Br. (Indian Sarsaparilla). *Herba Hungarica*, 16, 7–12.
Nadkarni, K.M. *Indian Materia Medica*. Vol I. Popular Prakashan, Bombay, India 1954.

9 Ashwagandha

Withania somnifera (L.) Dunal
Family: Solanaceae

It is also known as Indian ginseng.

THE PLANT AND ITS DISTRIBUTION

The herb grows as a weed in the drier part of India on waste land. A cultivar is being cultivated on a large scale in some parts of central India. The plant is an evergreen shrub, 1–2 m high, with the whole body covered with star shaped hairs. Leaves (Fig. 4A) are simple, petiolate, ovate, and glabrous. Flowers are inconspicuous, in axillary clusters, light green or pale yellow, calyx membraneous. Berries are small, globose, orange red when mature with numerous yellow reniform seed. In wild forms the roots (Fig. 4B) are thick, fibrous, brown to dark brown and may even get twisted with age, with very little starch. However, in the cultivated plants, the root (Fig. 4C) is pale white, cylindrical and starchy.

Four chemotypes of *W. somnifera* have been recognised so far within the plant's natural population. The biological activity of these cultivars varies significantly and their biochemical heterogenity has been established. The cultivated variety, which probably originated near the town Nagaur in Rajasthan (India) and was hence known as *Asgandh Nagori*, became popular because of the starchy nature of its root. *Asgandh Nagori* is sown in the rainy season and the roots are ready for harvesting in winter. There is a controversy about the botanical nature of this plant. Some authors are of the opinion that it is a cultivated variety of *Withania*, while others identify it as a distinct species, *W. ashwagandha* Kaul. Further details on this and other aspects of *Withania* can be had from the book on this herb by Sandhya Singh and Sushil Kumar (1998).

USES IN FOLKLORE AND AYURVEDA

Since ancient times *ashwagandha* has been considered a nervine tonic, alterative, aphrodisiac, deobstruent (having the property of removing obstruction in any system of the human body) and a sedative. It has been used in rheumatism, consumption and in debility. The Indian name *ashwagandha* (*ashwa-* horse, *gandha-* smell), now commonly

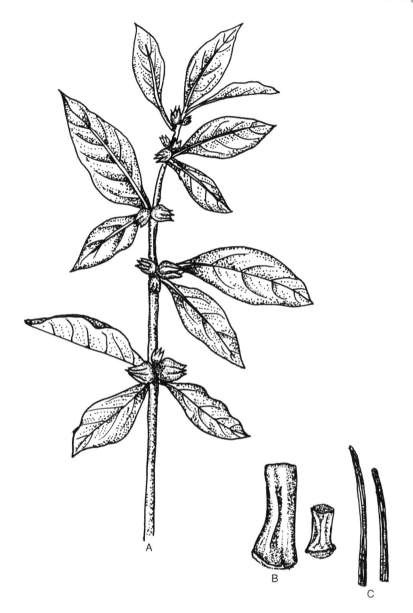

Figure 4 Withania somnifera **A** twig, **B** dry root from wild plants, **C** dry root from
cultivated plants.

called *asgandh* or *asgand*, is due to the smell that arises from the fresh root. In Ayurvedic
texts, it is mentioned that this herb imparts the power and (sexual) strength of horse
to a man.

Ashwagandha can be used by persons of both sexes, of all ages and at all stages of
their lives. In elders it provides energy, relieves inflammations, pains and aches of the
back, hand and feet, and in the generative system, nervous debility and diseases due to

vata. It is being prescribed as an anabolic agent, as an adaptogen and analgesic for the treatment of various arthropathies, certain forms of hypertension, insanity, etc. It imparts resistance to infection and stress. It stimulates sexual impulses and increases sperm counts. It is considered a *Rasayana*, for strength, vigour and for rejuvenation. The easiest way to use the root is to take one teaspoonful of the fine powder with sweetened milk, or mix the powder with *ghee*, lick the mixture followed by milk sweetened with sugar candy.

In gynecological practice it helps in sterility, leucorrhoea and inflammation of the vagina. It also helps breast development. For these purposes, take one teaspoonful of *ashwagandha* powder with half a teaspoonful of *ghee*, and honey before breakfast in the morning and before sleeping in the evening, followed by cold sweet milk. It must be taken for three months, particularly during winter.

Ayurvedic scholars consider the wild root to be a narcotic (the specific name *somnifera* means *sleep inducer* which implies its sedative nature) which should be applied externally to inflammation, boils, pimples and as an ingredient of massage oils. For internal consumption the wild root should be mitigated by boiling it in milk. *Asgandh Nagori* can be used as such.

Some of the important recipes of *ashwagandha* are as follows:

As a *Rasayana*

Method   Mix the powders of 100 g *Withania*, 50 g *Tinospora*, and 10 g of *Tinospora* (see *gaduchi*) starch.

Dose   Mix half a teaspoonful of this powder with half a teaspoon of *ghee* and two tea spoons of honey. Drink with cold sweetened milk twice daily for sixty days.

For infants and children, as a nutritive tonic, boil 1–2 g of this powder in a cup of milk, add to it 9–10 drops of *ghee* and give 1 teaspoonful of this warm milk to infants and two teaspoons to children.

Use   As a general tonic for all ages for vigour, vitality, nutrition, and stamina. It is a good nutritive tonic for malnourished men. It helps male sexual inadequacies (impotence, premature ejaculation, partial erection of penis, inability to perform the sex act, lack of libido and stamina, etc.).

For premature ejaculation

Pulverize 100 g each of *Withania*, *Argyreia*, *Hygrophila*, *Glycyrrhiza* and sugar candy. Take 10 g of this mixture with honey, and drink with milk.

In azoospermia

It is alleged that too much sexual indulgence through masturbation and other perverted sexual actions may lead to the collapse of vital body systems. For a cure, take in the morning on an empty stomach for 3–4 months, one teaspoon of *asgandh*, half a teaspoon of sugar candy, a quarter teaspoon of long pepper, half a teaspoon *ghee* and one and a half teaspoons of honey, followed by 200 ml milk boiled with one teaspoon of *Withania*, and one teaspoon of *ghee*.

During pregnancy

A decoction of 10 g *aswagandha* powder in a cup of water, when used for 2–3 months, provides nutrition to both the mother and foetus.

In leucorrhoea

I Take one teaspoon of *asgandh* powder and sugar with warm water for 3–4 months. It not only cures the disease but strengthens the body.

II Mix the fine powders of 100 g each of *asgandh* and *vidhara*, 20 g each of cardamom and eggshell ash, 10 g of processed tin and 150 g of sugar candy. Take 3 g of this powder, twice daily for four months.

For vata diseases

Due to indigestion and constipation, *vata* gets vitiated. For pacifying it, one tea spoonful of *Ashwagandhadi Ghrit* can be administered with a glass of water or make a mixture of equal quantities of *Withania and Asparagus* powders, with sugar candy. Take one teaspoon of this with milk twice daily.

In sterility

If conception is not possible due to improper ovum development, women should be prescribed 10 g *Withania* powder roasted in a small quantity of *ghee* on a low heat, followed by boiling it in a glass of milk for 15–20 minutes. This preparation should be taken for three days before and seven days after menstruation, freshly prepared and warm, in the morning on an empty stomach. Continue this treatment every month, until pregnant.

For sleeplessness

Take one teaspoon of *Withania* with *ghee* and honey every evening. If sleeplessness is due to *vata* add 2 g of long pepper to the above mixture.

As a galactagogue

For increasing milk during lactation, make a fine powder of equal quantities of *Withania*, *Asparagus*, *Pueraria tuberosa* and liquorice. This powder is taken twice daily.

AYURVEDIC PREPARATIONS

Ashwagandhadi Churn

Method   Pulverize 100 g *Withania* root, 100 g *Argyreia speciosa* root.

Dose   5 g twice daily with sweet milk or moisten the powder with *ghee* (butter oil), chew the mixture and swallow, followed by milk after 20 minutes or so. The powder can be administered with water but milk is preferred.

Use   *A. speciosa* fortifies the effect of *ashwagandha*. It should be drunk with milk. This *churn* strengthens physical, mental and sexual systems, particularly those of lean and thin persons. It builds resistance against infection, helps sleeplessness, nervous breakdown, memory, wrinkles on the face and premature ageing.

Asgandh pak

Method   1 kg *Aswagandh* powder, 500 g dry ginger, 250 g *Piper longum*, 112 g black pepper, 16 litre milk, 2 kg *ghee* (butter oil), ten g each of cinnamon, *Cinnamomum* spp. leaves, *Mesua ferrea*, cardamom, clove, *Piper longum* root, nutmeg, valerian, sandalwood, *Cyperus scariosus. Emblica officinalis*, bamboo manna (silicic acid), catechu, *Plumbago zeylanicum* root bark, *Asparagus racemosus* and *Pavonia odorata* powders. Syrup from 4 kg icing sugar.

Boil milk until reduced to half, add powders of *Withania*, ginger, long pepper and black pepper to it. Concentrate further until solid. Roast this condensed milk in *ghee* and add syrup made from the sugar, heat further and add fine powders of all the remaining items. When still warm, make balls of 10 g each.

Dose   10 g twice daily.

Use   A general tonic for all ages.

Ashwagandha Ghrit

Method   *Asgandh* root, 500 g coarse powder and 100 g fine powder, 250 g *ghee*, 1 litre cow's milk.

Method   Boil coarse *asgandha* powder in 4 litres of water to obtain 1 litre of decoction. Separately make a paste of fine powder of *aswagandha* in water. Add this paste to the filtered decoction, followed by *ghee*, milk and heat until the fatty matter is free from moisture.

Dose   Half to one teaspoon with sugar candy and milk as per the digestive power of an individual.

Indications   *Ashwagandha Ghrit* is very beneficial to infants (dose 3–4 drops with milk) and to children (dose 3 g to half teaspoon). It is highly nutritious. It makes the body strong, sturdy and stimulates the nervous system. It gives strength, cures diseases due to *vata*, arthritis, back pain, weakness in any part of the body, sleeplessness, sexual debility, depression, and nervous tension.

THERAPEUTIC INDICATIONS AND PHARMACOLOGICAL STUDIES

Psychotropic effects

It showed barbiturate hypnosis potentiation effect and a decrease in locomotive activity. It reduced the depletion of acetylcholine and catecholmine in the brain (Singh *et al.* 1979). It affected drug-induced narcosis in female and male mice (Ahmuda *et al.* 1991b). The total alkaloids exhibited prolonged hypotensive, bradycardia, respiratory stimulation, relaxant and antispasmodic effects, similar to papaverine, on intestinal, uterine, bronchial, and vascular systems. In mice, these prolonged sleeping time, as well as having a nicotenolytic effect. They increased the levels of serotonin and histamine in brain tissue. The protective effect of *asgandh* extract against pentylenetet-razole (PTZ) has been seen to induce convulsions in mice. This was dose dependent (Kulkarni *et al.* 1993) and was comparable to diazepam in both chemical and electrical kindling (Kulkarni and George, 1995) and against amygdaloid kindling (Kulkarni *et al.* 1995). Root extract protected electrographic activity in a lithium-pilocarpine model of status epilepticus. Acute pre-treatment with the extract enhanced the antiepileptic effect of diazepam and clonazepam (Kulkarni *et al.* 1998).

As an anabolic agent

Ashwagandha increased body weight, total protein content and mean corpuscular hae-moglobin in children. A weight promoting effect in young children was observed, without any toxic effect, even after 8 months of continuous daily administration (Venkatraghavan *et al.* 1984). This anabolic effect of *Withania* may be due to the fact that:

1   It contains steroidal substances, which enhance liver glycogen.
2   It stimulates the appetite by exhibiting anti-serotonergic activity, like cyprohep-tidine, with maximum effect in children.
3   It reduces adenocortical activity and has a sedative effect.
4   The depressant action produced by this herb may reduce metabolic rate leading to diminished calorie utilization and tendency towards weight gain. *Ashwagandha*-fed animals showed a reduction of 1.5°C in body temperature, which signifies lower metabolic rate and underutilization of glycogen.
5   It promotes growth by enhancing the growth of tissue components, with and without the release of growth hormones.
6   It increases liver weight, with no histopathological aberrations of cellular structures.

Immunomodulator activity

The important constituents of *ashwagandha*, withaferin A and withanolide D, induced significant immunosuppressive activity (Shobat *et al.* 1978). It was an immunomodulator and chemoprotector against cyclophosphamide (Praveen Kumar *et al.* 1994, Davis and Kuttan, 1998). It had the potential to alleviate the adverse effects of morphine and the attendant immunodepression (Ramarao *et al.* 1995). A significant modulation of immune activity was observed in three animal models used. It prevented myelosuppres-sion of mice treated with all three immunosuppresive drugs tested, with significant increase in haemolytic antibody response towards human erythrocytes (Ziauddin *et al.* 1996).

Anticancerous activity

Withania was able to arrest cell division, produce mitotic abnormality in meta-phase block and chromosome breakage in tissue culture of tumours. Cells in the resting stage were undamaged but the active cells degenerated. Withaferin A from the root exhibited significant retardation of tumour growth against sarcoma 180 and KB human carcinoma cells (Palyi *et al.* 1969). It also had antineoplastic activity. It prevented urethane-induced decreases in body weight, increased mortality and induced lung adenomas in albino mice. Simultaneous oral administration of *asgandha* in a dose of 200 mg/kg along with urethane protected the animals from the tumour inducing effect of this compound (Singh *et al.* 1986). Budhiraja and Sudhir (1987) also observed antitumour property from withanolides. Uma Devi *et al.* (1992, 1993, 1996) tried alcohol extract of *ashwagandha* and withaferin A and found that both had *in vivo* inhibitory effect on transplantable mouse tumour Sarcoma 180. Ganasoundri *et al.* (1997) and Sheena *et al.* (1998) confirmed this research. Dhuley (1997) studied the effect of *W. somnifera* on the function of the macrophages obtained from the mice treated with the carcinogen ochratoxin A. The chemotactic activity of murine macrophages was significantly decreased compared with the control. Production of interlukin-1 and tumour necrosis factor was also markedly reduced.

As an adjuvant to cancer therapy

Ashwagandha showed a radiosensitizing effect. It increased the effect of radiation on tumour regression and delayed the growth of tumours. When it was administered for ten days, with exposure to gamma radiation followed by hyperthermia, there was a significant increase in tumour cure (Uma Devi *et al.* 1993). A 75 per cent methanol extract of the herb significants increased the total blood cell count, bone marrow cellularity and lymphocyte. Leucopenia, induced by sub-lethal dose of gamma radiation, was reduced. It normalized the ratio of norchromatic and polychromatic erythrocytes after radiation exposure (Anand and Kuttan, 1995; Kuttan, 1996). Beneficial effects were seen when this drug was given before and after radiation (Bhattathiri *et al.* 1995). Uma Devi (1996) and Uma Devi *et al.* (1996) confirmed that withaferin is a good, natural source of a safe radiosensitizing agent.

Antistress activity

Withania improved mental functions by reducing stress (Shukla, 1981) due to its mild depressant action on the body. It induced a state of non-specific increase in resistance during stress (Sankara Subramanian, 1982). This antistress activity is useful in the prevention of stress-induced gastric ulcer, liver toxicity, leucocytosis, carcinoma, leucopenia, and hypertension, etc. (Singh *et al.* 1982). It influenced the dopaminergic system, which has been implicated in stress (Saksena *et al.* 1989). It was tried in 25 cases of depressive illness for two months. It showed notable symptomatic improvement, decrease in degree of anxiety and depression (Singh and Murthy, 1989; Singh *et al.* 1990). The root extract which had CNS depressant properties showed an antianxiety effect in the patients with anxiety neurosis (Gandhi, 1994). It helped in stress-induced response from anxiety, depression, analgesia, thermic changes, gastric ulcers, convulsions, and restored stress-induced depletion of the adrenals and ascorbic acid (Sandhya Singh and Sushil Kumar, 1998).

Looking into the central nervous system depressant action of this root, Pande and Sharma, (1992) suggested its use as an anaesthesia.

Gandhi *et al.* (1995) tested anabolic activity and endurance time by feeding mice with ginseng and *ashwagandha*. Both herbs were effective but *ashwagandha* had a better weight gaining capacity.

In cervical spondylosis

Withania (4 g) and *Smilax china* decoction was tried on 25 radiological confirmed cases of cervical spondylosis for 30 days. This herbal combination was as effective as Brufen and was without side effects (Shareef, 1993).

As an adaptogen

Singh (1982) studied the adaptogenic property of *ashwagandha*. It increased swimming endurance in mice and prevented gastric ulcers-induced chemically by stress in rats. Bhattacharya *et al.* (1987) isolated the compounds which were uniformly active in attenuating stress-induced responses ranging from anxiety, depression, analgesia, thermic changes, gastric ulcers, convulsions, tribulin activity and adrenocortical activation. Roy *et al.* (1992a, b) and Srivastava (1995) studied the changes in the psychophysiological status of trainee mountaineers by altitude gain up to 7,000 m and then descending. *Ashwagandh*, administered 500 mg daily, altered behaviour including sleep pattern, alertness, state of awareness, along with other physical capabilities.

As a geriatric tonic

When studied for its effect on the ageing process in healthy male adults, it showed significant increases in haemoglobin count and hair melanin, with decreases in nail calcium, serum cholesterol and erythrocyte sedimentation (Kuppurajan *et al.* 1980; Ahmuda *et al.* 1991a, b). Bhattacharya *et al.* (1995) studied the effect of glycowithanolides on animal models of Alzheimer's disease and perturbed central cholinergic markers of cognition in rats. The effects validated its use as a promoter of learning and memory.

Intake of a herbal capsule consisting of *Withania*, *Tribulus* and ginseng with milk enhanced certain aspects of psychomotor performance. An increase in strength, viability process and endurance time was shown (Karnick, 1992).

As an antiulcerogenic agent

It had a significant dose-dependent effect on aspirin-induced gastric ulcers. It reduced the ulcer index and caused the healing of ulcers (Sahni and Srivastava, 1993, 1994).

As an antiinflammatory agent

Bector (1968) studied the role of *ashwgandha* on various types of arthritis. Immuno electrophoresis studies revealed that this herb changed the concentration of various serum proteins. A therapeutic dose of 100 mg/kg body weight showed 46 per cent anti-inflammatory activity on paw volumes in rats (Anbalgan and Sadique, 1981a, b). A compound withaferin A inhibited adjuvant arthritis (Bahr and Hansel, 1982). Budhiraja *et al.* (1984) observed the marked effect of another compound from the root in sub acute inflammation. A comparison showed it to be better than phenylbutazone and hydrocortisone. Administration of *Withania* to inflamed rats caused a significant reduction in the level of alpha-2-macroglobulin and enhanced the synthesis of total serum protein (Anbalagan and Sadique, 1985). Hazeena Begum and Sadique (1988) studied long term effects of the herb on induced arthritis in rats. It prevented body-weight loss during the arthritic conditions and reduced paw swellings during the secondary lesions. Radiographic observations revealed that it prevented bone degeneration and compared well with hydrocortisone. Al-Hindawi *et al.* (1992), Sahni and Srivastava (1994, 1995) and Nanshine *et al.* (1995) confirmed anti-inflammatory effect of this root.

Kulkarni *et al.* (1991, 1992) tried an Ayurvedic preparation containing *Withania, Boswellia* and *Curcuma*. It relieved pain, morning stiffness, and caused a drop in erythrocyte sedimentation.

In skin problems

For keratitis and rough skin Gupta *et al.* (1994) prescribed *Ashwagandha Rasayana*, by concentrating *ashwagandha* powder seven times with *ashwagandha* decoction until completely dry and prescribed it in a dose 3 g twice daily. This preparation also stopped female hair loss after childbirth.

In liver diseases

The protective effect of withanolides against carbon tetrachloride-induced hepatotoxicity is well known (Budhiraja *et al.* 1986). Some of the modern drugs are known to cause hepatotoxicity. *Ashwagandha* can be an important adjuvant to these types of chemicals (Chhajed *et al.* 1991). When used with long pepper, it produced marked histopathological changes in induced hepatotoxicity. *Withania*, with other herbs, acted as a free radical scavenging agent for pancreatic islets (Bhattacharya *et al.* 1997a).

As an antioxidant

Dhuley (1998) evaluated the effect of *ashwagndha* on lipid peroxidation in stress-induced animals. It prevented the rise in lipid peroxidation. This antioxidant activity of glycowithanolids (sitoindosides VII-X, and withaferin A) was investigated for their effects on rat brain. These withanolides had a dose-dependent effect. This antioxidant effect may, at least in part, explain the antistress, immunomodulatory, cognition-facilitating, anti-inflammatory and anti-ageing effects of this herb reported in earlier studies (Bhattacharya *et al.* 1997b).

Sunanda Panda *et al.* (1997) investigated the effect of root extract containing 1.75 per cent withanolides in mice treated with cadmium chloride. *Ashwagndha* treatment attenuated lipid peroxidation induced by cadmium.

Chemical studies

During the earlier studies Sankara Subramanian (1982) found that the total alkaloids in the root are 0.13–0.32 per cent. Besides alkaloids, steroidal lactones under the generic name, withanolides, have been reported. Chemical studies of the four chemotypes of this plant showed that the main constituent of chemotype I is withaferin A, and that of chemotype II withanolide D, chemotype III is characterized by the presence of two groups of compounds: withanolide G & H and E & F. The chemotype IV is rich in withaferin A and withanone.

Toxicological studies

When withaferin A was studied for acute toxicity, a single injection of 50 mg/kg body weight did not cause any deaths. Higher doses of 100 mg/kg and above produced diarrhoea and severe weight loss. A single intraperitoneal injection of 1,100 mg/kg of the extract in mice did not cause any deaths within 24 hours. The LD50 value was calculated as 1,260 mg/kg body weight. Sub acute toxicity studies with repeated injections of extract at a dose of 100 mg/kg body weight for 30 days, in rats of either sex, did not result in any mortality or changes in peripheral blood constituents (Sharada *et al.* 1993a, b). It was devoid of side effects even after 8 months of use.

References

Ahumada, F., Aspee, F., Wikman, G., Hancke, J. (1991a) *Withania somnifera* extract. Its effect on arterial blood pressure in anaesthesized dogs. *Phytotherapy Research*, 5, 111–114.

Ahumada, F., Trincado, M.A., Arellano, J.A., Hancke, J., Wikman, G. (1991b) Effect of certain adaptogenic plant extracts on drug-induced necrosis in female and male mice. *Phytotherapy Research*, 5, 29–31.

Al-Hindawi, M.K., Al-Khafaji, S.H., Abdul Nabi, M.H. (1992) Anti-granuloma activity of Iraqi Withania somnifera. *Journal of Ethnopharmacology*, 37, 113–116.

Anand, I.V., Kuttan, G. (1995) Use of *Withania somnifera* as an adjuvant during radiation therapy. *Amala Research Bulletin*, 15, 83–87.

Anbalagan, K., Sadique, J. (1981a) Influence of an Indian medicine (Ashwgandha) on acute phase reactants in inflammation. *Indian Journal of Experimental Biology*, 19, 245–249.

Anbalagan, K., Sadique, J. (1981b) Response of alpha-1 globulins of serum during inflammation. *Current Science*, 50, 88–89.

Anbalagan, K., Sadique, J. (1985) *Withania somnifera* (Ashwagandha): a rejuvenating herbal drug which controls alpha-2 micro-globulin synthesis during inflammation. *International Journal of Crude Drug Research*, 23, 177–183.

Bahr, V., Hansel, R. (1982) Immunomodulating properties of 5,20 α ® dihydroxy 6 χ7 α epoxy-1-oxo(s a) with a-2,24 dieolide and solasodine. *Planta Medica*, 44, 32–33.

Bector, N.P. (1968) Role of *Withania somnifera* (Ashwagandha) in various types of arthropathies. *Indian Journal of Medical Research*, 56, 1581–1583.

Bhattacharya, S.K., Ashok Kumar, Ghoshal, S. (1995) Effects of glycowithanolides from *Withania somnifera* on an animal model of Alzheimer's disease and perturbed central cholinergic markers of cognition in rats. *Phytotherapy Research*, 9, 110–113.

Bhattacharya, S.K., Goel, R.K., Ravinder Kaur, Ghoshal, Shibnatha (1987) Anti stress activity of sitoindosides VII and VIII. New acylsteryl glucosides from *Withania* group. *Phytotherapy Research*, 1, 32–38.

Bhattacharya, S.K., Satyan, K.S., Chakraborti, A. (1997a) Effect of Trasina, an Ayurvedic herbal formulation, on pancreatic islet superoxide dismutase activity in rats. *Indian Journal of Experimental Biology*, 35, 297–299.

Bhattacharya, S.K., Satyan, K.S., Ghoshal, Shibnath (1997b) Antioxidant activity of glycowithanolides from *Withania somnifera*. *Indian Journal of Experimental Biology*, 35, 236–239.

Bhattathiri, V.N., Uma Devi, P., Sreelekha, T., Remani, P., Vijaykumar, T., Nair M.K. (1995) Biochemical modulation of GSH by ashwagnadha: relation to its usefulness as a radiosensitizer. *International Conference on Current Progress in Medicinal and Aromatic Plant Research*, Calcutta, India. 30 December 1994–1 January 1995.

Budhiraja, R.D., Garg, K.N., Sudhir, S., Arora, B. (1986) Protective effect of 3-β hydroxy-2, 3 dihydrowithanolide F against CCl4-induced hepatotoxicity. *Planta Medica*, 52, 28–29.

Budhiraja, R.D., Sudhir, S. (1987) Review of biological activity of withanolides. *Journal of Scientifc and Industrial Research*, 46, 488–491.

Budhiraja, R.D., Sandhu, S., Garg, K.N. (1984) Anti-inflammatory activity of 3β hydroxy-2, 3-dihyro withanolide F. *Planta Medica*, 50, 134.

Chhajed, S., Baghel, M.S., Ravishankar, B., Singh, G. (1991) Evaluation of hepatoprotective effect of *Piper longum* (Pippali) and *Withania somnifera* in hepatotoxicity induced by antitubercular drugs in mice. *Journal of Research and Education in Indian Medicine*, 10, 9–12.

Davis, L., Kuttan, G. (1998) Suppressive effect of cyclophosphamaide-induced toxicity by *Withania somnifera* extract in mice. *Journal of Ethnopharmacology*, 62, 209–214.

Dhuley, J.N. (1997) Effect of some Indian herbs on macrophage functions in ochratoxin A treated mice. *Journal of Ethnopharmacology*, 58, 15–20.

Dhuley, J.N. (1998) Effect of ashwagandha on lipid peroxidation in stress-induced animals. *Journal of Ethnopharmacology*, 60, 173–178.

Ganasoundari, A., Zare, S.M., Uma Devi, P. (1997) Modification of bone marrow radiosensitivity by medicinal plant extracts. *British Journal of Radiology*, 70, 599–602.

Gandhi, A., Mujumdar, A.M., Patwardhan, B. (1995) A comparative pharmacological investigation of Ashwgandha and ginseng. *Journal of Ethnopharmacology*, 44, 131–135.

Gandhi, S.S. (1994) The potential of *Withania somnifera* as an antistress agent. *Update Ayurveda–94*, Bombay, India. 24 to 26 February 1994.

Gupta, O.P., Dube, C.B., Ansari, Z. (1994) A clinical study of ashwagandha rasayana in patients of keratin and rough skin. *National Seminar on the use of Traditional Medicinal Plants in Skin care*, CIMAP, Lucknow, 25–26 November 1994.

Hazeena Begum, V., Sadique, J. (1988) Long term effect of herbal drug *Withania somnifera* on adjuvant-induced arthritis in rats. *Indian Journal of Experimental Biology*, 26, 877–882.

Karnick, C.R. (1992) Clinical observation on the effect of composite herbal drugs of *Withania somnifera, Panax ginseng* and *Tribulus terrestris* on psychomotor performance in healthy volunteers. *Indian Medicine*, 4, 1–4.

Kulkarni, R.R., Patki, P.S., Jog, V.P., Gandage, S.P., Patwardhan, B. (1991) Treatment of osteoarthritis with herbomineral formulation: a double blind, placebo controlled cross over study. *Journal of Ethnopharmacology*, 33, 91–95.

Kulkarni, R.R., Patki, P.S., Jog, V.P., Gandage, S.P., Patwardhan, B. (1992) Efficacy of an Ayurvedic formulation in rheumatoid arthritis: A double blind placebo controlled cross over study. *Indian Journal of Pharmacology*, 24, 98–101.

Kulkarni, S.K., George, B. (1995) GABA receptor modulation by herbal preparation (invited lecture) *International Seminar on Recent Trends in Pharmaceutical Sciences*, Ootacamund, 18–20 Feb. 1995.

Kulkarni, S.K., George, B., Mathur, R. (1998) Protective effect of *Withania somnifera* root extract on electrographic activity in a lithium-pilocarpine model of status epilepticus. *Phytotherapy Research*, 12, 451–453.

Kulkarni, S.K., George, B., Nayar, U. (1995) Amygdaloid kindling in rats: Protective effect of *Withania somnifera* (Ashwagandha) root extract. *Indian Drugs*, 32, 37–49.

Kulkarni, S.K., Sharma, A., Verma, A., Ticku, M.K. (1993) GABA receptor mediated anticonvulsant action of *Withania somnifera* root extract. *Indian Drugs*, 30, 305–312.

Kumar, P., Kuttan, R., Kuttan, G. (1994) Usefulness of Rasayana as immunomodulators and chemoprotectors against cyclophosphamide-induced toxicity. *Amala Research Bulletin*, 14, 49–51.

Kuppurajan, K., Rajagopalan, S.S., Sitaraman, R., Rajagopalan V., Janaki, K., Revathi, R., Venkatraghavan, S. (1980) Effect of Aswagandha (*Withania sonmnifera* Dunal) on the process of ageing in human volunteers. *Journal of Research in Ayurveda and Siddha*, 1, 247–208.

Kuttan G. (1996) Use of *Withania somnifera* Dunal as an adjuvant during radiation therapy. *Indian Journal of Experimental Biology*, 14, 854–856.

Nashine, K., Srivastava, D.N., Shani, I. (1995) Role of inflammatory mediators in anti-inflammatory activity of *Withania somnifera*. *Indian Veterinary Medical Journal*, 19, 268–288.

Palyi, I., Tyihak, E., Palyi, V. (1969) Cytological effects of compounds isolated from *Withania somnifera*. *Herba Hungarica*, 8, 73–76.

Panda, S., Gupta, P., Kar, A. (1997) Protective role of ashwagandha in cadmium-induced hepatotoxicity and nephrotoxicity in male mouse. *Current Science*, 72, 546–547.

Pande, S.B., Sharma, S. (1992) Role of ashwagandha in Sangyabaran (Anaesthesia): an experimental study. *International Seminar-Traditional Medicine*, Calcutta, 7–9 November 1992.

Ramarao, P., Rao, K.T., Srivastava, R.S., Ghosal, S. (1995) Effects of glycowithanolides from *Withania somnifera* on morphine-induced inhibition of intestinal motility and tolerance of analgesia in mice. *Phytotherapy Research*, 9, 66–68

Roy, A.S., Acharya, S.B., De, A.K., Debnath, P.K. (1992a) Mountain medicine: Effect of Aswgandha (*Withania somnifera*) on the changes of psychophysiological status of trainee mountaineers by altitude gain. *International Seminar-Traditional Medicine*, Calcutta, 7–9 November 1992.

Roy, U., Mukhopadhyay, S., Poddar, M.K., Mukherjee, B.P. (1992b) Evaluation of antistress activity of Indian medicinal plants, *Withania somnifera* and *Ocimum sanctum* with special reference to stress-induced stomach ulcer in albino rats. *International Seminar-Traditional Medicine*, Calcutta. 7–9 November 1992.

Sandhya Singh, Sushil Kumar, *The Indian Ginseng, Ashwagandha*. CIMAP, Lucknow, India 1998.

Sahni, Y.P., Srivastava, D.N. (1993) *Withania somnifera*: an indigenous anti-ulcerogenic drug. *Indian Journal of Indigenous Medicine*, 10, 53–56.

Sahni, Y.P., Srivastava, D.N. (1994) Anti-inflammatory and anti-ulcerogenic activity of *Withania somnifera*. *Update Ayurveda 94*, Bombay, India. 24–26 November 1994.

Sahni, Y.P., Srivastava, D.N. (1995) Role of inflammatory mediators in anti-inflammatory activity of *Withania somnifera* on chronic inflammatory reactions. *Indian Veterinary Medical Journal*, 19, 150–153.

Saksena, A.K., Singh, S.P., Dixit, K.S., Singh, N., Seth, K., Seth, P.K., Gupta, G.P. (1989) Effect of *Withania somnifera* and *Panax ginseng* on dopaminergic receptors in rat brain during stress. *Planta Medica*, 55, 95.

Sankara Subramanian, S. (1982) Ashwagandha an ancient Ayurvedic drug. *Arogya-Journal of Health Science*, 8, 135.

Sharada, A.C., Solomon, F.E., Uma Devi, P. (1993a) Toxicity of *Withania somnifera* root extract in rats and mice. *International Journal of Pharmacognosy*, 31, 205–212.

Sharada, A.C., Solomon, F.E., Uma Devi, P., Srinivasan, K.K., Udupa, N. (1993b) Withaferin A and plumbagin. Isolation and acute toxicity studies. *Amala Research Bulletin*. 13th August 1993.

Shareef, M.A. (1993) Management of cervical spondylitis through herbal drugs, *Withania somnifera* and *Smilax china*. A preliminary clinical study. *Medicinal Plants: New Vistas and Research*, 97–101.

Sharma, S., Dahunkar, S., Karandhikar, S.M. (1985) Effects of long term administration of the roots of Ashwagandha (*Withania somnifera*) and Shatavari (*Asparagus racemosus*) in rats. *Indian Drugs*, 23, 133–139.

Sheena, I.P., Singh, U.V., Kamath, R., Uma Devi, P., Udupa, N. (1998) Niosomal withaferin A with better antitumour efficacy. *Indian Journal of Pharmaceutical Sciences*, 60, 45–48.

Shobat, B., Kirson, I., Lavie, D. (1978) Immunodepressive properties of withaferin and withanolide D. *Biomedicine*, 28, 18.

Shukla, S.P. (1981) Anti-anxiety agent of plant origin. *Probe*, 20, 201–208.

Singh, N., Nath, R., Lata, A., Singh, S.P., Kohli, R.P., Bhargava, K.P. (1982) *Withania somnifera* (Ashwagandha), a rejuvenating herbal drug which enhances survival during stress (an adaptogen). *International Journal of Crude Drug Research*, 20, 29–35.

Singh, N. *et al.* (1986) Prevention of urethane-induced lung adenomas by *Withania somnifera* (L) Dunal in albino mice. *International Journal of Crude Drug Research*, 24, 90–100.

Singh, R.H., Nath, S.K., Behere, P.B. (1990) Depressive illness a therapeutic evaluation with herbal drugs. *Journal of Research in Ayurveda and Siddha*, 11, 1–6.

Singh, R.H. *et al.* (1979) Studies on psychotropic effect of indigenous drug Ashwaganda (*Withania somnifera*). II. Experimental studies. *Journal of Research in Indian Medicine, Yoga and Homeopathy*, 14, 49–54.

Singh, R.H., Murthy, A.R.V. (1989) Medhya rasayana therapy in the management of apsmara vis-a-vis epilepsies. *Journal of Research and Education in Indian Medicine*, 8, 13–16.

Srivastava, K.K. (1995) Adaptogen in high mountains. *Indian Journal of Natural Products*, 11, 13–19.

Uma Devi, P. (1996) *Withania somnifera* Dunal (Ashwagandha), potential plant source of promising drug for cancer chemotherapy and radiosensitisation. *Indian Journal of Experimental Biology*, 34, 927–932.

Uma Devi, P., Akagi, K., Ostapenko, V., Tanaka, Y., Sugahara, T. (1996) Withaferin A: a new radiosensitiser from the Indian medicinal plant *Withania somnifera*. *International Journal of Radiation Biology*, 69, 193–197.

Uma Devi, P., Sharada, A.C., Solomon, F.E. (1993) Antitumour and radiosensitising effects of *Withania somnifera* (Ashwagandha) on a transplantable mouse tumour, Sarcoma –180. *Indian Journal of Experimental Biology*, 31, 607–611.

Uma Devi, P., Sharada, A.C., Soloman, F.E. (1994) Anticancer potential of ashwagandha roots. *Update Ayurveda* 94, Bombay, India. 24–26 February 1994.

Uma Devi, P., Sharada, A.C., Solomon, F.E., Kamath, M.S. (1992) In vivo growth inhibitory effect of *Withania somnifera* (Ashwagandha) on a transplantable mouse tumour, sarcoma 180. *Indian Journal of Experimental Biology*, 30, 169–172.

Venkataraghavan, S., Seshadri, C., Sundersan, T.P., Ravathi, R., Rajgopalan, V., Janaki, K. (1984) The comparative effect of milk fortified with Aswagandha, and Punernava in children: a double blind study. *Journal of Research in Ayurveda and Siddha*, 1, 370–385.

Ziauddin, M., Phansalkar, N., Patki, P., Patwardhan, B. (1996) Studies on the immunomodulatory effects of Ashwagandha. *Journal of Ethnopharmacology*, 50, 69–76.

10 Badam

Prunus amygdalus Batsch
Syn: *Amygdalus communis* L. var. *dulce*
Family: Rosaceae

THE PLANT AND ITS DISTRIBUTION

It is a tree of the temperate zone with dry summers, naturalized in the Mediterranean Basin and is cultivated in Kashmir (India) Baluchistan (Pakistan), Afghanistan, Iran, Cyprus, Turkey, Spain and California (USA). According to Ayurvedic scholars almond from Iran is the best and that from the USA is of the lowest quality.

The plant is a small tree, 5–6 m high, purplish bark, bright green leaves, pale pink or white flowers. The drupe fruit is ovate, 5 cm long and 2.5 cm broad. Its seed is brown in colour, 17–15 mm long, 10–13 mm broad, oblong lanceolate and its brown outer covering can be removed by soaking the seed in water.

Several varieties of almond are known but broadly it can be classified into two varieties, bitter and sweet. Earlier there used to be occasional mixing of bitter almonds with the sweet one but now it is rare. The bitter almond is poisonous and should be used for external purposes only. Almond seed kernel is often adulterated with that of apricot, but the two can be easily differentiated by the small size and different shape of apricot kernel.

The seed should be stored, after completely drying them, to avoid the decomposition of amygdalin and fixed oil. Adding a few cloves to storage bins of almond delays this decomposition.

USES IN FOLKLORE AND AYURVEDA

As per the Ayurvedic concept, dry fruits generally provide nutrition and vital energy to the body. Out of all dry fruits, almond is said to provide maximum benefit. It suppresses *pita* and *vata*. It is oily and causes phlegm so it is harmful to the patients of *rakt pita*. Almond should be consumed as per the digestive power of an individual. During its consumption, if there is a loss of appetite or any other stomach trouble, then the quantity of almonds should be reduced but it should not be stopped altogether. Do not use almond with honey and hot milk. If honey is to be used, use cold milk. Almond kernel contains heat sensitive compounds so should not be heated while making any of its preparations.

In India, almond is generally considered a nutritive for the brain and nervous system. It is also said to improve eyesight. In a book on medical secrets of food, it is mentioned that more than 10,000 Jain monks in Karnataka (India) attribute their high intellectual level and longevity to the consumption of almond. As per their concept, the longevity of an individual is neither due to a strong body nor an active nervous system but due to thin sense fibres (*gyantantu*) which arise from the brain and pass through neck. Almond provides nutrition to these sense fibres. The other major uses of almond are:

As a general tonic

Almond is hard to digest by individuals with weak digestive powers, so the best method is to soak the almond kernel in water overnight. In the morning separate the outer brownish seed coat and mash the white kernel in a blender to get a thick milky paste. In this way, it is easily assimilated into the digestive system and does not cause indigestion. As a general tonic, to start with, take half a teaspoonful of almond paste, twice daily in the morning and evening, in a cup of milk, add honey according to taste. Increase the dose of almond paste everyday until unable to digest it. For additional effects, for males give 5 g *ashwagandha* powder and for ladies, 5 g of *shatawari* powder, along with the above almond paste. Continue this treatment for 40–60 days.

For delaying premature ejaculation

Soak one almond kernel in water, as above, and form a paste. To this paste add the powder of 4–5 black peppers, 2 g ginger powder and sugar as per taste. Lick this mixture, followed by milk for 60 days.

For gaining weight

Eat as much almond as possible for two months, or make a mixture of almond paste with butter and use along with bread.

For bronchial problems, and strengthening the male urino-genital system

Take almond kernel, *ashwagandha, pippli*, in equal quantities, with milk, sugar and honey.

In gynaecological problems

For relief of backache and leucorrhoea, almond is prescribed to women with *ashwagandha, pippali*. The paste of bitter almond is applied on generative organs. For women rendered weak after childbirth, a paste of 3–6 almonds should be given every day.

For mentally retarded children

The paste of 3–6 almonds with milk is beneficial if given every day.

Almond oil

It is light yellow in colour, with a mild, pleasing odour and a bland taste. It is known as *Roghan Badam* in India. It is extracted by a cold process. Adulterations in the oil can be detected by subjecting it to cold temperature; it is clear at −10°C but congeals at −20°C. The oil is commonly adulterated or substituted with peach and apricot oil, and, as a matter of fact, most of the oil sold as bitter almond oil is from the bitter kernels of apricot. To detect any adulterations, shake 2 parts of oil with one part of fuming nitric acid and one part distilled water. The mixture should not have any colour (peach and apricot oil will give a red colour, while sesame and cottonseed oil will give brown colour) (Culbreth, 1927).

Sweet almond oil is considered a nutritive, aphrodisiac (increases libido), mild laxative and is used for relieving headaches. Arabic women massage their breasts with almond oil after breastfeeding their infants.

Nutritive household preparations

Sardai

It is a cooling drink, made from soaking 2–3 almond kernels, 25 g poppy seed, a few black peppers and rose petals until soft. Make a paste of these in a blender. Suspend the paste in 250 ml water and filter to remove the water-insoluble portion. Ice, honey or sugar may be added to the drink as per taste (earlier *Cannabis* leaves were also used in the mixture). This drink is said to compensate for energy depletion arising from exposure to summer heat.

Almond nut cream

As a brain tonic, steep in water, orange or lime juice 3 parts almond, 2 parts walnut, 2 parts pine kernel until soft and make a cream in a blender (Nadkarni, 1954).

Nutritive candy balls

Take 100 g each of walnut, almond, poppy seed, melon seed kernel, *Trapa bispinosa* powder, with 250 g *ghee*, 260 g icing sugar, 2 g nutmeg, 1 g saffron, 20–22 cardamom seeds. Blanch the almond and other kernels. Wash the poppy seeds and macerate them in water to form a pulp. Mix this pulp with blanched nuts and roast them in *ghee* along with *Trapa bispinosa* flour, constantly stirring. When the whole mass turns brown, remove it from the heat, add sugar, followed by powders of nutmeg, saffron and cardamom. When warm make candy balls by hand.

It is a good tonic for the brain and physical strength.

Nutritive dessert

Separately soak two teaspoonsful of black beans (*Phaseolus mungo*), and one of almond kernel. When soft, remove seed coat and make a paste of both separately. Fry the bean paste with *ghee* until brown. Boil it in a cup of milk and, on cooling, add almond paste and sugar as per taste. Take this preparation for one month. It is specially recommended for those who use their brain a lot. It provides physical strength to both males and females for sexual acts, and may be used by diabetics. It also provides desired nutrition to pregnant women.

THERAPEUTIC INDICATIONS AND PHARMACOLOGICAL STUDIES

As an anti-inflammatory agent

Nagamoto (1988) isolated anti-inflammatory and analgesic compounds from almond. Kubo *et al.* (1990) tried it on adjuvant-induced arthritis, and the pepsin hydrolysis product inhibited the acetic acid-induced writhing in mice and cotton pellet-induced granuloma in rats.

As an immunity booster

Kim *et al.* (1996) observed that, following oral administration of amygdalin isolated from almond, it significantly increased body weight of rats, along with that of liver and thymus. Oral administration of amygdalin in non-dose dependent manner suppressed humoral and cell mediated immunity and the high doses increased phagocytic activity significantly.

As an anti-hepatotoxic agent

Matsuda *et al.* (1990) tried pepsin hydrolysis products of the water soluble portion of almond in experimental hepatitis. It suppressed the increase of connective tissue in the liver.

Chemical studies

The seed kernel has 58.9 per cent fat, 20.8 per cent protein, 2.9 per cent minerals, mainly calcium, phosphorus and iron. Other constituents are oxalic acid, vitamin B and folic acid. It is one of the richest sources of vitamin E. It has high concentration of glutamic acid, arginine, asparagine and aspartic acid. Bitter almond has more protein and less fat. It has 2.5 to 3.5 per cent amygadalin, which after hydrolysis produces hydrocyanic acid, which is poisonous.

Toxicological studies

The bitter variety contains hydrocyanic acid in its essential oil. About 60 seeds of these are enough to kill an adult. The sweeter variety contains a very low concentration of cyanides and hence it is safe.

References

Culbreth, D.M.R. *A Manual of Materia Medica and Pharmacology.* Lea and Febiger, Philadelphia, USA 1927.
Kim, J.H., Kang, T.W., Park, C.B., Cha, K.L., Ahn, Y.K. (1996) Immunobiological studies on route of administration of amygdalin. *Yak Hoeji*, 40, 202–211.

Kubo, M., Matsuda, H., Shiomoto, H., Namba, K. (1990) Effect of pepsin hydrolysis product of water soluble portion from almond on adjuvant-induced arthritis. *Shoyakugaku Zasshi*, 44, 101–117.

Matsuda, H., Shiomoto, H., Nanba, K., Kubo, M. (1990) Effect of pepsin hydrolysis products of water soluble portion from almonds on experimental hepatitis. *Shoyakugaku Zasshi*, 44, 112–116.

Nadkarni, K.M. *Indian Materia Medica*. Vol. I Popular Prakashan, Bombay, India 1954.

Nagamoto, N., Noguchi, H., Nanba, K., Nakamura, H., Mizuno, M. (1988) Active components having anti-inflammatory activities and analgesic activities from Armeniaceae semen, Pruni japonicae semen and almond seeds. *Shoyakugaku Zasshi*, 42, 81–88.

11 Bala

Sida acuta Burm. F
Syn. *S. caprinifolia* Mast
S. cordifolia L
S. grewioides Gvill and Perr.
S. ovata Forsk.
S. rhombifolia L
S. spinosa L
S. veronicaefolia Lam.
Syn. *S. humilis* Cav.
Family: Malvaceae

On the basis of the detailed literature survey, in addition to the above herbs, it has been observed that the following plants are also considered to be one or other form of *bala*:

Abutilin indicum Atibala or *Kangi* in trade
Sida alba, S. althaefolia, S. alnifolia, S. herbacea, S. lanceolata, S. orientalis, S. retusa, S. rotundifolia, and *S. rhomboidea*.
Grewia hirsuta, G. populifolia, and *G. tenax*
Triumfetta rotundifolia

THE PLANTS AND THEIR DISTRIBUTION

Bala means *strength* in Sanskrit. Commonly *Sida cordifolia* (Figs. 5A and B), is considered the source of this drug. *Atibala* is definitely *Abutilon* (Chunekar and Pandey, 1969). Yellow flowered *S. rhombifolia* (Figs. 5C and D) is also a strong candidate for *bala* while white flowered *S. rhomboidea* is *mahabala*, *S. veronicaefola* syn. *S. humilis* and *S. spinosa* is *nagbala* (Nag is Sanskrit for snake and also for spine, hence both the prostate and spiny species come under this category). *Grewia hirsuta* and *G. populifolia* are also considered *nagbala* by some authors but in trade they are known by the name *Gangeran*. Sometimes *S. spinosa* is further split into two species, *S. alba* if it has white flowers and *S. alnifolia* if it has coloured flowers.

Some scholars have formed a separate group of five *Sida* spp., which they call *Panch bala* (five *balas*). These are:

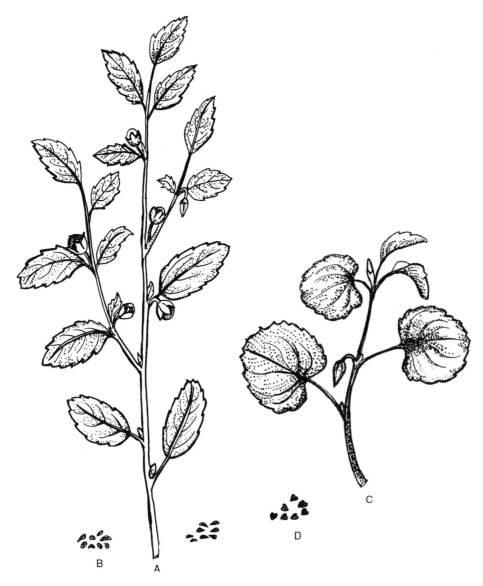

Figure 5 Sida cordifolia: **A** twig, **B** seed, *S. rhombifolia*: **C** twig, **D** seed.

Bala	*S. cordifolia* or *S. herbacea*, *S. rotundifiola*, *S. althaefolia*
Mahbala	*S. rhomboidea* var. *rhomboidea*
Nagbala	*S. spinosa* syn. *S. alba* and *S. alnifolia*
Atibala	*S. rhombifolia*, *S. rhomboidea*, *S. retusa*, and *S. orientalis*
Bala Phanjivika	*S. caprinifolia* Syn. *S. acuta* and *S. lanceolata*
Bhumibala	*S. humilis* or *S. veronicifolia*

Some other scholars on the basis of the number of *bala* used in a composition, form different groups, which are as follows:

Baladivya	*Bala* and *Atibala*
Balatriya	*Bala*, *Atibala* and *Nagbala*
Balachaturya	*Bala*, *Atibalal*, *Nagbala*, and *Mahabala*
Balapanchak	when *Bhumibala* is added to above four species.

In commerce the whole herb of *Sida* spp. is known as *Kharanti*, and usually no distinction is made between the various types of *bala* mentioned above. The seeds of these are called *Beejband* and those of *Abutilin indicum* are called *Kanghi*.

USES IN FOLKLORE AND AYURVEDA

Bala is used in the diseases of *rakta pitta* origin and is considered a healer of all malfunctions of the body. It is mainly used for following:

As a general tonic

For nervous debility, loss of memory, virility and as an aphrodisiac. In general weakness it is said to protect the inner vital energy of the body *ojas* and keep away old age. The herbs are well esteemed for strengthening the urinogenital systems of both males and females. These help sexual inadequacies and infectious diseases, particularly those transmitted sexually.

In gynaecological practices

1   In threatened abortion, strengthens placental retention in expectant mothers.
2   As per Ayurvedic concept leucorrhoea in females develops due to weakness in the body. One teaspoonful of fine *bala* powder prescribed twice daily, provides the desired strength.
3   In the case of inflammation of the ovary, a compound preparation of *bala*, *Balaydighrit* is given to the mother and to the newborn infant.

In Malaysia, *S. veornicaefolia* is used as a galactagogue and as an aid for labour parturition (Lutterodt *et al.* 1995).

As an anti-inflammatory agent

1   For suppuration of boils formed from pus, a poultice of tender leaves is applied to the boils. Cold water is sprinkled on occasionally. In this way the boil bursts without surgery.
2   The juice of the bark is anti-inflammatory and is used in urtica, scorpion sting, etc.

3   In burning micturition and polyurea, a fine powder of root and seed with *ghee* and sugar reduces inflammation.
4   In hoarseness of voice caused by too much cold, singing or crying loudly, half a spoon of *bala* powder with honey clears the throat.
5   The decoction of the root gives relief to alcoholics, who feel dryness of mouth, excessive thirst and burning sensation in the throat after consuming alcohol.

As a blood coagulant

In bleeding piles, where blood is passed with faeces and the problem is aggravated by indigestion and constipation, 10 g of *bala* powder, boiled with 80 ml of water until reduced to 20 ml is strained. One cup of mile is added to the filtrate. This mixture is taken in the morning. It not only helps with haemorrhoids but coagulates blood in the other parts of the body, such as nose and mouth.

As a stimulant

The flowers of *S. acuta* and *S. rhombifolia* are smoked as a stimulant and substituted for marihuana along the Gulf coastal region of Mexico. Ephedrine has been reported from these species (Shultes and Hofmann, 1979).

In sexual inadequacies

In males, 5 to 6 g of root powder in the morning on an empty stomach increases the viscosity of semen and prevents its involuntary discharge. In swollen testes, a decoction of *bala*, 4 teaspoons along with 2 teaspoons of castor oil, is prescribed.

Ayurvedic preparations

Bala oil

Method   Make a 400 ml decoction of each of *bala* root, *Dashmul* (see under *amalaki*), barley, *Zizyphus* fruit, *Dolichos biflorus* seed. Pulverize *Tinospora*, *Pistacia* galls, bamboo manna, *Prunus paddam*, dry black grapes, *Leptadenia reticulata*, *Glycyrrhiza* and any or all the members of *Ashtvarga* (see under *amalaki*), rock salt, *Aquillaria agallocha*, oleogum resin of *Pinus* and *Cedrus*, *Rubia cordifolia*, *Santalum album*, *Elettaria cardamomum*, *Ichnocarpus fruitescence*, *Hemidesmus indicus*, *Nardostachys grandiflora*, aromatic lichens, *Cinnamomum* spp. leaves, *Valeriana*, *Asparagus*, *Withania*, dill, *Boerhaavia*, and take cow's milk 4 litre, sesame oil 0.5 litre.

Make a paste of all the pulverized herbs with decoctions, milk and oil. Boil the whole mass, until the water evaporates and only the dehydrated oil is left. Filter the oil.

Use   Massaging the body with this oil before taking bath keeps away all the *vata* diseases, hastens healing, aids conception and increases sperm count. It makes the skin healthy and wrinkle free. When used along with other *bala* preparations, massaging with this oil fortifies the effect of these preparations.

Baladighrit

Method   Make a coarse powder of 500 g each of *S. cordifolia* root, *S. spinosa* stem, bark of *Terminalia arjuna*, and boil them in 8 litres of water until reduced to about 2 litres. To this decoction add 750 g *ghee*, heat again until all the water evaporates and only fatty matter is left.

Dose   One spoonful with sugar twice daily.

Use   For heart problems, dry coughs and the other diseases attributable to *vata*.

THERAPEUTIC INDICATIONS AND PHARMACOLOGICAL STUDIES

As an immunomodulator

Out of many plants considered as *bala*, three plants, *Abutilon indicum*, *Sida rhombifolia*, and *S. cordifolia*, are preferred. To find out which of the three herbs has a *Rasayana*-like activity, a comparative study was conducted by Dixit *et al.* (1978) on these for the following:

1   Hormonal antibody enhancing response against *Salmonella typhi* O antigens in rabbits.
2   Protective effect against *Staphylococcus aureus*.
3   Direct antibacterial activity against *S. aureus*.
4   Immunoglobulin changes in the serum following the administration of herbs.

Out of these herbs, *Abutilon indicum* was the most effective for prolonging the life-span of animals against virulent *S. aureus*. The gain in body weight was also significant. *A. indicum* did not have any direct antibacterial activity. Its effect was due to anabolism and immunostimulation of the body systems.

As an adaptogen

In a study, Sharma (1981) used *S. spinosa* for patients suffering from loss of vigour. There was a good response to physical and mental conditions, with increases in energy and weight. It made the patients happy and confident and increased their digestive power and appetite, whilst regulating bowel movements. The patients slept well with good dreams. It helped the proper development of secondary sexual characters and increased libido.

Hormonal effects

Venkitaraman and Radhkrishnan (1976) observed myotrophic and androgenic activity in the steroidal fraction of the root of *S. retusa* and *S. rhombifolia* in castrated rats. Lutterodt *et al.* (1995) found that when methanol extract of leaves of *S. veronicifolia* was administered to pregnant and non pregnant rats, the extract-induced the release of oxytocin after 5 minutes of administration but it was not statistically significant in pregnant rats.

Anti-inflammatory activity

The petroleum ether fraction from *A. indicum* root had an analgesic effect due to gallic acid (Bagi *et al.* 1985), while Lutterodt (1988) noted a muscarine-like activity in *S. veronicifolia.*

In poliomyelitis

Nair *et al.* (1980) observed a positive effect of *Sida* spp. in chronic cases of poliomyelitis.

As an antibacterial agent

Alcoholic extracts of *S. cordifolia*, *S. rhomboidea* and *Triumfetta rotundifolia* exhibited antibacterial activity against bacteria (Alam *et al.* 1991b). In another study by Bhatt *et al.* (1985) fatty acids of petroleum ether fraction showed good antibacterial activity against *Staphylococcus aureus* and fairly good against *Escherichia coli.*

Antihepatotoxic activity

The powder and different extracts of the whole plant showed anti-hepatotoxic activity comparable with silymarin (Rao and Mishra, 1998). Earlier Alam *et al.* (1991a) studied the effect of alcohol extracts of *S. cordifolia*, *S. rhomboidea* and *Triumfetta rotundifolia.* These extracts reduced serum and liver proteins. Muanza (1995) evaluated anticancer and anti-HIV activities and observed cytotoxic effects in the methanol extract of *S. cordifolia* leaves.

Kshirdhara

It is a special treatment, which is carried out by Ayurvedic physicians in the state of Kerala, south India. In *kshirdhara* (*kshir* is milk and *dhara* is uniform flow of a fluid) medicated milky emulsion is allowed to fall on the forehead of the patients. Ramu *et al.* (1982) treated the patients of anxiety neurosis by subjecting them to this treatment for 15 days. The authors prepared a decoction by boiling 50 g each of *Glycyrrhiza glabra*, *Nardostachys grandiflora* and *Sida cordifolia* in 6 litres of water, until the water was reduced to 2 litres. This decoction was mixed with 1.5 litres of milk. This mixture was poured into a pot with a hole at the bottom, in the centre. The pot was hung just above the head of the patients, in such a way that the liquid fell on the forehead. This treatment gave relief to 80 per cent patients of anxiety neurosis.

Chemical studies

The main compounds reported from the plants used as *bala* are: asparagine, vascine, vasicinone, pseudoephedrine, cryptolerine, hypaphorine, phenylethylamine, carboxylated tryptamines. Saponins and true tannins are absent but pseudotannins, oligosaccharides, flavonoids, choline, fructsopeptides, histidine glucine, tyrosine, oxalic acid, and phenolic acids are present (Lutterodt, 1988). Gallic acid is reported by Sharma *et al.* (1989). The biological activity of the herb is due to ephedrine and ephedrine-like compounds.

Toxicology

S. cordofolia was non-toxic. LD 50 value was higher than 10 g/kg in rats (Rao and Mishra, 1998).

References

Alam, M., Joy, S., Ali, U.S. (1991a) Screening of *Sida cordifolia* Linn., *Sida rhombifolia* Linn., and *Triumfetta rotundifolia* Lam. for anti-inflammatory and antipyretic activities. *Indian Drugs*, 28, 397–400.

Alam, M., Joy, S., Ali, U.S. (1991b) Antibacterial activity of *Sida cordifolia* Linn, *Sida rhomboidea* Roxb, and *Triumfetta rotundifolia* Lam. *Indian Drugs*, 28, 570–572

Bagi, K., Kalyani, G.A., Dennis J., Kumar, K.A., Kakrani, H.K. (1985) A preliminary phramacological screening of *Abutilon indicum*. I. Analgesic activity. *Fitoterapia*, 56, 169–171.

Bhatt, D.J., Baxi, A.J., Parikh, A.R. (1983) Chemical investigations of the leaves of *Sida rhombifolia* Linn. *Journal of Indian Chemical Society*, 60, 98.

Dixit, S.P., Tewari, P.V., Gupta, R.M. (1978) Experimental studies on the immunological aspects of Atibala (*Abutilon indicum* Linn.), Mahabala (*Sida rhombifoila* Linn), Bala (*Sida cordifolia* Linn.) and Bhumibala (*Sida veronicaefolia* Lam.). *Journal of Research in Indian Medicine, Yoga and Homoeopathy*, 13, 62–66.

Lutterodt, G.D. (1988) Responses of a gastrointestinal smooth muscles preparation to a muscarine principle present in *Sida veronicaefolia*. *Journal of Ethnopharmacology*, 23, 313–322.

Lutterodt, G.D., Okere, C., Liu C.X., Takashi, H. (1995) Induction of oxytocin release at various stages of pregnancy in rats by methanolic extractives of *Sida veronicaefolia*. *Asia Pacific Journal of Pharmacology*, 10(Supp.), 33–36.

Muanza, D.N., Euler, K.L., Williams, L., Newman, D.J. (1995) Screening for antitumour and anti- HIV activities of nine medicinal plants from Zaire. *International Journal of Pharmacognosy*, 33, 98–106.

Nair, P.R., Vijayan, N.P., Pillai, B.K.R., Bhagavathy Amma, K.C. (1980) Treatment of chronic cases of Saisaveeya vata (Poliomyelitis) II. *Journal of Research in Ayurveda and Siddha*, 1, 438–446.

Ramu, K.G., Janakiramiah, N., Sanapati, N.M., Shankara, M.R., Murthy, V.S.N. (1982) Ksirdhara on anxiety neurosis (Cittodvega): a pilot study. *Journal of Research in Ayurveda and Siddha*, 3, 126–132.

Rao, K.S., Mishra, S.H. (1998) Antihepatotoxic activity of *Sida cordifolia* whole plant. *Fitoterpia*, 69, 20–33.

Schultes, R.E., Hofmann, A. *Plants of the Gods*. Healing Arts Press, Vermont, USA 1979.

Sharma, P.V., Ahmed, Z.A., Sharma, V.V. (1989) Analgesic constituents of *Abutilon indicum*. *Indian Drugs*, 26, 333.

Sharma, S. *Rasayana* effect of herbs. *Sachitter* Ayurveda (in Hindi), July, 1981: 27–29.

Venkitaraman, S., Radhakrishinan, N. (1976) Myotrophic and androgenic activities of the steroidal fraction isolated from the roots of Sida retusa var. Sida rhombifolia Linn. (Bala). *Nagarjun*, 19, 26–27.

12 Banslochan

Syn: *Tabashir*
Melocanna bambusoides Trin.

It is a bluish, translucent, silicious concretion. The genuine material is obtained from the bamboo which was earlier identified as *Bambusa arundinacea* Willd., but studies by Puri (1984) have shown that the real source of *banslochan* is *Melocanna bambusoides* Trin. In this bamboo, the internodal region of the young female plant fills with sap. This sap is considered very nutritious and invigorating by inhabitants of the area and is drunk on exhaustion and for quenching thirst. When the plant matures the sap gets dried, and deposited inside the nodal region in the form of concretion. These *banslochan*-containing bamboo produce a rattling sound with the movement of wind or on shaking, and thus can be easily distinguished from non-concretion-containing plants. The concretion is collected by splitting bamboo longitudinally. The natural *banslochan* is very hard to obtain and is very expensive. It is very commonly substituted by synthetic silica.

USES IN FOLKLORE AND AYUREVEDA

Tabashir is mainly used for curing diseases of the region under the ribs, such as the thorax, lungs, intestine, etc. and for debility. It is an ingredient of a number of polyherbal and polymineral formulations. The common recipe for debility diseases of infants and young children consists of fine powders of long pepper 1/2 part, cardamom grain 1/4 part, cinnamon 1/8 part, *tabashir* 1 part and sugar 2 parts.

THERAPEUTIC INDICATIONS AND PHARMACOLOGICAL STUDIES

As a nutrient for the bones and the cartilages

Banslochan mainly consists of silica, which is one of the important components of connective tissue, cartilage, articulation tendons, arterial walls, skin, hair and nails. It has an effective remineralisation action in painful joints, fragility of the cartilage, osteoporosis and atherosclerosis. It stimulates the natural defence of the body during growth, pregnancy, repair of fractures, senescence, etc. Silica helps in calcium fixation by bones and improves the texture of collagen. As soon as the silica level in body tissue decreases, the calcium level goes up and elasticity is reduced. It helps in the assimilation of phosphorus for osteoporosis. Silica supplemented bones have 100 per cent increase in collagen over low silica bones. It is instrumental in faster healing of bones, and is a component of both the connective tissue and the fluid, which lubricate the joints. The lubricated joints move friction free, thus lessening the chances of inflammation.

In coronary heart problems

In areas where water contains low silica levels, the incidence of heart diseases are higher. Levels of silicon in the arterial wall decrease with the development of atherosclerosis. With silica deficiency, the arterial walls become non-elastic and are unable to accommodate variation in blood pressure.

As an antibacterial agent

Banslochan inhibited the growth of bacteria, probably due to the deposition of silica on the bacterial cell wall, which may have blocked the passage of nutrients from the medium into the bacterial body, or may have been due to its interaction with the proteinaceous cell wall, which produces an effect similar to that of silicosis. A comparative study on the binding of *tabashir* and silicic acid on the bacterial cell wall showed that in the two cases the nature of binding was similar (Malik and Shakil Ahmed, 1973).

In hormonal imbalance

Hormonal disturbance in the human organisms is sometimes due to calcium–magnesium imbalance. Silica can restore this balance.

As an immunostimulant

The skin, aorta and thymus (which activates the immune system) show a marked reduction in silica as we age. A deficiency of silica in the body exposes it to many diseases and makes it vulnerable to injury.

In degenerative diseases

Silica counteracts the effects of aluminium on the body and thus prevents Alzheimer's disease. The regenerative power of silica acts as a biological catalyst for tissues to regain their tone and elasticity.

Chemical studies

It consists of silicic acid (96.9 per cent), iron, calcium, choline and betaine.

References

Malik, W.U., Ahmed S. (1973) Studies on the effect of some indigenous drugs (Bhasamas and Tabashir) on the growth behaviour of *Escherichia coli* B. *Journal of Research in Indian Medicine*, 8, 35–39.

Puri, H.S. (1983) Medicinal Plants of Tezpur (Assam). *Bulletin Medico-Ethno-Botanical Research*, 4, 1–13.

13 Bhalatak

Semecarpus anacardium L.f.
Anacardiaceae

It is known as 'marking nut' because the black oil contained in the seed's pericarp was previously used by washer men for making a permanent identification mark on the cloth.

THE TREE AND ITS DISTRIBUTION

It is a middle sized deciduous tree, growing in the outer Himalayas, and in other warmer areas of India. Leaves are (Fig. 6A) 20–60 cm long, and 10–30 cm wide. Flowers are greenish yellow, in terminal panicle. The fruit is (Fig. 6B) 2.5 cm long, drupe, ovoid, and smooth lustrous black. The oil is highly vesicant. The kernel of the fruit is almond-like inside, but causes cutaneous eruptions if eaten (Wealth of India, 1972).

USES IN FOLKLORE AND AYURVEDA

The seed has *Rasayana*-like action but has a hot effect. It is considered beneficial for strength, vigour, vitality, in nervous disorders due to sexual exhaustion and in senile decay. In Indian medicine it is used in the treatment of arthritis and several other free radical mediated diseases, facial paralysis and in sciatica. Its continuous use combats ageing and those who have used it have wrinkle-free skin and black hair. It is considered so important that in the Indian state of Uttar Pradesh, in a village near Faizabad, a special fair called *Bhela ka Mela* is held, in which patients of various diseases are treated with this nut (Ahmed *et al.* 1993). The nut is not used as such but is mitigated, or treated using various methods to reduce the toxicity, as follows:

Purification of *Bhalatak*

Before purification the nuts are immersed in water. The fruits which sink are kept for processing, whilst floating ones are discarded. The juice from the pericarp is very corrosive, so precaution is taken so that the seed does not touch any part of body. The nuts, after removal of the crown, are mixed with a fine powder of bricks in a cotton bag. These are rubbed against brick powder until they are scraped enough to release

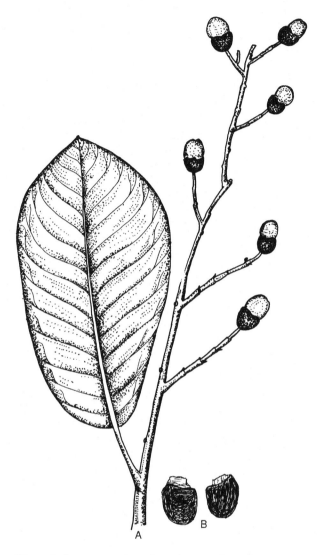

Figure 6 Semecarpus anacardium **A** twig, **B** seed.

the vesicant oil. When the brick powder has absorbed all the oil, the seeds are washed in hot water.

In Kerala, a state in south India, the nuts are first crushed to separate the kernels. These are then immersed in cow's urine for three days. During the day the seeds are taken out and exposed to sun. After this treatment for three days, the kernels are boiled in a decoction of *Terminalia bellirica* and then in a solution of cow dung, before being dried and washed with rice gruel (Shanvaskhan *et al*. 1997).

If blisters are formed during handling of the nut, they may be treated with the juice of *Amaranthus polygamous*, or a paste of *Terminalia chebula* or sesame seed in butter or milk. Alternatively a paste of macerated almond and coconut oil or coriander seed may be used or the juice of the leaves of *Cassia tora* or *C. fistula.* If poisonous symptoms develop during the administration of this seed, the patient is given a decoction of *T. chebula* or *Sesamum indicum* along with seed powder of *Embelia ribes* (Shanavaskhan *et al.* 1997).

Methods of using *Bhalatak* as *Rasayana* without toxicity
(Vaidya, 1998).

1   Fill seven earthen pots with soil in which 1 kg of pounded *bhalatak* are mixed and fenugreek grown in it. For irrigation do not use pure water but a decoction, made from 3 kg of crushed nuts. In winter, when the fenugreek crop is ready, cook and eat the leaves of one pot daily. Continue this for seven days. During the treatment spices and pepper should be avoided but bitters and a bit of salt may be used. This fenugreek is hot in effect, so hot spicy, non-vegetarian food and sexual intercourse should be avoided

2   Take 35 kg of nuts, after crushing them, use them as manure in a quarter acre of land to cultivate fenugreek. Eat the fresh leaves as salad for three months. Do not cook them. Radish can be grown in place of fenugreek and eaten raw.

3   Remove the crown from one marking nut and heat it in 25 g of butter until smoke starts coming out of it. Make an omelette with this butter. Discard both the nut and omelette but use the butter for vitality.

4   Remove the crown from 1 kg of nuts and boil them in 20 litres of milk. Separate the cream of the milk and make butter from it. Take about 3 g of this butter every day. To provide strength to the sexual organs massage them with this butter.

5   Boil one crushed *bhalatak* nut in 16 times water, until water is reduced to half. Measure the quantity of decoction obtained, add eight times as much milk to it and boil it again until the whole mass is condensed to half. Lubricate the mouth and throat with butter and swallow 12–25 g of this milk.

6   For acute inflammation arising from an accident, take one processed *bhalatak*, fry it in *ghee*, make *halwa* (porridge) and eat as much as possible.

External applications

For cracking soles and feet, an ointment is applied which is made by boiling *bhalatak* seed with rosin, bees wax and sesame oil.

When the body is massaged with *bhalatak* oil, it makes a person immune to all kinds of skin diseases and it turns grey hair black.

Ayurvedic preparations

Bhalatak Rasayana

Method   Pulverize equal quantities of ginger, *Embelia ribes*, processed iron, and *bhalatak*.

Dose   1 g with *ghee* and honey for three months.

Use   It increases blood, strength, youth and vigour. Use with care in anaemic patients.

Bhalatakadi Modka

Method Pulverize equal quantities of *bhalatak*, *haritaki* and sesame seed, mix these powders in raw sugar as per taste and make small candy balls.

Dose and Use As in *Bhalatak Rasayana*.

THERAPEUTIC INDICATIONS AND PHARMACOLOGICAL STUDIES

In various types of cancer

The extracts of the fruit were effective against human epidermoid carcinoma of the naso-pharynx. Oral administration of nut juice to cancer patients, particularly those suffering from mouth cancer, provided symptomatic relief. It also extended the survival time (Wealth of India, 1972). Anti-tumour activity of the chloroform soluble fraction was tested on a spectrum of experimental neoplasms. The fraction showed a significant increase in percent lifespan of leukaemia L12120, P388 resistant either to adriamycin and/or vincristine (Chitnis *et al.* 1980). The cytotoxic effects of acetylated oil on P388 lymphocytic leukaemia cell was tested *in vitro*. The oil inhibited biosynthesis of DNA, RNA and protein (The oil was acetylated because pure oil gets oxidized easily) (Phatak, 1983). Smit *et al.* (1995) confirmed the strong cytotoxic effect of the nut, which may be of use in cancer. Premlatha *et al.* (1997) studied the effect of *Anacardium* nut milk extract on hepatocellular carcinoma. A marked increase in liver peroxide livels and a concomitant decrease in enzymatic antioxidant levels were observed in rat liver cancer. Tripathi *et al.* (1998) studied the effect of this drug on the cell cycle and cell viability of transformed prostate cells. The plant extract significantly arrested the cell cycle. At higher concentrations, it affected cell viability. The response was dose dependent.

As an anti-inflammatory agent

The alcoholic extract of the nut protected the animals against electrically-induced convulsions but was not effective against chemical convulsions. An extract from the nut, containing catechin and epicatechin, helped in sciatica and was effective in ankylostomiasis. Catechin increased capillary resistance. When studied for inflammation, epicatechin produced a significant reduction in rat paw oedema (Mujumdar, 1977). Upadhyay *et al.* (1986) used the drug for anti-inflammatory and anti-arthritic effects. Of patients given 5–10 g *bhalatak* twice daily, 40 per cent showed complete remission, 20 per cent showed improvement and the rest minor effects. It also helped body pain, appetite, indigestion and the haemoglobin content in patients' blood. Sharma and Singh (1986) conducted a clinical trial of a preparation *Amrita Bhallataka* on patients suffering from rheumatoid arthritis. A significant symptomatic relief was seen with less need for analgesics.

A Siddha preparation *Serankottai Nei* made from the milk extract of the nuts, said to have a good anti-arthritic effect, was studied by Vijayalakshmi *et al.* (1996, 1997). After administering this preparation, the lysosomal enzyme activity and protein-bound carbohydrate component levels became significantly normal. It was effective at a dose of 150 mg/kg in rats with adjuvant-induced arthritis. The lysosomal membrane fragility of drug-treated animals was reduced.

Hypocholesterolic effect

The nut shell extract is hypocholesterolaemic in its action and prevents cholesterol-induced atheroma (Sharma *et al.* 1995).

Chemical studies

Major constituents are mono- and di-hydroxycatechols and tannins. The vesicant juice is rich in phenols (Thakur *et al.* 1989).

Toxicological studies

Many people are sensitive to it and after its consumption may pass darker urine with or without blood. There may be skin eruptions, itching, hot flushes, diarrhoea and even delirium. To counteract these side effects, the tender kernel of coconut fruit or fat and butter should be given.

References

Ahmed, A., Rahman, H.S.Z., Amin, K.M.Y., Khan, N.A. Evaluation of *Baladur* (*Semecarpus anacardium*) on the basis of literature and folk information. *Proceedings Ist National Seminar on Ilmul Advia, Beenapura*, India, 23–25 April 1993.

Chitnis, M.P., Bhatia, K.G., Phatak, M.K., Kesava Rao, K.V. (1980) Antitumour activity of the extract of *Semecarpus anacardium* L. nuts in experimental tumour models. *Indian Journal of Experimental Biology*, 18, 6–8.

Mujumdar, A.M. (1977) Central nervous system actions of *Semecarpus anacardium* Linn. *Journal University of Poona, Science and Technology*, 50, 147–150.

Phatak, M.K., Ambaya, R.Y., Indap, M.A., Bhatia, K.G. (1983) Cytotoxicity of the acetylated oil of *Semecarpus anacardium* Linn. *Indian Journal of Physiology and Pharmacology*, 27, 166–170.

Premlatha, B., Muthulakashmi, V., Vijayalakshmi, T., Sachanandam, P. (1997) *Semecarpus anacardium* nut extract-induced changes in enzymic antioxidants studied in aflatoxin B_1 caused hepatocellular carcinoma bearing Wistar rats. *International Journal of Pharmacognosy*, 35, 161–166.

Shanavaskhan, A.E., Binu, S., Unnithan, M.D., Santhoshkumar, E.S., Pushpagandan, P. (1997) Detoxification techniques of traditional physicians of Kerala, India, on some toxic herbal drugs. *Fitoterapia*, 68, 69–74.

Sharma, A., Mathur, R., Dixit, V.P. (1995) Hypocholesterolemic activity of nut shell extract of *Semecarpus anacardium* (Bhilawa) in cholesterol fed rabbits. *Indian Journal of Experimental Biology*, 33, 444–448.

Sharma, A.K., Singh, R.H. (1986) A clinical study on Amrita Bhallataka as a Naimittika Rasayan in the mangement of rheumatoid arthritis (amvata). *Rheumatism*, 21, 51–60.

Smit, H.F., Woerdenbag, H.J., Singh, R.H., Meulenbeld, G.J., Labadie, R.P., Zwaving, J.H. (1995) Ayurvedic herbal drugs with possible cytostatic activity. *Journal of Ethnopharmacology*, 47, 75–84.

Thakur, R.S., Puri, H.S., Akhtar Hussain (1989) *Major Medicinal Plants of India*. Central Institute of Medicinal and Aromatic Plants, Lucknow, India 1989.

Tripathi, Y.B., Tripathi, P., Reddy, M.V.R., Dutt, S., Tewari, D.S., Reddy, E.P. (1998) Effect of *Semicarpus anacardium* on the cell cycle of DU-145 cells. *Phytomedicine*, 5, 383–388.

Upadhyay, B.N., Singh, T.N., Tewari, C.M., Jaiswal, L.C., Tripathi, S.N. (1986) Experimental and clinical evaluation of *Semecarpus anacardium* nut (Bhallatak) in the treatment of Amavata (rheumatoid arthritis). *Rheumatism*, 21(3), 70–87.

Vaidya, A.R. *The Ancient Indian System of Rejuvenation and Longevity*. Indian Book Center, Delhi, India 1998.

Vijayalakshmi, T., Muthulakshmi, V., Sachdanandam, P. (1996) Effect of the milk extract of *Semecarpus anacardium* nut on adjuvant arthritis: a dose dependent study in Wistar albino rats. *General Pharmacology*, 27, 1223–1226.

Vijayalakshmi, T., Muthulakshmi, V., Sachdanandam, P. (1997) Effect of milk extract of *Semercarpus anacardium* nuts on glycohydrolases and lysosomal stability in adjuvant arthritis in rats. *Journal of Ethnopharmacology*, 58, 1–18.

Wealth of India: Raw materials. Vol IX. Council of Scientific and Industrial Research, New Delhi, India 1972.

14 Bhringraj

Eclipta prostrata L. Syn. *E. alba* (L.) Hassk.
Family: Asteraceae (Compositae)

THE PLANT AND ITS DISTRIBUTION

Bhringraj grows wild alongside streams in hot areas and on humid soil. It is an erect or prostate herb (Fig. 7A), leaves 2.5 to 7.5 cm, with white hairs. Floral heads are 6–8 mm in diameter, solitary and white. Seed is black in colour, achene and compressed.

It is often called white *bhringraj* or white *bhangra* to differentiate it from another plant *Wedelia calendulacea* Less. (Fig. 7B) which has yellow flowers and is also known as yellow *bhangra*. Whereas *E. alba* grows all over the country *W. calendulacea* is found only in some parts of east and south India (Bhargava and Seshadri, 1974). A brief account of *W. calendulacea* is given in the end of this chapter.

USES IN FOLKLORE AND AYURVEDA

For digestive problems

Bhringraj is used as an antihepatotoxic agent and for spleen enlargement. Root is emetic and purgative. In jaundice 20 g of fresh leaves with 7 black peppers are administered daily for 5–6 days.

For gynaecological problems

The herb is used to prevent abortion and miscarriage. It gives relief in cases of uterine pains and uterine haemorrhage, after the delivery.

As an antiinflammatory agent

The paste of the herb is applied externally as an antiinflammatory agent. Decoction of the plant is used as a tonic for arthritis.

For cold

Juice of the herb with honey is used for catarrh in children.

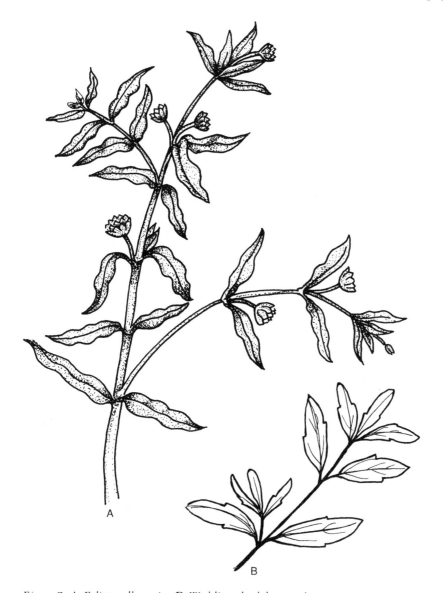

Figure 7 **A** *Eclipta alba* twig, **B** *Wedelia calendulacea* twig.

For hair growth

An oil made with leaf juice, boiled with sesame or coconut oil, is used for hair growth, delaying premature greying of hair and headaches.

For healing wounds

The fresh plant or its juice is applied for toothache. It is considered an antiseptic and applied to ulcers and wounds in cattle. The pounded plant is used to stop bleeding.

As a *Rasayana*

It is considered a *medhya* (nervine tonic) and a *Rasayana*. The seed (1 to 3 g) is used as an aphrodisiac. The juice (5–10 ml) is prescribed for one month as a part of *Rasayana* treatment. While administering the juice, the patient should survive only on milk.

In Chinese traditional medicine

It is used as an astringent for various types of haemorrhages, for example of the intestine (the vomiting of blood), haematuria, lumbago, epistaxis, cystitis and hepatitis.

THERAPEUTIC INDICATION AND PHARMACOLOGICAL STUDIES

Antihepatotoxic activity

Samana and Ramaswamy (1976) confirmed the protective effect of the herb against liver damage in dogs. Dixit and Achar (1979) tried a fine powder of herb for infective hepatitis. In 75 per cent cases there was recovery. In another study Dixit and Achar (1981) tried the powder of 50 mg/kg of the herb in 3 doses for jaundice in children and in the majority of cases it showed complete clinical and biochemical recovery in 1 to 5 weeks. It was concluded that this antihepatotoxic activity may be due to the anti-viral and anti-microbial activity of the herb. Devinder Kumar *et al.* (1981), through biochemical and histopathological studies, observed that the aqueous extract, equivalent to 5 g of dry herb, regularized liver abnormalities caused by carbon tetrachloride. Dube *et al.* (1982) used 50 mg of the extract three times a day for hepatocellular jaundice. It cured 55 per cent cases of jaundice within 3–4 weeks of treatment. Thyagarajan *et al.* (1982) observed immunoactive property in *Eclipta* against the surface antigen of hepatic B-virus. Wagner *et al.* (1986) detected coumestans as the active principle. *Eclipta*, when tried against various ailments of liver and gall bladder, exhibited significant stimulatory effects on liver cell enlargement. Raut *et al.* (1986) studied the effect of the herb on peptic ulcers, non-ulcer dyspepsia and the liver. When given along with Indian thyme (*Ptychotis ajwain* DC) a cholagogue property was observed in patients with derangement of the liver and gall bladder. Kumar and Tripathi (1987) also tried the herb for managing liver diseases. Chandra *et al.* (1987) studied the effect of herb on inflammation and liver injury and found that it counteracted liver weight and hepatic lipid peroxidation. Alcoholic extract using 50 mg/kg once a day for 7 days was found to be antihepatotoxic (Mogre *et al.* 1988). Singh *et al.* (1993) and Murthy *et al.* (1993) also found a hepatoprotective effect. Lin (1996) observed a hepatoprotective effect in an extract of herb against carbon tetrachloride, acetaminophen and beta-D-galactosamine-induced liver damage.

Premilla (1995) reviewed the antihepatotoxic activity of the herb.

Antihaemorrhagic activity

Kosuge *et al.* (1981) studied antihaemorrhagic principles of herb for homeostatic action.

Cardiovascular effect

Gupta *et al.* (1976) observed cardiovascular (cardiodepressant) activity in it when used for hepatic congestion, venous enlargement and turgidity. The water soluble fraction of the leaves produced a hypotensive effect unrelated to histaminergic and cholinergic mechanism. The polypeptide mixture had a tranquillizing effect. It induced rapid onset of pentobarbitone sodium's hypnotic activity. The average sleeping time was almost doubled by a crude extract dose of 2.5 mg/kg. Hypotensive effect was immediate and it lasted for 10–15 minutes. When clinical trials were undertaken using a decoction from 25 g of powder daily for 3 weeks, 73 per cent of hypertensive patients showed a good response. There were no headaches, insomnia or palpitations but urine output increased. Rashid *et al.* (1992) also observed antihypertensive activity in ethanol extract. The active constituent detected was culumbin.

In ulcers

Tewari (personal communication, 1979) tried 10 g of whole plant powder three times a day on 35 patients with non-ulcer dyspepsia and 25 patients with peptic ulcer dyspepsia for 3 months. A complete symptomatic relief in epigastric pain, nausea and vomiting was seen. There was a reduction in flatulence and the amount of free gastric acid. Eighty per cent of the patients of non-ulcer dyspepsia responded well, with relief in acid secretion, nocturnal pain, nausea and vomiting. In 48 per cent of patients with duodenal ulcer the results were excellent while in 75 per cent of cases there was radiological improvement. Raut *et al.* (1986) tried the herb for ulcers and peptic ulcers. Das (1992) studied the effect of the herb on gastritis by administering 12 g of pulverized herb daily, in three divided doses, for 45 days. In 52 per cent of cases of gastritis the results were excellent. In hyperchlorhydria there was total relief.

Antiinflammatory effect

Reddy *et al.* (1990) observed that *Eclipta* exhibited anti-inflammatory activity. It inhibited the higher levels of histamine due to chronic inflammation by 58.67 per cent.

Antivenomous effect

Melo *et al.* (1994) tested the aqueous extract of the herb and the three constituents, wadelolactone, stigmasterol and sitosterol, for protective effects against three crotalid venoms and three crotalid myotoxins. All the herbal preparations inhibited the myotoxic effects of the snake venom. Wadelolactone was an effective antagonist of the myotoxins. The aqueous extract and wadelolactone also inhibited haemorrhagic lesions.

Antimicrobial property

The alcohol extract had anti-viral activity. Polyacetylenes of the herb, in antibiotic tests, were strongly phototoxic (UV mediated) to microorganisms. A Chinese study has also shown that thiophenes in the herb are phototoxic to bacteria, fungi, nematodes and yeast.

Chemical studies

The main constituent is wadelolactone, a complex coumarin, alkaloid, with nicotine 0.08 per cent and nicotinic acid. The root contains polyacetylenes substituted thiophene derivatives and free triterpenoids.

Toxicological studies

In acute and sub-acute toxicity the behaviour of rats was normal, but in chronic toxicity they become dull and lethargic. The water intake was reduced and they were indifferent to their surroundings. There were no appreciable changes in the body weight of organs. No side or toxic effects were observed after the study of biochemical parameters and histopathology of liver, kidney, spleen and heart (Rashid *et al.* 1992).

Wedelia calendulacea Less

As mentioned earlier, *Eclipta* is sometimes substituted by this herb. The chemical and pharmacological studies have shown that this substitution is appropriate, as both have the same types of chemical constituents and effect.

In this herb coumestans was found to be the main active principle for liver protection (Wagner 1986). Sharma *et al.* (1989) noted that 50 per cent alcohol extract of the herb had a heptoprotective effect. It protected the functional and structural activity of the liver. Gopalkrishnan *et al.* (1989) also observed anti-hepatotoxic activity in it. It counteracted the increase in liver weight, hepatic liver peroxidation and serum alkaline phosphates induced by carbon tetrachloride. Hegde *et al.* (1994) noted that herb had a wound healing effect on rats.

References

Bhargava, K.K., Seshadri, T.R. (1974) Chemistry of medicinal plants: *Eclipta alba* and *Wedelia calandulacea*. *Journal of Research in Indian Medicine*, 9, 9–15.

Chandra, T., Sadiqui, J., Somasundram, S. (1987) Effect of *Eclipta alba* on inflammation and liver injury. *Fitoterapia*, 58, 23–32.

Chow, L.-S., Jung, Y.-C., Ching, L.-C., Yunho L. (1996) Hepatoprotective activity of Taiwan folk medicine: *Eclipta prostrata* Linn. against various hepatotoxins-induced acute hepatotoxicity. *Phytotherapy Research*, 10, 483–496.

Das, S. (1992) Effect of *Eclipta alba* on gastritis. *International Seminar-Traditional Medicine*, Calcutta, 7–9 November 1992.

Dixit, S.P., Achar, M.P. (1979) Bhringraja (*Eclipta alba* L) in the treatment of infective hepatitis. *Current Medical Practice*, 23, 237–242.

Dixit, S.P., Achar, M.P. (1981) Study of Bhringraja (*Eclipta alba*) therapy in jaundice in cholera. *Journal of Scientific Research in Plants and Medicine*, 2, 96–100.

Dube, C.B., Devendkumar, Srivastava, P.S. (1982) A trial of Bhringraja Ghansatva on the patients of Kostha-Shakaraista-Kamala (with special reference to hepatocellular jaundice). *Journal National Integrated Medical Association*, 24, 265–269.

Gopalakrishnan, S., Sadique, J., Chandra, T. (1989) Antihepatotoxic activity of *Wedelia calendulacea* in rats. *Fitoterapia*, 60, 456–459.

Gupta, S.C., Bajaj, U.K., Sharma, V.N. (1976) Cardiovascular effect of *Eclipta alba* (Hassk.) Bhringraja. *Journal of Research in Indian Medicine and Homoeopathy*, 11, 91–92.

Hegde, D.A., Khosa, R.L., Chansuria, J.P.N. (1994) A study of the effect of *Wedelia calendulacea* Less on wound healing in rats. *Phytotherapy Research*. 8, 439–440.

Kosuge, T. *et al.* (1981) Studies on anti-haemorrhagic principles in the crude drug for hemostatics: on hemostatic activity of the crude drugs for hemostatics. *Yakugaku Zasshi*, 101, 501–503.

Kumar, D., Dube, C.B., Srivastava, P.S. (1981) Controlled experimental study of Bhringraja Ghansatva. *Journal of Research in Ayurveda and Siddha*, 2, 32–41.

Kumar, S., Tripathi, S.N. (1987) Role of certain Ayurvedic medicines in the management of liver disease. *Journal of the National Integrated Medical Association*, 29, 7–14.

Melo, P.A., Nascimento, M.C., Mors, W.B., Suarez-Kurtz, G. (1994) Inhibition of the myotoxic and hemorrhagic activities of crotalid venoms by *Eclipta prostrata* (Asteraceae) extracts and constituents. *Toxicon* (Oxford) 32, 595–603.

Mogre, K., Vohra, K.K., Seth, U.K. (1988) Protective effect of *Picrorrhiza kurroa* and *Eclipta alba* on Na+. K+ Atphase in hepatic injury by hepatotoxic agents. *Indian Journal of Pharmacy*, 13, 253–259.

Murthy, T.S., Rao, B.G., Satyanaryana, T., Rao, R.V.K. (1993) Hepatoprotective activity of *Eclipta alba*. *Journal of Research and Education in Indian Medicine*, 12, 41–43.

Premilla, M.S. (1995) Emerging frontiers in the area of hepatoprotective herbal drugs. *Indian Journal of Natural Products*. 11, 9.

Sharma, A.K., Anand, K.K., Pushpangadan, P., Chandan, B.K., Chopra, C.L., Prabhakar, Y.S., Damodaran, N.P. (1989) Hepatoprotective effects of *Wedelia calendulacea*. *Journal of Ethnopharmacology*, 25, 93–102.

Singh, B., Saxena, A.K., Chandan, B.K., Agarwal, S.G., Bhatia, M.S., Anand, K.K. (1993) Hepatoprotective effect of ethanolic extract of *Eclipta alba* on experimental liver damage in rats and mice. *Phytotherapy Research*, 7, 154–158.

Rashid, M.D., Karim, V., Ahmed, M., Choudhury, A.R. (1992) Antihypertensive activity of *Eclipita alba*. *International Seminar-Traditional Medicine, Calcutta*, 7–9 November, 1992.

Raut, A.A., Tewari, S.K., Kumar, S. (1986) *Eclipta alba* – a scientific appraisal with special reference to its effect on peptic ulcer, non-ulcer dyspepsia and liver. *Journal of NIMA*, April 1986, 17–23.

Reddy, K.R.K., Tehara, S.S., Goud, P.V., Alikhan, M.M. (1990) Comparison of the antiinflammatory activity of *Eclipta alba* (Bhangra) and *Solanum nigrum* (Mako Khushk) in rat. *Journal of Research and Education in Indian Medicine*, 9, 43–46.

Samana, H.C., Ramaswamy, V.M. (1976) Protective effect of *Eclipta alba* in experimentally induced liver damage in dogs. *Cheiron*, 5, 96–98.

Thyagarajan *et al.* (1982) In vitro activation of Hb. Ag by *Eclipta alba* Hassk and *Phyllanthus niruri*. *Indian Journal of Medical Research*, 76, 124–130.

Wagner, H., Geyer, B., Kiso, Y., Hikino, H., Rao, G.S. (1986) Coumestans as the main active principles of the liver drugs *Eclipta alba* and *Wedelia calendulacea*, *Planta Medica*, 5, 370–374.

15 Bhuiamla

Phyllanthus amarus Aschum. & Thonn.
P. debile Klein ex. Willd
P. fraternus Webster
P. niruri L
P. urinaria L
P. virgatus Forst, Syn. *P. simplex* Retz.
Family: Euphorbiaceae

THE PLANTS AND THEIR DISTRIBUTION

The plant species given above are called *bhuiamalaki* in Ayurveda because the leaves in these have a superficial resemblance to those of the *amalaki* (*Emblica officinalis*) tree and the small fruits in these prostate herbs grow along the soil. *Bhuiamalaki* thus means a prostate *amalaki* and the corrupted form of this name is *bhuiamla*.

The herb is probably a native of tropical America. In nearly all the earlier literature, the herb *bhuiamla* was identified as *Phyllanthus niruri* and it is reported as such in most of the Indian floras, but recent studies have shown *bhuiamla* to be a mixture of at least three species: P. *amarus*, P. *fraternus*, and P. *debilis*. There is a possibility that other allied species are identified as *bhuiamla*. The true P. *niruri* is endemic to the West Indies and has not been found to occur in India (Thakur *et al.* 1989). P. *debilis* is confined to the coastal areas of India, while the other two species are widespread throughout the plains. The other species which can be considered as the source of *bhuiamala* is P. *maderaspatensis* (Singh *et al.* 1994). Keeping in view the medicinal importance of this genera, studies were carried out in the allied species. In P. *urinaria* there were significant differences amongst the intraspecific accessions. Accessions of P. *amarus* from various locations were not significantly different (Unander and Blumberg, 1991).

Herbal *Phyllanthus* species (Fig. 8) are small annual, creeping or erect plants, growing in moist, shady places in most parts of India. Leaves are elliptic oblong, obovate oblong or obtuse, varying in different species. Flowers are axillary, unisexual or bisexual. Capsules are round and vary in shape and size. All these species are characterized by the fruits growing along the underside of the leaves

The four important species of Indian *Phyllanthus* spp. growing in the plains of India, on the basis of a dichotomous key given by Bagchi *et al.* (1992), can be identified as follows:

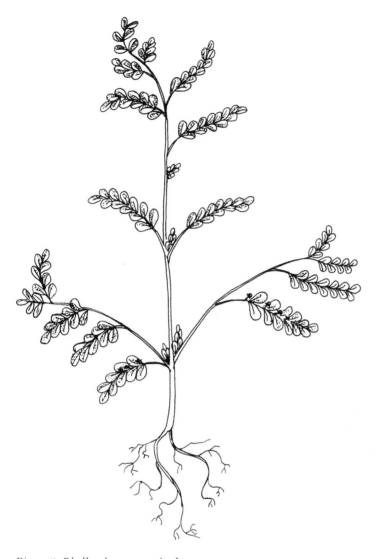

Figure 8   Phyllanthus amarus herb.

1	Plants prostate and parenchymatous cells are full of starch grains	*P. virgatus*
2	Plants erect and parenchymatous cells have few or no starch grains	3/4
3	Capsule verrucose and fiber cells are not present in branchlets	*P. urinaria*
4	Capsule smooth and fiber cells are present in branchlets	5/6
5	Cymules bisexual, calyx lobes 5, druse crystals are present	*P. amarus*
6	Cymules unisexual, calyx lobes 6, druse crystals are absent	*P. fraternus*

USES IN FOLKLORE AND AYURVEDA

It is considered bitter, astringent, stomachic and a febrifuge.
The uses of this herb are:

In jaundice

Fifteen grams of the crushed herb with a cup of milk is given in the morning and evening. Dry leaves, in powder form, may also be prescribed (Nadakarni, 1954).

For jaundice in Silent Valley (Kerala), 10 g of this herb, with 10 g of the root bark of *Cassia auriculata* L. is made into paste and administered with cow's milk for three days, on an empty stomach in the morning (Bhatt *et al.* 1981).

THERAPEUTIC INDICATIONS AND PHARMACOLOGICAL STUDIES

According to Bagchi *et al.* (1992) much of the earlier botanical, phytochemical and pharmacological work previously reported from India on *P. niruri* was apparently done on *P. fraternus*, *P. amarus* or *P. debilis*. The summary of these findings is as follows:

Immunomodulator activity

The crude extract, as well as the red pigment of the herb, had immunoactivating ability against HBsAg (Thakur *et al.*, 1989).

Effect on the liver

Children suffering from jaundice were given the herb in powder form. In the majority of cases, hepatic tenderness disappeared with improvement in appetite (Dixit and Achar, 1983). It also helped in alcohol-induced fatty liver development (Umarani *et al.* 1985) and was used in jaundice due to liver damage by Shyamsunder *et al.* (1985). The effect of alcohol-induced liver cell damage in non-hepatectomised rats was studied by Agarwal *et al.* (1986). It protected induced cytotoxicity in primary cultured hepatocytes and also provided protection against cytotoxicity induced by lead, aluminium salts (Dhir *et al.* 1990) and by nickel chloride (Agarwal *et al.* 1992). *P. niruri* was found effective in induced hepatotoxicity in calves (Kohale *et al.* 1993). According to Satyan *et al.* (1994) both *P. niruri* and *P. urinaria*, provided protection to the liver due to a major bioactive lignan, phyllanthin. *P. urinaria* lacked phyllanthin, so the protective effect was less in this case. For comparison, Sane (1995) studied the hepatoprotective effect of both *P. amarus* and *P. debilis* on the liver by bringing about a change in the various constituents of serum by carbon tetrachloride. *P. debilis* was more potent than *P. amarus*. Polya *et al.* (1995) found that hydrolyzable tannins from *P. amarus* were the most specific potent inhibitors of the rat cyclic AMP dependent protein kinase catalytic sub unit.

Effect on Hepatitis B virus: This study is important because a relationship between hepatoma and hepatitis B virus (HBV) infection exists. Definite immune inactive properties of *Phyllanthus* against the surface antigen of hepatitis B virus was reported by Thygarajan *et al.* (1982). These authors (Thygarajan *et al.* 1988) observed that *P. amarus* clears the chronic state of the B virus. Venkateswaran *et al.* (1987) studied the effect of an extract of *P. niruri* on hepatitis B and woodchuck hepatitis viruses. It inhibited woodchuck hepatitis virus DNA polymerase and surface antigen expression. Jayaram *et al.* (1987) also confirmed anti-hepatitis B virus properties of this herb after clinical trials. The treatment was found quite safe, with no mortality, weight loss or behavioural changes. Jayram *et al.* (1997) treated 28 chronic cases of HBV by using *P. amarus*, for up to three months. Clearance was observed in 20 per cent of cases. The study proposed a dose of 500 mg of the herb three times a day for six months. Munshi (1993) found this herb a good agent for post exposure prophylaxis in neonatal duck hepatitis B virus (DHBV) infection. Milne (1994) standardized the extract of *P. amarus* to contain 200 mg of geraniin. The results indicated that this extract had no effect on New Zealand hepatitis B carriers. Alonso *et al.* (1995) tried an alcohol extract of *Phyllanthus* spp. and the flavonoids of the herb inactivated the surface antigen *in vitro* in HBV. Unamder *et al.* (1995), after a review, concluded that the herb has some use as an anti-viral agent to treat jaundice and liver diseases. It acted as a liver tonic in the case of non-hepatitis B virus diseases. The effects on chronic infection with HBV or related viruses have generally been negative. Ott *et al.* (1997) observed that *P. amarus* suppresses hepatitis B virus by interrupting interactions between HBV enhancer I and cellular transcriptase factors. Jayram *et al.* (1997) carried out clinical trials on the patients of acute viral hepatitis A, B, and non-A, and non-B. After four weeks, significant biochemical and clinical normalcy in hepatic virus A infected patients was observed. It seemed to accelerate the clearance of the majority of HBV patients. Karin (1999) isolated seven ellagitannins from *P. urinaria*, which had strong activity against Epstein Barr virus.

Antidiabetic effect

Hukeri *et al.* (1988) confirmed hypoglycaemic activity of *P. fraternus* in rats. Sivaprakasam *et al.* (1995) tried *P. amarus* in 25 diabetic patients. Statistically significant lowering of blood sugar levels was observed with a dose of 1 g, thrice daily for three months. Srividya and Periwal (1995) observed diuretic, hypotensive and hypoglycaemic effects of the herb. Blood glucose was significantly reduced without any side effects. It also lowered the cystolic blood pressure in non-diabetic, hypertensive females. Moshi *et al.* (1997) confirmed non-insulin dependent hypoglycaemic activity in *P. amarus*.

Effect on fat metabolism

The herb caused increased depletion of triglycerides, cholesterol and phospholipids found in liver, heart and kidney and brought them down to normal levels (Umarani, 1985).

Effect on vascular system

An angiotensin converting enzyme inhibitor from *P. niruri* was isolated (Ueno *et al.* 1988). Endothelin is a potent vasoconstrictor peptide and could be involved in the development of hypertension in man. A non-peptide endothelial antagonist has been reported from *P. niruri* (Hussain, 1995).

Anti-bacterial property

Cruz (1994) observed that a hexane fraction of *P. urinaria* leaves have an antibacterial effect. Unander (1995) confirmed it.

Anti-nociceptive activity

This activity was observed from an extract of the herb. It failed to inhibit formalin-induced paw oedema (Santos *et al.* 1995).

Antioxidant property

Three compounds isolated from *P. niruri*, were six times more potent than quercitin for inhibiting aldose reductase (Shimizu *et al.* 1989). *P. niruri* caused a 50 per cent inhibition of superoxide scavenging activity, and potent inhibition of lipid peroxide formation. It was a scavenger of hydroxyl radical in vitro, which shows it to be a good antioxidant (Joy and Kuttan, 1995).

Anti-spasmodic activity

P. urinaria extract had a relaxant effect on isolated trachea (Paulino *et al.* 1996).

Anti-fungal activity

This activity of the herb against *Helminthosporium sativum* and *Alternaria alternata* has been reported (Thakur *et al.* 1989).

Chemical studies

Many lignanas have been isolated from various species. Phyllanthin is a major bioactive lignan but it is absent in *P. urinaria* (Satyan *et al.* 1994). Five flavonoids, four leucodelphins and two alkaloids have also been reported. (Thakur *et al.* 1989). From the alcoholic extract of *P. niruri* Ueno *et al.* (1988) isolated ellagic acid, gallic acid and geraniin. These exhibited angiotensin converting enzyme activity.

References

Agarwal, K., Dhir, H., Sharma, A., Talukdar, G. (1992) The efficacy of two species of *Phyllanthus* in counteracting nickel clastogenicity. *Fitoterapia*, 63, 49–54.

Agarwal, S.S., Garg, A., Agarwal, S. (1986) Screening of *Phyllanthus niruri* Linn and *Riccinus communis* Linn on alcohol-induced liver cell damage in non-hepatectomised rats. *Indian Journal of Pharmacology*, 18, 211–214.

Alonso, G.D.B., Perez, O.C., Chevalier, P. (1995) In vitro inactivation of Ags HB by plant extracts of *Phyllanthus* genus. *Revista Cubana de Medicina Tropical*, 47, 127–130.

Bagchi, G.D., Srivastava, G.N., Singh, S.C. (1992) Distinguishing features of medicinal herbaceous species of *Phyllanthus* occuring in Lucknow District (U.P.) India. *International Journal of Pharmacognosy*, 30, 161–168.

Bhatt, A.V., Nair, K.V., Nair, C.A.A. (1981) Ethnobotanical studies in the Silent Valley and the adjoining areas. *Bulletin of Medico-Ethno-Botanical Research*, 3, 153–161.

Chandra, T., Sadique, J. (1987) A new recipe for liver injury. *Ancient Science of Life*, 7, 99–103.

Cruz, A.B., Moretto, E., Cechinel Filho, V, Niero, R., Montanari, J.L., Yunes, R.A. (1994) Antibacterial activity of *Phyllanthus urinaria*. *Fitoterapia*, 65, 461–462.

Dhir, H., Roy, A.K., Sharma, A., Talukdar,G. (1990) Protection afforded by aqueous extracts of *Phyllanthus* species by lead and aluminum salts. *Phytotherapy Research*, 4, 172–176.

Dixit, S.P., Achar, M.P. (1983) Bhunyamlaki (*Phyllanthus niruri*) and jaundice in children. *Journal National Integrated Medical Association*, 25, 269–272.

Hukeri, V.I., Kalyam, G.A., Kakrani, H.K. (1988) Hypoglycaemic activity of flavonoids of Phyllanthus fraternus in rats. *Fitoterapia*, 59, 68–70.

Hussain, R.A., Dickey, J.K., Rosser, M.P., Matson, J.A., Kozlowski, M.R., Brittain, R.J., Webb, M.L., Rose, P.M., Fernandes, P. (1995) A novel class of non-peptidic endothelin anatgonists isolated from the medicinal herb *Phyllanthus niruri*. *Journal of Natural Products*, 58, 1515–1520.

Jayaram, S., Thyagarajan, S.P., Panchanadam, M., Subramanian, S.S. (1987) Anti-hepatitis B virus properties of *Phyllanthus niruri* Linn. and *Eclipta alba* Haussk: in vitro and in vivo safety studies *Biomedicine*, 7, 9–16.

Jayaram, S., Thyagarajan, S.P., Sumathi, S, Manjula, S., Malathi, S., Madangopalan, N. (1997) Efficacy of *Phyllanthus amarus* treatment in acute viral hepatitis A, B, and non A and non B: an open clinical trial. *Indian Journal of Virology*, 13, 59–64.

Jayaram, S., Valliammai, T., Thyagrajan, S.P., Pal, V.G., Jayaraman, K., Madangopalan, N. (1990) Study on HBV markers in chronic HbsAg carriers while on treatment with *Phyllanthus amarus* using ELISA and DOT biohybridisation method VIR 3. *XIV National Congress of the Indian Association of Medical Microbiologist*, Vellore, TN, October 25–27, 1990.

John, G., Krishnamurthy, S. (1993) Some biochemical effects of *Phyllanthus niruri*: an ayurvedic drug for hepatitis in rats. *Medical and Nutritional Research Communication*, 1, 40–46.

Joy, K.L., Kuttan, R. (1995) Anti-oxidant activity of selected plant extracts. *Amala Research Bulletin*. 15, 68–71.

Karin, C.S., Liu, C., Lin, M.-T., Lee, S.-S., Faen, C.J., Ren, S., Lien, E.J. (1999) Antiviral tannins from two *Phyllanthus* species. *Planta Medica*, 65, 43–46.

Kohale, K.N., Bijwal, D.L., Patnaik, B.S., Sadekar, R.D., Moele, S.G. (1993) Efficacy of *Phyllanthus niruri* Linn in experimentally induced hepatotoxicity in crossbred calves. *Indian Journal of Veterinary Medicine*. 13, 16–17.

Milne, A., Lucas, C.R., Waldon, J., Foo, F. (1994) Failure of New Zealand hepatitis B carriers to respond to *Phyllanthus amarus*. *New Zealand Medical Journal*, 107, 243.

Moshi, M.J., Uiso, F.C., Mahunnali, R.L.A., Malele, S.R., Swai, A.B.M. (1997) A study of the effect of *Phyllanthus amarus* extract on blood glucose in rabbits. *International Journal of Pharmacognosy*, 35, 167–173.

Munshi, A., Mehrotra, R., Panda, S.K. (1993) Evaluation of *Phyllanthus amarus* and *Phyllanthus maderasptensis* as agent for post exposure prophylaxis in neonatal duck hepatitis B virus infection. *Journal of Medical Virology*, 40, 53–58.

Nadkarmi, K.M. *Indian Materia Medica*, Vol. I. Popular Prakashan, Bombay, India 1954.

Ott, M., Thygarajan, S.P., Gupta, S. (1997) *Phyllanthus amarus* suppresses hepatitis B virus by interrupting interactions between HBV enhancer I and cellulose transcriptase factors. *European Journal of Clinical Investigations*, 27, 908–915.

Paulino, N., Cechinel Filho, V., Yunes, R.A., Calixto, J.B. (1996) The relaxant effect of extract of *Phyllanthus urinaria* in the guinea-pig isolated trachea. Evidence for involvement of ATP-sensitive potassium channels. *Journal of Pharmacy and Pharmacology*, 48, 1158–1163.

Polya, G.M., Wang, B.H., Foo, L.Y. (1995) Inhibition of signal regulated protein kinases by plant derived hydrolysable tannins. *Phytochemistry*, 38, 307–314.

Prakash, A, Satyan, K.S, Wahi, S.P., Singh, K.P. (1995) Comparative hepatoprotective activity of three *Phyllanthus* species, *P. urinaria*, *P. niruri* and *P. simplex* on carbon tetrachloride-induced liver injury in the rat. *Phytotherapy Research*, 9, 594–596.

Reddy, B.P., Murthy, V.N., Venkateshwarlu, V., Kokate, C.K., Rambhau, D. (1993) Antihepatotoxic activity of *Phyllanthus niruri*, *Tinospora cordofolia* and *Ricinus communis*. *Indian Drugs*, 30, 338–341.

Sane, R.T., Kuber, V.V., Chalissery, M.S., Menon, S. (1995) Hepatoprotection by *Phyllanthus amarus* and *Phyllanthus debilis* in Ccl4-induced liver dysfunction. *Current Science* 68, 1243–1246.

Santos, A.R.S., Cechinel Filho, V., Yunes, R.A., Calixto, J.B. (1995) Further studies on the antinociceptive action of the hydroalcoholic extracts from plants of the genus *Phyllanthus*. *Journal of Pharmacy and Pharmacology*, 47, 66–71.

Satyan, K.S., Nand Prakash, Singh, R.P., Wahi, S.P. (1994) Chemical and hepatoprotective activity of *Phyllanthus* Linn. Species; Family: Euphorbiaceae. *Proceedings of 46th Annual Indian Pharmaceutical Congress*. Chandigarh, 28–30 December 1994.

Shimizu, M., Horie, S., Terashima, S., Ueno, H., Hayashi, T., Ariswa, M, Suzuki, S., Yoshizaki, M. Morita, N. (1989) Studies on aldose reductase inhibitors from natural products II. Active components of a Paraguayan crude drug *Para-parai mi*, *Phyllanthus niruri*. *Chemical and Pharmaceutical Bulletin*, 37, 2531–2532.

Shyamsunder, Kodakandla Venkata, Bikram Singh, Raghunath Singh Thakur, Akhtar Hussain, Yoshunobu Kiso, Hiroshi Hikino (1985) Anti-hepatotoxic principles of *Phyllanthus niruri* herb. *Journal of Ethnopharmacology*, 14, 41–44.

Singh, R.T., Sharma, A., Handa, S.S. (1994) Standardisation of *Phyllanthus amarus* Schum. & Thonn. *Proceedings of 46th Annual Indian Pharmaceutical Congress*, Chandigarh, 28–30 December 1994.

Sivaprakasam, K., Yasodha, R., Sivandanam, G., Veluchamy, G. (1995) Clinical evaluation of *Phyllanthus amarus* Schum & Thonn in diabetic mellitus. *Seminar on Research in Ayurveda and Siddha CCRAS*, New Delhi, 20–22 March 1995.

Somanabandhu, A., Nityangkuras, S., Mahidol, C., Ruchirawat, S., Likhit-wityayawind, K., Shieh, H., Chai H., Pezznto and Cordell, G.A. (1993) 1H and 13C NMR assignment of phyllanthin and hypophyllanthin. Lignans that evidence cytotoxic response with cultured multi drug resistant cells. *Journal of Natural Products*, 56, 233–239.

Srividya, N., Periwal, S. (1995) Diuretic, hypotensive and hypoglycaemic effect of Phyllanthus amarus. *Indian Journal of Experimental Biology*, 33, 861–864.

Thakur, R.S., Puri, H.S., Hussain, A. *Major Medicinal Plants of India*. Central Institute of Medicinal and Aromatic Plants, Lucknow, India 1989.

Thyagrajan, S.P. (1982) In vitro inactivation of Hb, Ag by *Eclipta alba* Haussk and *Phyllanthus nirurri*. *Indian Journal of Medical Research*, 76, 124–130.

Thyagarajan, S.P., Jayaram, S., Satyasekaran, M., Madangopalan, N. (1990) Efficacy of *Phyllanthus amarus* v/s *Essentiale* in acute viral hepatitis. VIR 5. *XIV National Congress of the Indian Association of Medical Microbiologists*, Vellore, TN. October 25–27, 1990.

Thyagarajan, S.P., Subramanian, S., Thirunalasundri, T., Venkateswaran, P.S., Blumberg, B.S. (1988) Effect of Phyllanthus amarus on chronic carriers of hepatitis B virus. *Lancet*, II (8614), 764–766.

Tripathi, S.C., Patnaik, G.K., Visen, P.K.S., Saraswat, B., Kulshreshtha, D.K., Dhawan, B.N. (1992) Evaluation of hepatoprotective activity of *Phyllanthus amarus* against experimentally induced liver damage in rat. *Proceedings of 25th Indian Pharmacological Society Conference*, Muzzafarpur, Bihar, India. 5–8 December 1992.

Ueno, H., Horie, S., Nishi, Y., Shogwa, H., Kawasaki, M., Suzuki, S., Hayashi, T., Arisawa M., Shimizu, M., Yoshizaki, M., Morita, N., Bergenza, L.H., Ferro, E., Bagua, Wo, I. (1988) Chemical and pharmaceutical studies on medicinal plants in Paraguay, geraniin an angiotensin-converting enzyme inhibitor from *Paraparai Mi Phylanthus nirurui*. *Journal of Natural Products*, 51, 357–365.

Umarani, D., Devaki, T., Govindraju, P., Shanmugasundram, K.R. (1985) Ethanol-induced metabolic alternations and the effect of *Phyllanthus niruri* in their reversal. *Ancient Science of Life*, 4, 174–180.

Unander, D.W., Blumberg, B.S. (1991) In vitro activity of *Phyllanthus* (Euphorbiaceae) species against the DNA polymerase of hepatitis viruses: effect of growing environment and inter and intra-specific differences. *Economic Botany*, 45, 225–242.

Unander, D.W., Webster, G.L., Blumberg, B.S. (1995) Usage and bioassays in *Phyllanthus* (Euphorbiaceae). IV Clustering of antiviral uses and other effects. *Journal of Ethnopharmacology*, 45, 1–18.

Venkateswaran, P.S., Millman, I., Blumberg, B.S. (1987) Effect of an extract of *Phyllanthus niruri* on hepatitis B and woodchuk hepatitis viruses: in vitro and in vivo studies. *Proceedings National Academy of Sciences* USA, 84, 274–278.

Zhibao, M., Shan, C.H., Xitan, Z., Wu, S.X., Zhuang, L., Xioming, W. (1995) Duck hepatitis B virus model for screening of antiviral agents from medicinal herbs. *Chinese Medical Journal*, 108, 660–664.

16 Brahmi

Bacopa monnieri (L.) Penn.
Syn. *Herpestis monniera* (L.) H.B.K.
Bacopa monniera Wettst.
Moniera cuneifolia Michx.
Family: Scorphulariaceae

THE PLANT AND ITS DISTRIBUTION

It is a small prostate herb (Fig. 9A,B) with ascending branches and serrate, entire, oblong or obovate, 2.5 long and 0.6 cm wide leaves. The flower is solitary and the fruit is an ovoid capsule with persistent style. The plant grows in damp places and marshy grounds on the majority of the Indian plains.

USES IN FOLKLORE AND AYURVEDA

Earlier *Centella asiatica* was known as *brahmi* to distinguish it from *Centella*; it is known in the trade as *jal brahmi* (*brahmi* growing along water) or *jal neem* (*neem* is *Azadirachta indica* and this herb is as bitter as *neem*, so it was called hygrophytic *neem*). Even now *Centella* is sometimes used in place of this herb.

The literal meaning of *brahmi* is *which expands consciousness*. According to Hindu mythology *Brahma* is one of the three gods of trinity, who controlled the world during its origin. The other names of this herb in ancient texts are: *Sureshta* – liked by gods, *Divy* – divine, *Saraswati, Sharad, Bharati* – goddesses of learning (the herb is named after these goddessess to show that it has a good effect on intellectuality), *Vayastha* – arrests old age, *Sharma* – charming and *Medhya* – good for mental work.

It is one of the three *medhya* herbs of Ayurveda, used for psychoactive diseases. It has a beneficial effect on intelligence and memory by reducing anxiety and tension. It is considered a nervine tonic for neurasthenia, epilepsy, insanity and for nervous breakdown. For learning and memory up to 30 ml of plant juice is given twice daily before breakfast in the morning and two hours after dinner. It is quite bitter so honey is added to it to make it palatable.

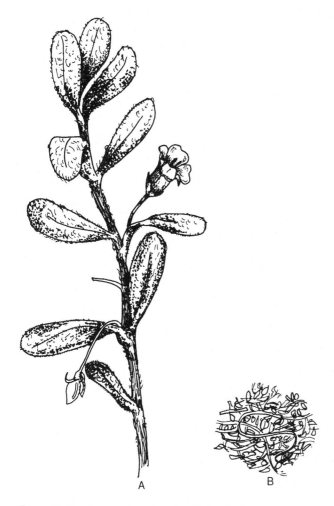

Figure 9 Bacopa monniera **A** twig, **B** dry herb.

THERAPEUTIC INDICATIONS AND PHARMACOLOGICAL STUDIES

Psychotropic effects

To confirm the identity of *brahmi*, Singh *et al.* (1975) studied the therapeutic activities of both *Centella* and *Bacopa* and concluded that *Bacopa* was the source of *brahmi*. This herb showed significant psychotropic action as evidenced by excessive sleep and conformation changes in the brain, as well as in the blood. A significant barbiturate hypnosis potentiation effect was observed, with reductions in the acetylcholine and cholinesterase content of the brain tissue and the blood.

Earlier studies had shown that the herb's alkaloid brahmine resembled strychnine in its stimulating action but was less toxic (Chopra *et al.* 1955). Deshpande and Lalta

Prasad (1978) observed sedation and nembutal hypnosis effect in the herb, which showed better effects than Luminal. It did not produce dizziness, nausea or vomiting and could be used for cardiac patients. When tried by Nair *et al.* (1976) on patients of tubercular meningitis, it could not prevent convulsions but reduced the severity and hastened recovery in the post-convulsive stage. To study its effect on memory, Dey *et al.* (1976) observed that this herb produced maximum improvement during maze learning by albino rats. Singh *et al.* (1979) observed an anti-anxiety effect in the alcoholic extract of the herb. The saponins showed a significant barbiturate potentiation effect. It was effective in anxiety neurosis after one month of treatment (Singh and Singh, 1980). There was significant relief in symptoms and quantitative reduction in the level of anxiety. It had an adaptogenic effect also. Khanna and Ahmed (1992) used the herb in the treatment of epilepsy and postulated that it acted through β-adrenergic receptors. Martis *et al.* (1992) experimented with the aqueous and alcoholic extracts of the herb. The extracts did not produce sedation or muscle incordination and they had no anti-depressant action. Singh and Dhawan (1994) carried out pre-clinical neuropsy-chopharmaceutical investigations on the active constituents of the herb bacoside. It was found to be nootropic and a memory enhancer. Dar and Channa (1997) observed a complete relaxant effect with the alcohol extract of the herb. Vohora *et al.* (1997) isolated a new triterpene bacosine from the herb, which was opioidergic in nature. It exhibited moderate analgesic effects. For the study of anxiolytic activity, the standard-ised extract of the herb was compared with lorazepam, a benzodiazepine anxiolytic agent. The standardised extract produced a dose related anxiolytic activity, which, in certain respects was better than lorazepam (Bhattacharya and Ghoshal, 1998).

Abhang (1993) tried a herbal preparation containing *Bacopa* on the intelligence quotient of 10–13 year old boys. The preparation caused a statistically significant increase in intelligence. A polyherbal preparation *Brahmi rasyana* containing *Bacopa*, clove, long pepper and cardamom seed showed anti-inflammatory activity (Jain *et al.* 1994) comparable to that of indomethacin. This preparation may act by interfering with prostaglandin synthesis and by stabilizing the lysosomal membrane.

Anti-cancerous activity

The ethanol extract exhibited anti-cancerous activity in Sarcoma 180 cell culture (Elangovan *et al.* 1995). Kiri and Khan (1996) tested the active constituents for genotoxic activity and no chromosomal aberration was observed.

Antioxidant effect

The alcohol extract of the herb had an antioxidant effect, which showed protection against lipid peroxidation. The memory enhancing, mild sedative effects as well as relief in epilepsy and insomnia of this herb may be due to this antioxidant activity (Tripathi *et al.* 1996).

Chemical studies

Earlier brahmine, hespestine and a mixture of three alkaloids were isolated but the therapeutic activity of the herb has been found to be due to saponins, bacosides A and B.

A preparation containing these bacosides has been commercialized as a memory enhancer.

References

Abhang, R. (1993) Study to evaluate the effect of a micro (suksma) medicine derived from brahmi (*Herpestis monierra*) on students of average intelligence. *Journal of Research in Ayurveda and Sidha*, 14, 10–21.

Bhattacharya, S.K., Ghoshal, S. (1998) Anxiolytic activity of a standardised extract of *Bacopa monniera*: an experimental study. *Phytomedicine*, 5, 77–82.

Chopra, R.N., Nayar, S.L., Chopra, I.C. *Glossary of Indian Medicinal Plants*. Council of Scientific and Industrial Research, New Delhi, India 1955.

Dar, A., Channa, S. (1997) Relaxant effect of ethanol extract of *Bacopa monniera* on trachae, pulmonary activity and aorta from rabbits and guinea pigs. *Phytotherapy Research*, 11, 323–325.

Deshpande, P.J., Lalta Prasad (1978) Role of indigenous drugs as preanaesthetic agents. *Journal of Research in Indian Medicine, Yoga and Homoeopathy*, 13, 1–8.

Dey, C.D., Bose, S., Mitra, S. (1976) Effect of some centrally active phyto products on maze learning of albino rats. *Indian Journal of Physiology and Allied Sciences*, 30, 88–97.

Elangovan, V., Govindasamy, S., Ramamoorthy, N., Balasubramanian, K. (1995) In vitro studies on the anticancer activity of *Bacopa monnieri*. *Fitoterapia*, 66, 211–215.

Jain, P., Khanna, N.K., Pendse, V.K., Godhwani, J.L. (1994) Antiinflammatory effects of an Ayurvedic preparation, *Brahmi rasayana* in rodents. *Indian Journal of Experimental Biology*, 32, 633–636.

Khanna, T. Ahmad, B. (1992) Some beta adrenergic activity of saponins derived from ethanolic extract of *Bacopa monniera*. *Proceedings of Conference on Trends in Molecular and Cellular Cardiology*, Lucknow. 4–5 May, 1992.

Kiri, A.K., Khan, K.A. (1996) Chromosome aberrations, sister chromatid exchange and micronuclei formation analysis in mice after in vivo exposure to Bacoside A and B. *Cytologia*, 6, 99–103.

Martis, G., Rao, A., Karanth, K.S. (1992) Neuropharmacological activity of *Herpestis monniera*. *Fitoterapia*, 63, 399–404.

Nair, V., Sadanand, S., Athavalo, V.B. (1976) "Brahmi" as an anticonvulsant: trials in rats and in patients with tuberculous meningitis. *Pediatric Clinics India*, 11, 246–252.

Singh, H.K., Dhawan, B.N. (1994) Pre-clinical neuro-psychopharmacological investigations on bacosides: A nootropic memory enhancer. *Update Ayurveda 94*. Bombay, India, 24–26 February, 1994.

Singh, R. H., Singh, L. (1980) Studies on the anti-anxiety effect of the Medhya rasayna drug, Brahmi (*Bacopa monniera* Wettst). Part I. *Journal of Research in Ayurveda and Siddha*, 1, 133–148.

Singh, R.H., Singh, L., Sen, S.P. (1979) Studies on the anti-anxiety effect of the Medhya rasayana drug Brahmi (Bacopa monniera Linn). Part II. Experimental studies. *Journal of Research in Indian Medicine, Yoga and Homoeopathy*, 14, 1–6.

Singh, R.H., Sinha, A.N., Pandey, H.P. (1975) A comparative study on the psychotropic action of the Medhya drugs, Brahmi (*Bacopa monniera*) and Mandukaparni (*Hydrocotyl asiatica*). *Journal of Research in Indian Medicine*, 10, 108–110.

Tripathi, Y.B., Chaurasia, S., Tripathi., E, Upadhyaya, A., Dubey, G.P. (1996) *Bacopa monniera* Linn as an anti-oxidant mechanism of action. *Indian Journal of Experimental Biology*, 34, 523–526.

Vohora, S.B., Khanna, T., Athar, M., Bahar Ahmed (1997) Analgesic activity of bacosine, a new triterpene isolated from *Bacopa monnieri*. *Fitoterapia*, 68, 361–365.

17 Chitrak

Plumbago zeylanica L.
Syn: *P. rosea* L.
P. capensis Thunb.
P. indica L.
Family: Plumbaginaceae

THE PLANT AND ITS DISTRIBUTION

It grows in arid zones in most parts of India throughout the year. It is a wild growing herb (Fig. 10) and may be up to 1 metre tall. The stem is dark brown externally and white internally. Its leaves are 3 cm or so wide and about 5 cm long, deciduous in summer but with leaves in rainy season. Flowers are white with a pink tinge, or sky blue in colour but the white flowers are common and the coloured ones are rare.

The root is blackish brown, knotted with horny fracture. It tastes pungent and bitter, causing a tingling sensation. Fresh roots have been advised but usually the dry ones are used. In south India (Shanavaskhan, 1997) the roots are detoxified before use by treating chopped root pieces repeatedly with fresh lime water. With this treatment, the root turns red first, but with repeated washing the red colour fades away. In another method, root pieces are boiled in dilute cow dung solution. (The fresh root acts as a vesicant and cause inflammation and blisters. If this happen, an antidote of 5 g of *Asparagus* root with 200 ml of drinking yogurt is given.)

USES IN FOLKLORE AND AYURVEDA

As a *Rasayana*

Plants with sky blue flowers (*Plumbago capensis*) are preferred for this purpose. The root is dried, powdered and administered for one month with milk or water. It is said to impart a long disease-free life. It delays greying of hair, increases strength, intelligence and bestows beauty.

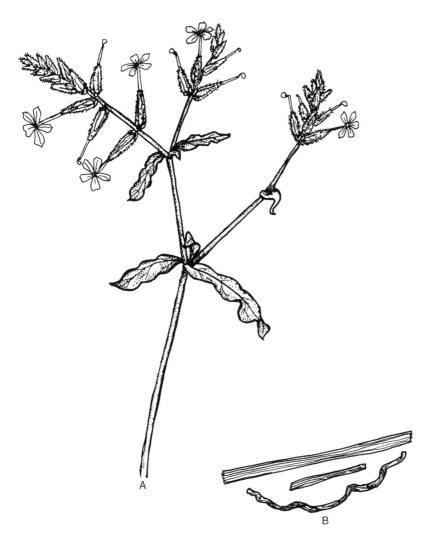

Figure 10 Plumbago zeylanica **A** twig, **B** dry root.

For indigestion

As per Ayurveda, this herb is considered pungent, hot, and said to increase the body's digestive fire (*agni*) manyfold. It stimulates the liver and spleen and is an antidote to the undesirable metabolites produced (*ama*) during digestion. Therefore it is prescribed in all diseases which arise from a disturbed digestive system, including those caused by microbes and worms. For digestive problems, a paste of the root made with water is heated in *ghee* and prescribed. A mixture of powders of equal parts of *Plumbago* root, rock salt, long pepper and *Terminalia chebula* is also used.

For liver problems

In hepatotoxicity due to chronic fever and in enlargement of liver and spleen, it is prescribed with yogurt.

For loose motions

In diarrhoea, dysentery and gastroenteritis, it is prescribed with *Embelia ribes* and *Cyperus scariosus*.

For chronic skin diseases

It is prescribed in the second stage of leprosy and syphilis.

In gynaecological practices

It causes the contraction of the uterus and may cause abortion.

Ayurvedic preparation

Shaddharna yoga

Method   Pulverize equal parts of *Plumbago zeylanica*, *Wrightia tinctria* seed, *Stephania hernandifolia*, *Picrorhiza kurrooa*, *Aconitum heterophyllum* and *Terminalia chebula*.

Dose   25 g.

Use   For flatulence.

THERAPEUTIC INDICATIONS AND PHARMACOLOGICAL STUDIES

Hypolipidaemic and antiatherosclerotic effects

The active constituent plumbagin increased the faecal excretion of cholesterol and phospholipids (Purushothaman *et al.* 1985). It prevented the accumulation of cholesterol and triglycerides in liver (Sharma *et al.* 1991).

Anti-tumour property

Chitrak showed the regression of experimental tumours (Purushothaman *et al.* 1985) due to plumbagin, which had a growth inhibitory and radiosensitizing effect on experimental mouse tumours. Uma Devi *et al.* (1994) observed that the extract of the herb significantly reduced tumour glutathione content. The results were better when lower doses of the herb were used with radiation and hyperthermia.

Hormonal effect

Plumbagin has strong antiprogestational, antifertility activity (Dhar *et al.* 1995).

Chemical studies

Mainly naphthaquinone derivatives like plumbagin have been reported.

Toxicological studies

In large doses, the herb is a narcotic. It causes dryness of mouth, nausea, diarrhoea and numbness of skin. In pregnant women it causes a burning sensation, bleeding, contraction and miscarriage. The active constituent, plumbagin, was studied for its sub-acute toxicity. It did not show any histopathological change or toxicity within the prescribed dose (Purushothaman *et al.* 1985). The oral administration of the above, 1,250 mg/kg of ethanol root extract, in rat and mice produced severe diarrhoea. In sub-acute studies when 50 mg/kg of the extract was injected daily for 30 days, no mortality was observed but there was no weight gain in the treated rats (Emerson Solomon, 1993). Another extract was toxic at 100 mg/kg (Ganasoundari *et al.* 1997).

References

Dhar, S.K., Rao, P.G. (1995) Hormonal profile of plumbagin. *Fitoterapia*, 66, 442–446.

Emerson Solomon, F., Sharda, A.C., Uma Devi, P. (1993) Toxic effects of crude root extract of *Plumbago rosea* (Rakta chitraka) on mice and rats. *Journal of Ethnopharmacology*, 38, 79–84.

Ganasoundari, A., Zare, S.M., Uma Devi, P. (1997) Modification of bone marrow radiosensitivity by medicinal plant extracts. *British Journal of Radiology*, 70, 599–602.

Purushothaman, K.K., Mohana, K., Susan, T. (1985) Biological profile of plumbagin. *Bulletin Medico Ethnobotanical Research*, 6, 177–188.

Shanavaskhan, A.E., Binu, S., Unnithan, M.D., Santhoshkumar, E.S., Pushpagandan, P. (1997) Detoxification techniques of traditional physicians of Kerala, India on some toxic herbal drugs. *Fitoterapia*, 68, 69–74.

Sharma I., Gusain D., Dixit V.P. (1991) Hypolidaemic and antiatherosclerotic effect of plumbagin in rabits. *Indian Journal of Physiology and Pharmacology*, 35, 10–14.

Uma Devi, P., Emerson Solomon, F., Sharada, A.C. (1994) In vivo tumour inhibitory and radiosensitising effects of an Indian medicinal plant, *Plumbago rosea*, on experimental mouse tumours. *Indian Journal of Experimental Biology*, 32, 523–528.

18 Chuara

Phoenix dactylifera L
Family: Palmae

THE PLANT AND ITS DISTRIBUTION

The plant mainly grows in Iraq and the other Arabian countries. It has unbranched, erect, tall, cylindrical stem, up to 20 m tall, crowned by long pinnate, fronds, from which spikes may arise. The other species, *P. sylvestris*, is found throughout drier parts of India but the fruit in this case has thinner pulp.

In India, the fresh mature fruit is known as *khajur* or *pind khajur*, while the dry form is called *chuara*. Fruits of *chuara* are up to 5 cm long, about 1 cm thick, cylindrical with slightly broad base, tapering towards the stalk end, brownish and wrinkled. The dry pulp, which is leathery and sweet, encloses the stone. The dry date palm is considered auspicious in marriage ceremonies and is given with milk on the nuptial night. It is considered essential for some religious functions. In Muslims, if the real date palm is not available, they make a sweetmeat with fat, sugar, and wheat flour in the shape of date palm and call it *chuara*, for breaking the fast of Ramdzan. Mahatama Gandhi used date palm soaked in water, for breakfast as part of his diet. The Indian date has the same but inferior effect.

In Indian commerce, three grades of dry date palm are recognized:

1. *Sakariya* (sugary) from Iraq and Muscat. It is considered the best.
2. *Chupchap* from Basra (Iraq). It is intermediate in quality.
3. *Zharakhlati*. It is of inferior grade.

USES IN FOLKLORE AND AYURVEDA

It is considered cooling in effect. (There is controversy amongst Ayurvedic scholars about the nature of the date. Some of them consider it to be hot in effect while others argue, since it is consumed by the people of hot areas (Arab deserts), if it had a hot effect it would not have been possible for Arabs to digest this fruit.)

The other uses of date palm fruits are:

As a general tonic

It is a demulcent, expectorant, nutrient, emetic, laxative, aphrodisiac, good for heart and satisfying (keeps contented). It increases vital fluids, strength and is prescribed for tuberculosis, gastroenteritis, dryness of mouth, coughs, respiratory diseases, unconsciousness, diseases due to alcoholism, asthma, chest complaints, fevers and gonorrhea. It is given wherever there is a loss of vital body energy, for general weakness, high blood pressure and fatigue. For physiological strength 10–15 pieces of dates (or as per the digestive capacity of an individual), should be chewed slowly, followed by milk. It not only makes the body strong but gives the skin a lustrous and healthy look. It prevents premature greying of hair and wrinkle formation. It probably has an anabolic and hormonal effect on the body. It increases vital energy so is given to physically weak children, adults and expectant mothers for strength, as follows.

I.   Boil 25 g date pulp in 250 ml milk, until the pulp is soft. Both the date and milk are consumed. Some people add a pinch of saffron to milk before boiling it.

II.   In the morning, when the stomach is empty, and before sleep in the evening, take two dry dates daily for the first two weeks, increase the dose to three in the third week and four pieces in the fourth week onwards. Do not eat more than four dates at one time. Follow this regime for at least three months. After this period boil dates in milk before use.

For infants

During teething trouble, date is given to infants for chewing. It hardens the gums and is also a mild laxative.

For sexual weakness

Remove the stone from date, replace with 4–5 pieces of saffron and tie the fruit with thread in such a way that saffron does not escape from inside. Boil the date in 250 ml of milk until it is reduced to half. Macerate the date in this condensed milk and discard milk-insoluble part. Drink by chewing the milk slowly. It invigorates the sexual systems of both sexes.

For asthma

Chew two dry dates in the morning every day. It gives strength to the lungs, and the body becomes immune to cold and allergies.

For colds

After two days of a cold attack, take four pieces of fresh date. Boil the minced pulp of these dates with four seeds of black pepper and one cardamom in 250 ml of milk. After brisk boiling, add one teaspoon of *ghee*. Chew and swallow the contents and drink the milk afterwards. This preparation not only cures colds, but if used for 3–4 nights, it helps headaches, heavy heads, dry coughs, lethargy, mild fever and loss of appetite.

Ayurvedic preparation

Cold drink

Date has been considered as an antifatigue and a thirst quencher. In Ayurvedic work *Sarangdhara* a recipe for a cold drink made from the infusion of equal parts of date, dry pomegranate seed (sour variety which grows wild in the western Himalayas), black grape, fruit of *Grewia asiatica*, tamarind, with salt and spices as per taste, is mentioned.

Chemical studies

The fruit contains protein (1.2 per cent), fat (0.4 per cent), carbohydrate (33.8 per cent), fibre (3.7 per cent), and the minerals calcium (1.7 per cent) and phosphorus (1.7 per cent).

19 Draksha

Vitis vinifera L.
Family: Vitaceae

THE PLANT AND ITS DISTRIBUTION

It is a climber with broad leaves, now cultivated in most of the temperate parts of the world. There are many varieties of grapes, but in Ayurveda dry, big, black grapes with seed are mainly used.

USES IN FOLKLORE AND AYURVEDA

Black grape is considered a nutritive, energizer, anti-inflammatory, diuretic, laxative and bronchiodilater. It is an important ingredient of most fermented Ayurvedic preparations (*asav* and *arishta*).

Medicated wine from grapes

Method Take 1kg black grapes (dry), 1kg sugar, 1kg honey, 125 g *Woodfordia fruticosa* and 10 g each of *Cinnamomum* spp. leaves, cardamom seed, *Mesua ferrea*, clove, nutmeg, black pepper, long pepper, *Plumbago zeylanica*, *Piper cubeba*, *Piper longum* root, *Piper chaba* and *Vitex negundo*. Wash grapes and boil them in 5 litres of water until the water is reduced to one-fourth, macerate the whole mass and filter through a coarse cloth to obtain the juice. Dissolve sugar and honey in this juice. Make a coarse powder of all the herbs and spices given above, mix them in this fluid and store them in a suitable container for fermentation for 45 days. The earlier method of fermentation was to use earthen pitchers, covering the mouth of pitcher with an earthen lid, sealed with coarse cloth followed by a layer of clay, but now for large-scale manufacturing wooden vats are used.

Dose Two rice/teaspoons with half a cup of water twice daily.

Use It is a nutrient for digestive problems, indigestion, fatigue and flatulence.

Drakshavleh

Method   Take 1kg dry black grapes, 200 g *ghee*, 2 kg sugar and 15 g each of nutmeg, mace, cardamom, bamboo manna (silicic acid), *Mesua ferrea* and 3 g saffron. Macerate the grapes after soaking them in water for one hour, heat them with *ghee* on a slow fire. Make a sugar syrup and add it to these heated grapes, followed by fine powder of all the herbs. Add water and allow the whole mixture to ferment for 45 days.

Dose   10–20 ml with milk twice daily.

Use   As a nutrient, in hyperacidity, constipation and cirrhosis of liver.

Draksharishta

The formulation of *Draksharishta* varies slightly as compared to *Drakshasavleh* and both of these can be substituted for each other.

Method: 1 kg dry black grapes, 4 kg raw sugar, 150 g *Woodfordia* flowers, and 20 g each of *Embelia ribes*, long pepper, cinnamon, cardamom seed, *Cinnamomum* spp. leaves, ginger, *Mesua ferrea* and black pepper. Follow the process of *Drakshasavleh*.

Use: As a laxative, for mental, physical fatigue and insomnia. It provides immediate energy to the body. It is of use to women for excessive bleeding during menstruation, leucorrhoea, etc.

THERAPEUTIC INDICATIONS AND PHARMACOLOGICAL STUDIES

Procyanidins from seed have an antimutagenic effect which counteracts spontaneous mutation of *Sacharomyces cerevisiac* both at mitochondrial and nuclear level (Liviero *et al.* 1994). Due to the antioxidant properties of procyanidins, it has potential use for the chemoprevention of several pathological situations.

On the combined basis of a large number of epidemological and clinical studies it was concluded that wine phenolics can reduce heart diseases and mortality (Waterhouse, 1995). This nutritional and pharmacological significance may be due to flavonoids (epicatechin, malvidin 3 glucosides, quercetin and procyanidins).

References

Liviero, L., Puglisi, P.P., Morazzoni, P., Bombardelli, E. (1994) Antimutagenic activity of procyanidins from *Vitis vinifera. Fitoterapia*, 65, 203–209.

Waterhouse, A.L. (1995) Wine and heart disease. *Chemistry and Industry*, No 9, 338–341.

20 Gaduchi

Tinospora cordifolia (Willd.) Miers ex Hook.f. and Thomas
T. malabarica (Lam.) Miers
Family: Menispermaceae

THE PLANT AND ITS DISTRIBUTION

It is often substituted by other wild or cultivated species of *Tinospora*. It is a household remedy, known as *giloe*, in most parts of India. *Giloe* climbing on *Azadirachta indica* tree, known as *neem*, is considered superior and is called *neem giloe*. It is said that, through its contact with the *neem* tree, it is able to absorb the therapeutic active constituents from it.

The plant (Fig. 11A) is a liana or a climber with a 1–3 cm thick stem and rough, corky bark. Leaves are glabrous, cordate, 5–10 cm wide, acute or acuminate. Male and female plants are separate. The flowers are small, yellow green in colour. The male flowers are in fascicles, while females are solitary. The fruit is red when ripe.

The green stem or small dry pieces (Fig. 11B), about 2–5 cm long, are used as medicine but the fresh stem is preferred. The dry pieces have an outer papery skin, brownish wrinkled surface and numerous pores along the sides. It has a bitter, mucilaginous taste.

USES IN FOLKLORE AND AYURVEDA

In Ayurveda it is called *Amrita* (nectar). The herb is considered bitter, hot in effect, nutritive and a *rasayana*. The major uses of this herb are:

As a *Rasayana*

a The juice is given with honey or raw sugar.
b Boil 10 g of paste of *gaduchi* with 10 g *Hemidesmus indicus* in 100 ml of water, in a covered pan for two hours on a low heat. Macerate the herbs in hot water and filter. The dose is 5–10 ml, three times a day. This decoction is a good diuretic and *Rasayana*. It is administered for leprosy, in the second stage of syphilis and to convalescent patients after chronic diseases to combat the disease.

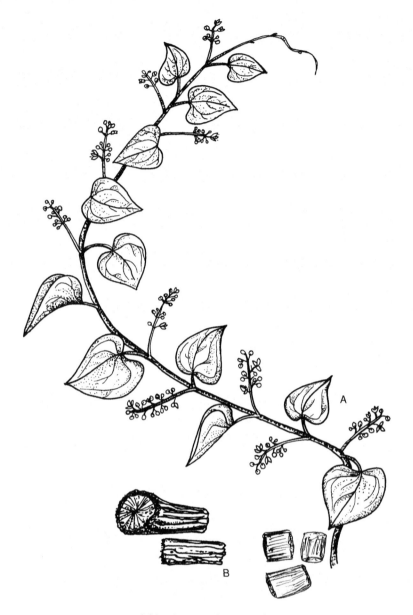

Figure 11 Tinospora cordifolia **A** twig, **B** stem pieces.

For urinogenital diseases

In sexually transmitted diseases, and in diabetes, etc., the herb's juice or powder is prescribed.

For malfunctioning of liver

The decoction of the herb with long pepper and honey is prescribed for lack of appetite due to malfunctioning of liver, and in high fevers. In cirrhosis, jaundice, indigestion, vomiting, mild stomach-ache, about 10 ml juice of the herb is given with honey.

For skin diseases

In both chronic and obstinate types, it is given along with *Commiphora, Azadirachta, Emblica*, turmeric and *Acacia nilotica*.

For menstruation problems

In South India, stem pieces are boiled in 2 cups of water and drunk during irregular and excessive menstruation.

T. crispa

In Indonesia, it is used for malaria, small pox, as a vermifuge, an appetizer, for cholera and for diabetes mellitus (Cavin *et al.* 1998).

Ayurvedic preparations

Amritadi kwath

Method   Make a coarse powder of equal quantities of *Cyperus rotundus, Tinospora, Adhatoda vasica, Acacia catechu* bark, *Azadirachta* leaves, turmeric, and *Berberis* bark.

Dose   Boil 20 g of the above powder in 200 ml of water until reduced to 50 ml. Filter and drink 50 ml or so of this decoction, as per capacity on an empty stomach in the morning.

Uses   For all digestive and liver problems as a blood purifier, an antidote to poisons in chicken pox, small pox, for small ulcers in the mouth, fevers, skin diseases and against all intestinal worms.

Amritarisht

Method   Boil the coarse powder of 1 kg *Tinospora* and 1 kg *Dashmul* (see a*malaki*) until reduced to one-fourth, macerate the herb and filter. When cool, add 3 kg raw sugar to the decoction in a pot, along with 160 g cumin, 20 g *Fumaria indica* herb, fine powders of 10 g each of *Alstonia scholaris* bark, ginger, black pepper, long pepper, *Cyperus rotundus, Mesua ferrea, Picrorhiza kurroa, Aconitum heterophyllum* and *Holarrhena antidysterica* seed. Seal the mouth of the pot with clay to make it air tight and let it ferment for 30 days. Filter the fermented liquor and pour into bottles.

Dose   2 dessertspoonfuls for adults and 2 teaspoonfuls for children, in 200 ml of water (one cup) after the meal, twice daily for a month.

Use   It is said to be cooling in effect. It helps indigestion, acidity, stomach problems, chronic fevers, fever after childbirth, colds, skin diseases, infectious hepatitis, polyurea due to diabetes and arthritic pains. It is useful for convalescing patients who are weak due to fevers. It protects the liver from jaundice and other diseases.

Pit shamak Rasayana churn

Method   Pulverize equal quantities of powders of *Tinospora, Pedalium murex, Emblica officinalis* and sugar.

Dose   One teaspoonful with *ghee* on an empty stomach in the morning and two hours after meals before retiring.

Use   It helps flatulence, hyperacidity, urinogenital diseases, polyurea, diabetes and sexual inadequacies. It is particularly useful as an antidote to toxins present in the body after the cure of sexually transmitted diseases.

Gaduchi satva

Method   It is a starch obtained from the plant by chopping and crushing twigs about 2 cm thick and immersing them in water. The crushed pieces are macerated by hand to separate the starch from the fibres. The starch settles down after some time. The water is decanted and the starch dried.

   This starch is said to be highly nutritive and is given to patients of chronic diarrhoea and dysentery, in seminal weakness and as a rejuvenator in general debility. Two grams of this starch with milk is given for burning urethras, following the passing of urine, and for urinary obstruction (enlarged prostate).

THERAPEUTIC INDICATIONS AND PHARMACOLOGICAL STUDIES

Anti-microbial property

The alkaloid berberine has anti-bacterial, anti-fungal, anti-viral and anti-protozoal properties.

Anti-ulcerogenic effect

Three indigenous preparations containing *gaduchi* had anti-ulcerogenic effect (Biswas *et al.* 1993). Sarma *et al.* (1995b) confirmed this activity.

As an anti-inflammatory agent

Shah and Pandya (1976) observed anti-inflammatory effects in the aqueous extract. Mhaiskar *et al.* (1976), after clinical evaluation, noted that about half the patients of arthritis and body pain received relief from this herb. Pendse *et al.* (1977) found anti-inflammatory and immunosuppressive effects in the water extract of *neem giloe*. Oral or intraperitoneal administration of water extract of the herb significantly inhibited acute inflammatory response. It also had an analgesic effect. It potentiated morphine but had no antipyretic effect. When Kishore *et al.* (1980) tried ginger with *gaduchi* in rheumatism and arthritis, the results were comparable with the other Ayurvedic preparations. Gulati *et al.* (1980) used this herb in rheumatoid arthritis. Gulati and Pandey (1982) confirmed its anti-inflammatory activity. Ansari and Gaur (1983) observed that *gaduchi* directly affects the metabolic activity of body and regulates heart beat. It helps in chronic and acute inflammation and rheumatism. When 22 sufferers of rheumatoid arthritis were treated with water extract of the herb, there was a significant improvement.

Amrutadiguggulu containing *Tinospora* with *Commiphora* gave good results in rheumatic patients (Deshmukh and Ranade 1995).

As a hepatoprotective agent

The herb prevented fibrous changes and regeneration of parenchymal tissue in albino rats (Rege *et al.* 1984). It caused modulation of immunosuppression in obstructive jaundice. The water extract 100 mg/kg for seven days improved cellular immune functions and the mortality rate of the rats was significantly reduced to 16.67 per cent (Rege *et al.* 1989). Peer *et al.* (1990) found this herb was quite effective in proper liver function in goats. *T. cordifolia* decoction showed improvement and regeneration of hepatic cells. Reddy *et al.* (1993) confirmed this activity.

Anticancerous activity

The effect of *T. cordifolia* on the functions of macrophages obtained from mice treated with the carcinogen ochratoxin A was investigated by Dhuley (1997). It decreased the chemotactic activity of murine macrophages and the production of interlukin and tumour necrosis factor.

Hypoglycaemic effect

Wadood *et al.* (1992) observed this activity in leaf extract. Prasad *et al.* (1992) studied hypoglycaemic and anti-hyperglycaemic effects of the extract. It showed synergistic effect with insulin, tolbutamide and propranol. A significant fall in glycaemic levels in rats with glucose-induced hyper-glycaemia occurred. It showed anti-hyperglycaemic effect in moderate alloxan diabetic rats but it was not effective in severe cases.

Noor and Ashroft (1989) and Cavin *et al.* (1998) noted that *T. crispa* aqueous extract exhibited hypoglycaemic activity in moderately diabetic rats. After two weeks of the treatment there was an improvement in glucose tolerance and an increase in plasma insulin levels, which showed improvement in diabetic conditions by virtue of its action on endocrine pancreas.

A polyherbal patent preparation containing *gaduchi* was also found effective in pancreatic islet superoxide dismutase activity in hyperglycaemic rats (*Bhattacharya et al.* 1997).

Immunomodulater activity

Dhanukar *et al.* (1988) studied the effect of this herb on the immunotherapeutic modification of abdominal sepsis induced by caecal ligation. The protective effect of pre-treatment with *T. cordifolia* against mixed abdominal infection was also studied. This pre-treatment reduced the mortality rate, which was comparable to metrinidazole and gentamycin. It also caused localization of infection. There was an increase in the peripheral neutrophil count and peritoneal macrophages, which was associated with increased phagocytic activity of macrophages. Pendse *et al.* (1977) and Rege *et al.* (1989) recorded immunosuppression activity. Deshmukh and Usha (1994) noted the potent immunostimulant activity in it. *Tinospora* stimulated percentage phagocytosis in neutrophils in a dose dependent fashion. Usha *et al.* (1994) postulated that immunomodulating potential produced leucocytosis in treated animals and protected them against experimental models of infection. The herb produced a dose dependent increase in bone marrow proliferation. Pokharankar and Nagarkatti (1994) observed modulation of alveolar macrophage function in tuberculosis. Koti *et al.* (1994) studied it in immunotherapy of multiple organ dysfunction in obstructive jaundice to bolster the defence and to decrease the incidence of septicaemia. It resulted in increased survival of patients. In experimental rats *T. cordifolia* 100 mg/kg/day for 5 weeks decreased renal damage, improved the fibrinogen level and reduced lead acetate-induced endo-toxaemia. It decreased renal ischaemia-induced mortality. The herb increased the number and function of neutrophils and monocyte macrophages. Dhawale (1994) studied the immunostimulant effect of the herb on T-lymphocytes by carrying out a thymocyte count. It was observed that pre- and post-treatment with *Tinospora* attenuated the lymphopenic effect of steroids and hastened the regeneration of thymocytes. Maurya *et al.* (1996) confirmed immunostimulant action of the herb.

As an anti-stress agent

The herb helped in stress-induced gastric damage (Tillu *et al.* 1994). Sipahimalani *et al.* (1994) isolated the adaptogen compounds to combat stress. Sarma *et al.* (1995a, 1996) studied the effect of 100 mg/kg of ethanol extract of *Tinospora* orally for 16 days on brain neurotransmitters in stressed rats.

A polyherbal preparation from *Rauvolfia serpentina*, *Nardostachys jatamansi* and *Tinospora cordifolia* was evaluated by Rani and Naidu (1998), for clinical efficacy and safety on the patients of insomnia by subjective and polysomnographic methods. The results were encouraging.

As an anti-allergic agent

The aqueous extract of the herb had this effect. It significantly decreased bronchiospasms, capillary permeability and reduced the number of disrupted mast cells in a number of animals (Nayampalli *et al.* 1988).

Antioxidant effects

Three compounds isolated from *T. crispa* exhibited antioxidant and radical scavenging properties (Cavin *et al.* 1998).

Anti-endotoxic property

Jayle *et al.* (1994) carried out these studies.

Diuretic effect

Oke *et al.* (1977) observed that it produced marked diuretic effect in rats and dogs and altered sodium, potassium and chlorine levels in urine.

Reviews

Sharma and Khosa (1993) reviewed chemistry and pharmacology and Pathak *et al.* (1995) reviewed a chemistry and biological activity. Siddiqui and Zafar (1995) reviewed phytochemical, pharmacological analysis and the formulations containing *Tinospora*.

Chemical studies

The plant contains quarternary alkaloids, such as protoberberine bases, palmatine, berberine, jattorrhizine and choline, phenylpropene, etc. (Bisset and Nwaiwu, 1983).

References

Ansari, M.S., Gaur, S.K. (1983) On the medicinal utility of Giloy. *Nagarjun*, 26, 12.

Bhattacharya, S.K., Satyan, K.S., Chakraborti, A. (1997) Effect of Trasina, an ayurvedic herbal formulation, on pancreatic islet superoxide dismutase activity in hyperglycaemic rats. *Indian Journal of Experimental Biology*, 35, 297–299.

Bisset, N.G., Nwaiwu, J. (1983) Quarternary alkaloids of *Tinospora* spp. *Planta Medica*, 48, 275.

Biswas, T.K., Chattopadhyaya, R.N., Dutta, S., Marjit, B., Maity, L.N. (1993) A preliminary study on antiulcerogenic effect of three indigenous drugs. *Indian Journal of Physiology and Allied Sciences*, 47, 170–175.

Cavin, A., Hostettmann, K., Dyatmyko, W., Potterat, O. (1998) Antioxidant and lipophilic constituents of *Tinospora crispa*. *Planta Medica*, 64, 393–396.

Deshmukh, A., Usha, D. In vitro effect of *Tinospora cordifolia* on PMN function. *Update Ayurveda 94*, Bombay, 24–26 February, 1994.

Deshmukh, R., Ranade, S.B. (1995) Sandhishoola-sandhishotha and Amrutadi guggulu, in Kulkarni, P.H., ed., *Advanced Research Papers*.

Dhamnskar, R.K., Tanksale, K.G., Ainapurne, S.S. Hypoglycaemic effect of *Tinospora cordifolia* with special reference to enzymes in glycolytic pathway. *Proceedings of 46th Annual Indian Pharmaceutical Congress*, Chandigarh, India. 28–30 December, 1994.

Dhanukar, S.A., Thatte, U.M., Pai, N., Move, B.B., Karandikar, S.M. (1988) Immunotherapeutic modification by *Tinospora cordifolia* of abdominal sepsis induced by caecal ligation in rats. *Indian Journal of Gastroentrology*, 7, 21–23.

Dhawale, D.P. Effect of *Tinospora cordifolia* on thymocyte counts in normal and lymphopenic mice. *Update Ayurveda-94*, Bombay India. 24–26 February, 1994.

Dhuley, J.N. (1997) Effect of some Indian herbs on macrophage functions in ochratoxin A treated mice. *Journal of Ethnopharmacology*, 58, 15–20.

Gulati, O.D., Pandey, D.C. (1982) Antiinflammatory activity of *Tinospora cordifolia*. *Rheumatism*, 17, 76–83.

Gulati, O.D., Shah, C.P., Kanani, R.C., Vaidya D.C., Shah, D.S. (1980) Clinical trial of *Tinospora cordifolia* in rheumatoid arthritis. *Rheumatism*, 15, 143–148.

Javle, H.S., Koti, R.S., Bapat, R.D. Antiendotoxic effect of *Tinospora cordifolia*. *Update Ayurveda-94*, Bombay, India. 24–26 February, 1994.

Kishore, P., Pandey, P.N., Ruhil (1980) Role of Sunthi-Gaduci in the treatment of amvata-rheumatoid arthritis. *Journal of Research in Ayurveda and Siddha*, 1, 417–420.

Koti, R.S., Rege, N.N., Javle, H.S., Desai, N.K., Bapat, R.D., Dahnukar, S.A *Tinospora cordifolia*: A boon in therapy of multiorgan dysfunction in obstructive jaundice. *Update Ayurveda* 94, Bombay, India, 24–26 February, 1994.

Mhaiskar, V.B., Pandey, D.C., Karmakar, K.B. (1976) Clinical evaluation of *Tinospora cordifolia* in amvata and sandhigatvata. *Rheumatism*, 11, 77–81.

Maurya, R., Wazir, V., Kapil, A., Kapil, S. (1996) Cordifoliosides A and B, two new phenylpropene disaccharides from *Tinospora cordifolia* possessing immunostimulant activity. *Natural Product Letters*, 8, 7–10.

Nayampalli, S.S., Desai, N.K., Ainapure, S.S. (1988) Antiallergic properties of *Tinospora cordifolia* in animal models. *Indian Journal of Pharmacology*, 18, 250–252.

Noor, N., Ashroft, S.J.H. (1989) Antidiabetic effects of *Tinospora crispa* in rats. *Journal of Ethnopharmacology*, 27, 149–161.

Oke, V.G., Ainapure, S.S., Molgiri, S.R., Shah, N.D., Dhar, H. L. Diuretic action of *Tinospora cordifolia* (Abstract). *9th Annual Conference of Indian Pharmacological Society*, Varanasi, Dec. 29–31, 1976. *Indian Journal of Pharmacology*, 9, 77. Abstr.92.

Pathak, A.K., Jain, D.C., Sharma, R.P. (1995) Chemistry and biological activities of the genera *Tinospora*. *International Journal of Pharmacognosy*, 33, 277–287.

Peer, F., Sharma, M.C., Prasad, M.C. (1990) Efficacy of Liv.52 and *Tinospora cordfolia* in experimental C Cl4 hepatopathy in goats. *Indian Journal of Animal Sciences*, 60, 526–531.

Pendse, V.K., Dadhich, A.P., Mathur, P.N., Bal, B.M.S., Madan, B.R. (1977) Antiinflammatory, immunosuppresive and some related pharmacological actions of the water extract of neem giloe (*Tinospora cordifolia*) a preliminary report. *Indian Journal of Pharmacology*, 9, 221–224.

Pokharankar, S.L., Nagarkatti, D.S. Modulation of alveolar macrophage function by antituberculous agents and *Tinospora cordifolia*. *Update Ayurveda-94*, Bombay, India, 24–26 Feb. 1994.

Prasad, H.C., Majumdar, R., Chakraborty, R. Hypoglycaemic and antihyperglycaemic effect of medicinal plants from Assam. *International Seminar-Traditional Medicine*, Calcutta, 7–9 November 1992.

Rani, P.U., Naidu, M.U.R. (1998) Subjective and polysomnographic evaluation of a herbal preparation in insomnia. *Phytomedicine*, 5, 253–257.

Reddy, B.P., Murthy, V.N., Venkateshwarlu, V., Kokate, C.K., Rambhau, D. (1993) Antiheptotoxic activity of *Phyllanthus niruri, Tinospora cordifolia* and *Ricinus communis*. *Indian Drugs*, 30, 338–341.

Rege, N., Dhanukar, S., Karndikar, S.M. (1984) Hepatoprotective effects of *Tinospora cordifolia* against carbon tetrachloride-induced liver damage. *Indian Drugs*, 21, 544–555.

Rege, N., Nazareth, H.M., Bapat, R.D., Dhanukar, S.A. (1989) Modulation of immunosuppression in obstructive jaundice by *Tinospora cordifolia*. *Indian Journal of Medical Research*, 90, 478–483.

Sarma, D.N.K., Khosa, R.L., Chansuria, J.P.N., Ray, A.K. (1995a) Effect of *Tinospora cordifolia* on brain neurotransmitters in stressed rats. *Fitoterapia*, 66, 421–422.

Sarma, D.N.K., Khosa, R.L., Chansuria, J.P.N., Sahai, M. (1995b) Anti-ulcer activity of *Tinopsora cordifolia* Miers and Centella asiatica Linn. extracts. *Phytotherapy Research*, 9, 589–590.

Sarma, D.N.K., Khosa, R.L., Chansuria, J.P.N., Sahai, M. (1996) Antistress activity of *Tinospora cordifolia* and *Centella asiatica* extracts. *Phytotherapy Research*, 10, 181–183.

Shah, D.S., Pandya, D.C. (1976) A preliminary study about the anti-inflammatory activity of *Tinospora cordifolia*. *Journal of Research in Indian Medicine, Yoga and Homoeopathy*, 11, 77–83.

Sharma, D.N.K., Khosa, R.L. (1993) Chemistry and pharmacology of *Tinospora cordifolia* Miers. *Indian Drugs*, 30, 549–554.

Siddiqui, A.A., Zafar, R. (1995) *Tinospora cordifolia* Miers. A review. *Hamdard Medicus*, 38, 85–90.

Sipahimalani, A., Norr, H., Wagner, H. (1994) Phenylpropanoid glycosides and tetrahydrofurofuran lignan glycosides from the adaptogenic plant drugs, *Tinospora cordifolia* and *Drypetes roxburghii*. *Planta Medica*, 60, 596–597.

Tillu, C.V. Comparative effects of plant products on stress-induced damage. *Update Ayurveda-94*, Bombay, India, 24–26 February, 1994.

Usha, D., Thatte, U.M., Joshi, D.S. Flow cytometry evaluation of bone marrow proliferation induced by *Tinospora cordifolia*. *Update Ayurveda-94*, Bombay, India, 24–26 February, 1994.

Wadood, N., Wadood, A., Shah, S.A.W. (1992) Effect of *Tinopsora cordifolia* on blood glucose and total lipid levels of normal and alloxan-diabetic rabbits. *Planta Medica*, 58, 131–136.

21 Gokshru

Tribulus terrestris L.
Family: Zygophyllaceae

The herb is known as *gokshru* (*go* is cow and *kshru* hoof) in Sanskrit because of the shape of each of the fruit's cocci, which resemble the hoof of a cow. The corrupted form of this name in Indian languages is *gokhru*. In the western countries it is commonly known as *Puncture Vine* or *Caltrop fruit*.

THE PLANT AND ITS DISTRIBUTION

It is a prostate spiny, hairy herb (Fig. 12A) with yellow flowers. Leaves are 2–4 cm long, paripinnate, with 6–10 oblong leaflets. The fruit is hemi-spherical, breaking into five cocci, with two types of spine: bigger and smaller. Sometimes the smaller spines are quite inconspicuous. Each cocci has five seeds (Fig. 12B). The seed is quite hard and woody but can be powdered easily. The powder is starchy and has a pleasant smell.

Tribulus terrestris is often called small *gokhru* and *Pedalium murex* (Fig. 12C) is known as big *gokhru* because its seeds are bigger (Fig. 12D). Whereas *T. terrestris* grows on dry and arid land, *P. murex* is found growing in dry and hot coastal areas.

USES IN FOLKLORE AND AYURVEDA

The fruit is mainly used as a single entity in various recipes, whereas the root is an ingredient of a preparation called *Dashmul* (see *amalaki*). In Ayurveda, the fruit is considered to be cooling in effect, having diuretic, tonic and aphrodisiac properties. It is mainly used in the form of an infusion for painful micturition, calculus affections, urethral discharges, impotence, gout, kidney diseases and kidney stones. Plant and dry spiny fruits are also used for spermatorrhea, phosphaturia, urinary incontinence, Bright's disease, nephritis and inflammation of the kidney. It has a diuretic effect similar to buchu and uva-ursi. It is mainly used for diseases of the urinogenital system as follows:

1   In impotence, the plant is boiled until mucilaginous and mixed with *Hyoscyamus* and opium.

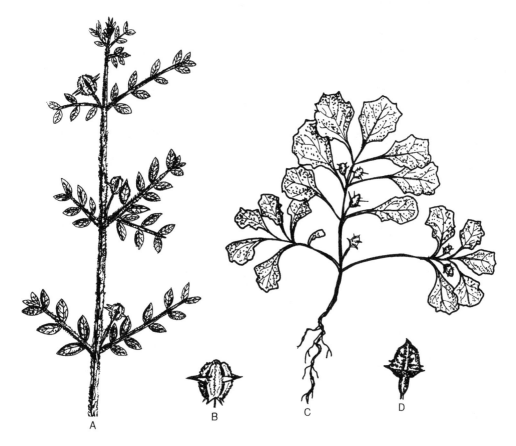

Figure 12 Tribulus terrestris: **A** twig, **B** fruit, *Pedalium murex*: **C** twig, **D** fruit.

2   Equal parts of *Tribulus* seed, sesame seed and goat milk cures impotence.
3   Take 2.5 kg of *T. terrestris* herb and boil it in 64 litres of water until reduced to one-fourth, strain, add 6 kg of sugar to it and boil again until a thick syrup is formed. To this syrup add the fine powder of ginger, long pepper, black pepper, cardamom, *Mesua ferrea*, *Cinnamomum* spp. leaves, nutmeg, *Terminalia arjuna*, and bamboo manna.

Dose   25 g twice daily.

Use   Stimulant tonic, for sexual debility and impotence.

4   Pulverize equal quantities of clove, cardamom and *Tribulus*.

Dose   10 g twice daily with milk and *ghee*.

Use   An elixir preparation for strength and long life.

5   Make an infusion of the whole plant by taking one part of the herb in 8 parts of water.

Dose   100 ml thrice daily.

Use   It relieves burning of the urethra whilst passing urine, cures nocturnal emission and impotence.

6   Take 40 g each of *Chlorophytum arundinaceum* root, *Tribulus* fruit, henna leaves, gum tragacanth, *Butea frondosa* gum, *Cydonia vulgaris* seed, soapstone and 60 g sugar candy. Make a fine powder of all these items and divide it into 40 doses.

Dose   Take two *Strychnos potatorum* seeds and grind them on stone with water until a fine paste is formed. Shake this paste in a glass of water and take it with one dose of powder prepared above, twice daily.

Use   It not only clears leucorrhoea but helps physiological weakness, body aches, etc. For better results use 10 g fried gum acacia along with milk sweetened with sugar.

7   The whole herb of *Tribulus* is collected at the pre-fruiting stage, dried in the shade, powdered and macerated for one day in fresh juice of *Tribulus*, dried again and powdered.

Dose   12 g with milk. Take rice as a staple diet.

Use   It makes the body strong, good looking, sexually active and imparts longevity.

In Chinese Medicine

It is considered a diuretic, aphrodisiac and a cardiotonic. It is included amongst the herbs used for curing liver wind and stopping tremors. It is used for eye, liver and cardiac diseases (Jian Xin Li, 1998), as an immunobuilder for restoration of normal body functions and for promoting blood circulation to remove blood stasis (Fang, 1999).

Ayurvedic preparations

Gokshuradi churn I

Ingredients   Pulverize 110 g *T. terrestris* and 40 g each of *Piper cubeba, Mesua ferrea, Rheum palmatum* and potassium nitrate.

Dose   10–20 g.

Use   For various urinary diseases.

Gokshuradi churn II

Ingredients   Pulverize 60 g each of *T. terrestris, Astercantha longifolia, Asparagus racemosus, Mucuna pruriens, Sida cordifolia*, and *Abutilon indicum*.

Dose   2–3 g with warm, sweet milk, one hour before retiring.

Use   As a nutritive tonic for increasing libido, and for curing premature ejaculation.

Gokshuradi churn III

Ingredients   Pulverize equal quantities of *Sida rhombifolia, S. spinosa, Mucuna pruriens* dry boiled seed, *Asparagus racemosus, Astercantha longifolia* and *Tribulus terrestris*.

Dose   One teaspoon two to three times a day with milk.

Use   It increases mental, physical and sexual power, particularly in the cases of premature ejaculation and spermatorrhoea, if used for 3–4 months. It is a good aphrodisiac if used one hour before intercourse.

Contraindication   Avoid acidic (sour) food substances.

Dhatu paushtik churn

Ingredients   3 g each of finely powdered *T. terrestris* and gum tragacanth.

Dose   Heat the above powder in two teaspoonfuls of clarified butter (*ghee*), use it along with warm milk first thing in the morning and have a meal after three hours. Similarly in the evening take this powder two hours after dinner as the last item consumed, so nothing should be eaten afterwards. Continue this treatment for minimum of two months.

Use   For proper function of the sexual system.

Contraindications   Avoid fried, spicy and sour food.

Narsimha churn

Ingredients   Equal parts of powdered *Emblica officinalis, Terminalia chebula, T. bellirica*, ginger, long pepper, black pepper, sesame seed and *Semecarpus anacardium*.

Dose   1–4 g powder with milk and *ghee*.

Indications   For sexual inadequacy.

THERAPEUTIC INDICATIONS AND PHARMACOLOGICAL STUDIES

As an anabolic agent

Some of the studies have indicated that *Tribulus* caused a 50 per cent increase in testosterone levels and improved reproductive function. The active constituents of the fruit had a stimulating effect on immune, sexual and reproductive systems, with improved muscle building, stamina and endurance. It also caused a reduction in cholesterol. It altered moods and imparted a feeling of well-being. *Tribulus* as a liver tonic breaks down the cholesterol and fats that inhibit healthy liver function. The cholesterol and fats are converted to hormones and energy, resulting in increased performance and stamina, which is very beneficial to body builders. It also causes a positive nitrogen balance and early recovery from muscular stress.

Diuretic activity

Earlier, diuretic activity of the herb was considered to be due to the nitrates present in it, but it may also be due to alkaloids (Santha and Iyer (1967). Deepak Prakash *et al.* (1985) and Singh *et al.* (1991) confirmed the diuretic activity of the herb. *Tribulus* alkaloid (harmine) increased blood pressure and renal perfusion.

Varunadi kwath, a decoction made from *Crataeva religiosa, Tribulus*, ginger, *Bergenia ligulata, Woodfordia fruticosa* and raw sugar, was given to patients with urinary complaints. Excellent results were obtained in 64 per cent cases (Suru and Kulkarni, 1991).

Nephroprotective potential

Simultaneous administration of 200 mg/kg/day of *Tribulus* extract and gentamycin to female rats decreased gentamycin-induced renal damage in both structural and functional terms. The effect was comparable to verpamil (Nagarkatti *et al.* 1994).

Antiurolithic effect

Various extracts of the herb showed significant dose-dependent protection against urolith, induced by glass bead implantation in albino rats. It also protected leucocytosis and elevation in serum urea levels. The anti-urolithic activity appeared to be due to the combined effects of several constituents present in the extracts (Anand *et al.* 1994). The therapeutic response of aqueous extract on hyperoxaluria in male adult rats was studied by Sangeeta *et al.* (1993). After 24 hours urinary oxalate excretion reversed to normal. These authors (Sangeeta *et al.* 1994) studied oxalate metabolism further and postulated that normalization of kidney LDH (lactate dehydrogenase) feeding was mainly due to increases in the LDH5 fraction as the LDH1 remained unchanged in the groups. It decreased the activities of glycolate oxidase and glycolate dehydrogenase in liver, but the activity of hepatic lactate dehydrogenase was unaltered. The ethanol extract was tested for experimentally induced urolithiasis in albino rats. It exhibited dose-dependent anti-urolithiatic activity and almost completely inhibited stone formation. Other biochemical parameters in urine and blood serum and the histopathology of the urinary bladder, which were altered during the process of stone formation, were also normalized by the plant extract (Anand *et al.* 1994).

As a sexual stimulant

A new preparation *Tribestan* had a stimulative effect on the sexual system. The active components are steroidal saponins of furostanoic type (Tomova, 1987). Oral administration of saponin terrestrioside F in male rats increased libido and sexual response. In females the compound potentiated oestrus and increased fertility (Anon., 1992).

Effect on cardiovascular system

The aqueous extract had a potent stimulant effect on heart muscles in a hypodynamic state (Seth and Jagadeesh, 1976). The aqueous extract, the ethanol water extract 30 per cent, and ethanol extract of the fruit produced hypotensive effect in anaesthetized animals (Anon., 1977). The total steroidal sapogenins have shown antisclerotic properties (Schreter, 1980). The alkaloid produced a slight rise in blood pressure and an increase in kidney secretions. When coronary heart disease patients were treated with saponins, the total efficacious rate of remission in angina pectoris was 82.3 per cent. The saponins dilated coronary arteries, improved coronary circulation and had the effect of improving ECG of myocardial ischaemia. It had no adverse effect on renal, blood or hepatic systems and thus is a drug of choice to treat angina pectoris (Bowen *et al.* 1990).

Effect on central nervous system

The activity of alkaloid is α-adrenergic, β-adrenergic and papaverine-like (Noogi *et al.* 1977). When 20 mg/kg of the drug was administered to rats, there was a sign of CNS excitation, characterised by increase in spontaneous motility, excitability and restlessness (Deepak Prakash *et al.* 1985).

As a hepatoprotective agent

Tribulus provided hepatoprotection to primary cultured hepatocytes (Lee *et al.* 1992). The compounds isolated from the herb significantly prevented cell death induced by α-galactosamine, tumour necrosis factor (Jian Xin Li, 1998).

Antibacterial activity

The extract of the herb inhibited the growth of *Staphylococcus aureus* and *Escherichia coli* (Anon., 1977).

Chemical studies

Quite a number of steroidal sapogenins have been reported. The important ones are diosgenin, hicogenin, ruscogenin, yamogenin, epismilagenin, tigogenin, neotigogenin, gitogenin and neogitogenin (Mahato *et al.* 1978, Miles *et al.* 1994). Five new steroidal saponins (terrestrosins A-E) were isolated by Wang Yan *et al.* (1996).

Toxicological studies

Due to grazing on the herb *Tribulus*, a disease called geeldikkop, which causes photo-sensitivity, has been reported in sheep (Miles *et al.* 1994). No such toxicity has been reported from the various experiments carried out in India.

Substitutes

Pedalium murex L.

It is known as big *gokhru* in commerce and is used in place of *T. terrestris*.

An infusion of the fresh herb, 1 part in 20 parts of water, dose 500 ml, is given daily in cases of spermatorrhoea and nocturnal emission. A decoction of dry fruit is used when the fresh plant is not available. Fresh leaves and young shoots, kept for a few minutes in boiling milk, give it a bitter taste and renders it mucilaginous. The milk so obtained is used as an aphrodisiac and is advised in sexual debility.

Tribulus alatus Del.

The fruit of this herb, which is pear-shaped winged, with two seeds, is known as *Gokhru Kalan*.

References

Anand, R., Patnaik, G.K., Srivastava, S., Kulshreshtha, D.K., Dhawan, B.N. (1994) Evaluation of antiurolithiatic activity of *Tribulus terrestris*. *International Journal of Pharmacognosy* 32, 217–224.

Anon. *Encyclopaedia of Chinese Medicinal Substances*. Shanghai People's Publishers, Shanghai, China 1977.

Anon. *Selected Medicinal Plants*. Chemxcil, Bombay, India 1992.

Bowen, W., Long'en, M. Tongku (1990) Clinical observation on 406 cases of angina pectoris of coronary heart disease treated with saponin of *Tribulus terrestris*. *Chinese Journal of Traditional and Western Medicine*, 10, 85–87.

Fang, S., Hao, C., Liu, Z., Song, F, Liu S. (1999) Application of electrospray ionisation, mass spectrometry techniques for the profiling of steroidal saponin mixture extract from *Tribulus terrestris*. *Planta Medica*, 65, 68–73.

Jian, Xin Li, Shi, Q., Xiong, G., Prasain, J.K., Tezuka, Y., Hareyama, T., Wang, Zlex, tanaka, K., Namba, T., Kadota, S. (1998) Tribulusamide A & B, new hepatoprotective lignamides from the fruits of *Tribulus terrestris*: Indication of cytoprotective activity in murine hepatocyte culture. *Planta Medica*, 64, 628–631.

Lee, J.W., Choi, J.H., Kang, S.M. (1992) Screening of medicinal plants having hepatoprotective activity. Effect with primary cultured hepatocytes intoxicated using carbon tetrachloride cytotoxicity. *Korean Journal of Pharmacognosy*, 23, 268–275.

Mahato, S.B., Sahu, N.P., Pal, B.C., Chakravarti, R.N., Chakravarti, D., Ghosh, A. (1978) Screening of *Tribulus terrestris* plants for diosgenin. *Journal Institute of Chemistry* (India), 50, 49–50.

Miles, C.O., Wilkins, A.L., Erasmus, G.L., Kellerman, T.S., Coetzer, J.A.W. (1994) Photosensitivity in South Africa. VII. Chemical composition of biliary crystals from a sheep with experimentally induced geeldikkop. *Onderstepoort Journal of Veterinay Research*, 61, 215–222.

Nagarkatti, D.S., Rege, N.N., Mittal, B.V., Uchil, D.A., Desai, N.K., Dahanukar, S.A. Avenue ahead: Nephroprotection by *Tribulus terrestris*. *Update Ayurveda-94*, Bombay, India 1994.

Noogi, N.C., Chakraborty, B., Sikadar, S., Ray, N.M. (1977) Investigations on the pharmaco-logoical properties of *Tribulus terrestris*. *Indian Medical Gazette*, 17, 174–176.

Prakash, Deepak, Singh, P.N., Wahi, S.P. (1985) An evaluation of *Tribulus terrestris* L. (chota gokhru). *Indian Drugs*, 22, 332–333.

Sangeeta, D., Sidhu, H., Thind, S.K., Nath, R., Vaidyanathan, S. (1993) Therapeutic response of *Tribulus terrestris* (Gokhru) aqueous extract on hyperoxaluria in male adult rats. *Phytotherapy Research*, 7, 116–119.

Sangeeta, D., Sidhu, H., Thind, S.K., Nath, R. (1994) Effect of *Tribulus terrestris* on oxalate metabolism in rats. *Journal of Ethnopharmacology*, 41, 61–66.

Santha, G., Iyer, G.Y.N. (1967) Preliminary studies on the diuretic effects of *Hygrophila spinosa* and *Tribulus terrestris*. *Indian Journal of Medical Research*, 55, 714–716.

Schreter, I.A. (1980) Distribution of *Tribulus terrestris* L. in the Soviet Union. *Rastitelnye Resursy*, 16, 513–523 (in Russian).

Seth, S.D., Jagdeesh, G. (1976) Cardiac action of *Tribulus terrestris*. *Indian Journal of Medical Research*, 64, 1821–1825.

Singh, R.G., Singh, R.P., Usha, Shukla, K.P., Singh, P. (1991) Experimental evaluation of diuretic action of herbal drug *Tribulus terrestris* on albino rats. *Journal of Research and Education in Indian Medicine*, 10, 19–21.

Suru, P.P, Kulkarni, P.H. (1991) Study of use of *Varunadi Kwath* in Mutrakruchchra. *Deerghayu International*, 7, 2–4.

Tomova, M. (1987) Tribestan (A preparation from *Tribulus terrestris*). *Farmatsiya* (in Russian), 37, 40–42.

Wang Yan, Ohtani, K., Kasai, R., Yamasaki, R. (1996) Steroidal saponins from fruits of *Tribulus terrestris*. *Phytochemistry*, 42, 1417–1422.

22 Guggal

Commiphora wightii (Arn.) Bhandari
Syn. *C. mukul* (Hook. ex Stocks) Engl.,
Balsamodendron roxburghii Stocks
Family: Burseraceae

THE PLANT AND ITS DISTRIBUTION

It is a woody shrub (Fig. 13A) up to 2 m tall with knotty, crooked, spiny, brown branches, growing in hot rocky areas of Indian deserts and adjoining areas in Pakistan. Leaflets 1–3, rhomboid-ovate serrate. Flowers are brownish red in fasciles of 2–3. There are 8–10 stamens which alternate between long and short, and are half the size of the petals. There are 8–10 lobed discs and the ovary is oblong-ovoid. The fruit is a red drupe, 6–8 mm in diameter.

For medicinal purposes oleo-gum resin (Fig. 13B) is used. It is exuded from the plant in winter or is collected by making cuts or by removing bark at some places. It is a lustrous pale brown, semi-solid mass. Application of inorganic acids to the stem increases the yield of gum but the plant dies after this treatment because of dehydration.

The quality of the gum depends on its colour and on the amount of foreign organic and inorganic matters present in it. The fresh good quality *guggal* is sticky, lustrous, yellowish, sweet smelling (cedarwood-like), where as old guggal is dull in colour, brownish black. The lump of gum, which has a greenish hue and superficially resembles the eye of a buffalo, is considered the best. The other grades of the gum are brownish with some wood chips, while inferior gum is a mixture of dirt and rocks. Earlier, the low-grade gum was used as floor plaster. The genuine gum can be differentiated from its common substitute *salai guggal* by flame test. *Guggal* near a flame bulges like a balloon and bursts, but *salai guggal* burns immediately. When macerated in water, *guggal* forms greenish white emulsion.

Purification of *Guggal*

As far as possible only fresh *guggal* should be used. For incorporation into herbal formulations, it is purified and cleaned to remove foreign organic and inorganic matters like pieces of wood, bark, stone, sand and soil. Various methods are followed for this purpose but usually the gum is put into a bag of thick coarse cloth and boiled in an aqueous medium such as pure water, cow's urine, decoction of *Triphala* or other

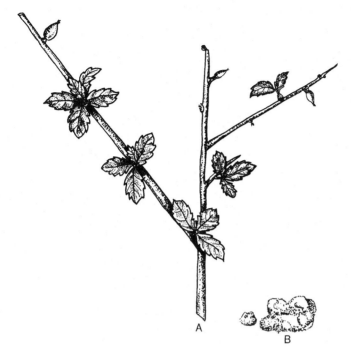

Figure 13   Commiphora wightii **A** twig, **B** gum.

herbs. Boiling is continued until the *guggal* turns soft. On a separate table, a wooden board is smeared with *ghee* and the molten gum is spread on the board with a spatula. All impurities are picked out by hand and the gum is allowed to dry in the air. The dried gum is fried in *ghee* and is powdered for medicinal purposes. In another method, a decoction is prepared from equal quantities of coarse powders of *Triphala* and *Tinospora*, with milk. The decoction is filtered to remove water insoluble matter. Raw *guggal* is put into a cloth bag and this bag is allowed to hang in this boiling decoction. Occasionally the cloth bag is pressed with big wooden spatula to extract molten *guggal* from the bag. When nearly all of the molten *guggal* has come out, the bag is discarded. The mixture of decoction and extracted *guggal* is heated further, in the presence of *ghee*, until dry. In south India (Shanavaskhan *et al.* 1997), crude gum is boiled in water containing 3 parts of *Azadirachta* leaves and one part of freshly harvested untreated turmeric (normally turmeric is boiled and dried before storage). The mixture is filtered through cheesecloth and the filtrate heated further until no water is left. The resulting gum residue is fried in *ghee* or castor oil and used. All these treatments cause the loss of essential oil, which has a therapeutic activity, so a better method is to first sort the gum by hand and then macerate it in hot *ghee*.

USES IN FOLKLORE AND AYURVEDA

Guggal has been mentioned in *Atheraveda* and in most of the other ancient Ayurvedic works. It is considered dry, pungent, aromatic, a *Rasayana*, anti-*tridosha*, nutritive, lubricant for the body systems, stimulant and digestant. This gum is so important in Ayurveda that it constitutes a separate group of preparations under the general name *guggal* in *materia medica*. It is not possible to mention the details of all these so only selected uses are given here.

For rheumatism

As per Ayurveda, *gum guggal* acts as an anti-inflammatory agent for all types of pains in the body because of its *hot* effects, particularly rheumatism, called *amavata* in Ayurveda. *Ama* is produced by improper digestion and metabolism and gets lodged in the joints to produce inflammation and pains. Usually the patients with diet irregularity and constipation are affected by *amavata*. To counteract it, a polyherbal and polymineral preparation *Mahayograja guggal* is often prescribed for these purposes, but it has been observed that *Simhanda guggal* is more useful for the patients suffering from constipation. If it causes a burning sensation then the dose may be reduced. If there is constipation, then a mild laxative like castor oil may be prescribed along with the pills.

For liver problems

Because of its dry nature *guggal* helps in sluggish liver.

For malaria

It helps in fever, when accompanied by shivering.

As an aphrodisiac

This effect, is probablys due to its power to dissolve fat from the arteries, which allow free flow of blood to sexual parts, and thus helps impotence, and in vaginal diseases.

For bronchial troubles

This effect is due to the gum's pungency and hotness. In chronic cases of bronchitis and in tuberculosis it dissolves sputum and clears the throat. Ten grams of a preparation made from equal quantities of long pepper, *Adhatoda* leaves, honey and *ghee* is prescribed for these purposes.

For cardiac problems

It is used for heart diseases, blood pressure problems , anaemia and other diseases of the blood, normally along with *pushkarmul*.

As a diuretic

Through its diuretic effect, it dissolves kidney stones.

For digestive problems

In indigestion, diarrhoea, dysentery, gastroenteritis, inflammation of the intestine, it acts as an intestinal antiseptic. It may be mixed with an equal quantity of aloe extract to make a dose of 5 g.

For sexually transmitted diseases

It reduces the inflammation of the urinogenital tract. In gonorrhoea, it is given with *Hemidesmus indicus*, and in syphilis with *Tinopsora*.

For fractures

Pills made with equal quantities of this gum and *shilajit* (a bituminous herbo-mineral compound) are prescribed during fractures. A plaster of the gum is applied externally.

In gynaecological practices

It has a beneficial effect on the female reproductive system. In general practice, pills made with *gum guggal* along with the extract of aloe and ferrous sulphate are given. In sterility due to leucorrhoea, *guggal* with *Berberis* extract is a drug of choice.

For skin diseases

In all types of skin diseases of unknown aetiology, a dose of 25–200 mg of gum *guggal* has been found to impart lustre to the skin, giving it a healthy look. It has given good results even in leprosy.

External applications

Because of anti-inflammatory, antiseptic and healing properties, external application of gum is useful in arthritis, rheumatic pains and piles. A gargle of alcoholic extract of the gum in water is effective for all mouth and throat problems, such as ulcers, inflammation, tonsillitis, dental caries and pyorrhoea. A drop of the gum in the mouth is also used as a lozenge.

It is an anti-microbial and deodorant, so it is used as a fumigant in obstinate ulcers and in chronic septic cases.

Contraindications

While using *guggal* preparations, avoid acidic foods, strong medicines, alcohol, heavy exercises, sunbathing, anger and sexual intercourse.

Side effects

It may cause rashes in some cases.

If not used in a proper way, it has a deleterious effect on the liver and lungs. Its use can cause excessive dryness of the body, impotence, giddiness and laziness. If any of these conditions exist then this gum should not be used for these and other related diseases.

Ayurvedic preparations

Mahayograja guggulu

Ingredients   1.12 g each of ginger, long pepper fruit and root, asafoetida, celery, cumin, mustard, calamus, *Piper chaba*, *Plumbago zeylanica*, *Wrightia tinctoria*, *Vitex agnus-castus*, *Cissampelos pareira*, *Embelia ribes*, *Scindapsus officinalis*, *Picrorhiza kurrooa*, *Aconitum heterophyllum*, *Clerodendrum serratum*, and *Senseveria roxburghiana*, 49.5 g *Triphala*, 65 g *guggul* gum, and 17.5 g each of processed tin, silver, lead, iron, mica, and red oxide of mercury.

Method   Macerate and heat the gum, add all the ingredients in powder form so the whole mass is homogenous. Moisten with water if necessary and make pills of 250 mg each.

Dose   250–500 mg.

Uses   In various rheumatic and arthritic conditions, neuritis, lumbago, sciatica, obesity, cardiac diseases, respiratory diseases such as asthma and in gastrointestinal disorders, such as colitis, etc.

  Mahayograj Guggal or its simpler form, *Yograja Guggal*, are manufactured by a large number of pharmacies. The ingredients and the quantities of the raw materials in these products vary in each case so Arora *et al.* (1973) prepared a standardized *Yograja Guggal*, as per classical Ayurvedic method, and tested it against arthritis produced by various agents. This product was not significantly effective. The various commercial products sold in the market were much less active compared with the standardized ones. Autarkar *et al.* (1984) studied side effects and tolerability of *Yograj Guggal*.

Medohar guggal

Ingredients   Five grams of finely powdered ginger, long pepper, black pepper, *Triphala*, *Plumbago zeylanica*, *Cyperus scariousus*, and *Embelia ribes*, 45 g *gum guggal* and 10 ml castor oil.

Preparation   Sprinkle castor oil on *gum guggal* and pound it. When soft add the fine powders of the above herbs and make pills of 250 mg from the homogenous mass.

Dose   2–4 pills twice daily with water. During this medication, eat light food regularly and do not remain hungry. Drink a minimum amount of water with meals, but as much as possible one to two hours after the meals. Drink water on an empty stomach in the morning.

Uses   In obesity use the above pills for 5–6 months.

Contraindications   Avoid sweet and fatty foods. Do mild exercise regularly.

Guglip

(Patent preparation) CIPLA, Bombay.

Ingredient   Each tablet contains 25 mg of guggalsterone.

Indications   In mixed hyperlipidaemia: total serum cholesterol > 220 mg/dl
total serum triglyceride > 170 mg/dl
In hypercholesterolaemia: total serum cholesterol > 220 mg/dl
In hypertriglyceridaemia: total serum triglyceride > 190 mg/dl

Dosage   1 tablet three times a day after the meals.

Precautions   Use under medical supervision in hepatic diseases, diarrhoea, dysentery, etc.

THERAPEUTIC INDICATIONS AND PHARMACOLOGICAL STUDIES

As a hypolipidaemic agent

Keeping in view the importance of *guggal* in Ayurvedic pharmacopoeia, after interpreting the ancient texts, extensive studies were carried out in Benaras Hindu University, Varanasi in India by Satyawati (1969, 1988) and others. It was seen that in *Sushsrut Sanhita*, it has been given for aetiology, pathogenesis, treatment of obesity, associated lipid disorders and the complications arising due to them. On the basis of this information, gum *guggal* was screened for possible hypolipidaemic, obesity and hypercholesterolaemic effects. It was seen that it protected animals against cholesterol-induced atherosclerosis. It reduced the body weight. When patients of various illnesses were administered 6–12 g of raw gum *guggal* in three divided doses for 15–30 days, there was a fall in serum cholesterol. The oral administration of crude *guggal*, the alcohol soluble and insoluble fractions brought about a fall in serum cholesterol and serum turbidity (high serum turbidity is associated with hypercholesterolaemia) due to steroids (Malhotra *et al.* 1970). The effect of crude *guggal* on serum lipids in obese bodies was studied by Kuppurajan *et al.* (1973). When used for three months it brought about a significant decrease in mean serum cholesterol levels. A patented preparation of *guggal* was found to be effective in obesity (Varadani, 1973). The petroleum ether extract of *guggal* prevented hyperlipidaemia caused by oestrogen. It did not allow the synthesis of fats in the body so body weight was reduced and amount of blood lipids became less. Histological changes indicated enhance activities in the thyroid. On the basis of this study Gupta *et al.* (1974) concluded that *guggal* was a good therapeutic agent to prevent and treat hyperlipidaemia and adiposity associated with oestrogen hyperactivity and with hypothyroidism. Tripathi *et al.* (1975) observed that the active principles of the gum showed regression of hyperlipidaemia. *Guggal* in general reduced body weight in the obese objects. The feeding of oleoresin to cholesterol-fed rats enhanced the faecal excretion of bile acids, with an increase in cholesterol excretion (Sidhu *et al.* 1976). Gupta *et al.* (1978) assessed the hypocholesterolaemic and hypolipid-aemic effects of the gum in patients suffering from lipid disorders. Singh *et al.* (1983) studied the effect of ether extract on experimental hypothyroidism by melatonin. It increased the weight and iodine uptake of the thyroid gland. Kotiyal *et al.* (1985) tried a fraction of the gum for obesity. Agrawal *et al.* (1986) and Gopal *et al.* (1986) carried out clinical trials of gugulipid (guggalsterone) isolated from gum *guggal* by ethyl acetate, in primary hypolipidaemia. According to Satyawati (1988) this fraction lowered serum lipids including cholesterol, triglyceride, phospholipid when tried on various animals and human beings. It protected LDL against the depletion of lipid constituents such as cholesterol, triglycerides and phospholipids as well as the conversion of cholesterol into oxygenated cholesterol. This protective action may be due to its free radical scavenging properties. This compound significantly inhibited the generation of hydoxyl radicals in enzymatic systems. Ahluwalia and Amma (1988) studied the effects of oral ingestion of the gum and its effect on the faecal excretion of cholesterol and bile acids in hypo- and hypercholesterolaemic rats. Sharma *et al.* (1988) investigated the effect of a mixture of alcohol extract of *Triphala* and petroleum ether extract of gum. Verma *et al.* (1988) tried it in the patients of hyperlipidaemia. Kulkarni and Paranjape (1990) and Kulkarni (1991) tried a preparation containing *guggal* with *Triphala* and minerals in obesity. Saukhala *et al.* (1992) used this gum in pre-venting diet-induced hypercholesterolaemia in rats. Duwiejua *et al.* (1993) studied anti-inflammatory activity in the oleoresins of the plant family Burseraceae. Bhatt *et al.* (1994) conducted a trial on obese patients by dividing the volunteers into two groups. One group just conducted standardized physical exercises, while the other group used *guggul* preparations whilst carrying out the physical exercises. After the study it was concluded that *guggal* has a definite effect on lowering the body weight. Patel *et al.* (1995) tried it in obese patients. Guggulsterone was found to be a potent hypolipidaemic agent, which prevented oxidation of low density lipoprotein (Kavita Singh *et al.* 1997).

As an anti-inflammatory agent

Chaurasia *et al.* (1995) carried out research on antioxidant and anti-inflammatory properties of the *guggal*-containing drug. The various uses documented are:

For sciatica   Nair *et al.* (1978), Tyagi and Prasad (1995).

For inflammatory pains   Purushottam Dev (1979).

For rheumatic arthritis   Pandit and Shukla (1981), Shukla *et al.* (1985), Pandey and Sharma (1986), Vyas and Shukla (1987) tried pure *guggal* whilst Majumdar (1984) used a polyherbal preparation and a *guggal* preparation containing gold. Kishore *et al.* (1987) carried out clinical studies with the preparation *Sunthi-guggal* containing *Commiphora* with ginger. Chandrasekharan *et al.* (1994) worked on an Ayurvedic preparation. Sannd and Kumari (1994) used a compound preparation in osteoarthritis.

For fractures   Panda (1990) prepared a plaster with lac and *guggal*.

In cervical spondylitis   Mehra and Gurdip Singh (1986).

In heart diseases

Guggal was evaluated for fibrinolytic activity and platelet aggregation in coronary artery disease (Bordia and Chuttani, 1979, Baldwa *et al.* 1980), as a cardioprotective agent in patients of coronary artery disease, hypertension and diabetes mellitus (Arora *et al.* 1995).

An Ayurvedic preparation *Pushkar Guggal*, in which *guggal* is used with *Inula racemosa*, was effective as an anti-anginal and hypolipidaemic agent in coronary heart disease (Singh *et al.* 1993, Dubey *et al.* 1995).

In skin diseases

Guggulipid gave good results when taken orally in acne vulgaris (Dogra *et al.* 1990).

Anthelmintic activity

Kakrani and Kalyani (1984) noted the anthelmintic activity of essential oils. Bagi *et al.* (1985) also carried out pharmacological studies on the essential oil.

In leucorrhoea

Rao *et al.* (1985) used a compound preparation of *Phyllanthus emblica* and *guggal*.

In thyroid stimulation

Tripathi *et al.* (1984), Singh *et al.* (1985), Tripathi *et al.* (1988) studied thyroid stimulation using a constituent obtained from the gum, z-guggalosterone.

In urinary tract infection

Gokshuradi Guggal made from a gum of *guggal*, *Tribulus terrestris* and other herbs was tried in urinary tract infections (Upadhyaya and Singh, 1979).

Review

Kakrani (1981) and Satyawati (1988) has reviewed this drug.

References

Agrawal, R.C., Singh, S.P., Saran, R.K., Das, S.K., Sinha, M., Asthana, O.P., Gupta, P.P., Nityanand, S., Dhawan, B.N., Agarwal, S.S. (1986) Clinical trials of guggulipid-a new hypolipidemic agent of plant origin in primary hypolipidaemia. *Indian Journal of Medical Research*, 84, 624–634.

Ahluwalia, P., Amma, M.K.P (1988) Effect of oral ingestion of oleo-resin of gum guggal on the fecal excretion of cholesterol and bile acids in hypo- and hypercholesterolemic rats. *Research Bulletin Panjab University*, 39, 53–55.

Arora, R.B., Gupta, L., Sharma, R.C., Gupta, S.K. (1973) A standardisation of Indian indigenous drugs and preparations. III Standardisation of Yogaraj Guggulu with reference to its anti–inflammatory activity. *Journal of Research in Indian Medicine*, 8, 20–24.

Arora, R.B., Sharma, J.N., Shastri, H. (1982) Beneficial effect of fraction of gum guggal in arthritic syndrome and liver function in clinical and experimental arthritis. *Rheumatism*, 18, 9–16.

Arora, R.C., Agarwal, N., Arora, S. (1995) Evaluation of CTI (cardioprotective drug) in subjects of coronary artery disease, hypertension and diabetes mellitus. *Flora and Fauna*, 1, 203–205.

Autarkar, D.S., Pande, R., Athavale, A.V., Saoji, S.R., Shah, K.N., Jakhmola, A.T., Vaddya, A.B. (1984) Phase I Tolerability study of Yogarajguggulu, a popular Ayurvedic drug. *Journal Postgraduate Medicine*, 30, 111–115.

Bagi, M.K., Kakrani, H.K., Kalyani, C.A., Datyanarayana, D., Manvi, F.V. (1985) Preliminary pharmacological studies of essential oil from *Commiphora mukul*. *Fitoterapia*, 56, 245–248.

Baldwa, V.S., Sharma, R.C., Ranka. P.C., Chittora, M.D. (1980) Effect of *Commiphora mukul* (guggal) on fibrinolytic activity and platelet aggregation in coronary artery disease. *Rajasthan Medical Journal*, 19, 84–86.

Bhatt, A.D., Dalal, D.G., Shah, S.J., Joshi, B.A., Gajjar, M.N., Vaidya, R.A., Vaidya, R.B., Autarkar, D.S. Challenge of assessing efficacy of guggulu in obesity. Pointers from a naturalistic trial. *Update-94, Ayurveda*, Bombay, 24–26 Feb., 1994.

Bordia, A., Chuttani, S.K. (1979) Effect of gum guggulu on fibrinolysis and platelet adhesiveness in coronary heart disease. *Indian Journal of Medical Research*, 70, 992–996.

Chandrasekharan, A.N., Porkodi, R., Radhamadhavan, Parthiban, M., Bhatt, N.S. (1994) Study of Ayurvedic drugs in rheumatoid arthritis compared to auranofin. *Indian Practitioner*, 57, 489–502.

Chaurasia, S., Tripathi, P., Tripathi, Y.B. (1995) Antioxidant and anti-inflammatory property of Sandhika: a compound herbal drug. *Indian Journal of Experimental Biology*, 33, 428–432.

Dogra, J., Aneja, N., Saxena, V.N. (1990) Oral gugulipid in acne vulgaris management. *Indian Journal of Dermatology, Venerology and Leprology*, 56, 381–383.

Dubey, G.P., Singh, S., Mishra, A.K. Effects of Pushkar-guggulu on body composition in CHD cases. *Seminar on Research in Ayurveda and Siddha, CCRAS*, New Delhi, India, 20–22 March, 1995.

Duwiejua, M., Zeitlin, I.J., Waterman, P.G., Chapman, J., Mhango, G.J., Proven G.J. (1993) Anti-inflammatory activity of resins from some species of the plant Burseraceae. *Planta Medica*, 59, 12–16.

Gopal, K., Saran, K.K., Nityanand, S., Gupta, P.P., Hasan, M., Das, M., Sinha, N., Agarwal, S.S. (1986) Clinical trials of ethyl acetate extract of gum guggal (guggulipid) in primary hyperlipidaemia. *Journal Association of Physicians of India*, 34, 249–251.

Gupta, M., Tripathi, S.N., Prasad, B. (1974) Effect of extract of gum guggulu on estrogen-induced hyperlipidemia in chicks. *Journal of Research in Indian Medicine*, 9, 4–11.

Gupta, M., Tripathi, S.N., Upadhyay, B.N. (1978) Assessment of hypocholestrolemic and hypolipidemic action of Commiphora mukul in human beings suffering from lipid disorders. *Antiseptic*, 75, 271–275.

Kakrani, H.K. (1981) Guggal – a review. *Indian Drugs*, 18, 417–421.

Kakrani, H.K., Kalyani, G.A. (1984) Anthelmintic activity of essential oil of *Commiphora mukul*. *Fitoterapia*, 55, 232–234.

Kishore, P., Devi Das. K.V., Banerjee, S. (1987) Clinical studies on the treatment of amvata-rheumatoid arthritis with sunthi-guggal. *Journal of Research in Ayurveda and Siddha*, 3, 133–146.

Kotiyal, J.P., Singh, D.S., Bisht, D.B. (1985) Gum guggulu (*Commiphora mukul*) fraction A in obesity – A double blind clinical trial. *Journal of Research in Ayurveda and Siddha*, 1, 20–35.

Kulkarni, P.H. (1991) Clinical study of effect of sookshma (subtle) Triphala Guggulu (TG3X) in obesity. *Deerghayu International*, 7, 17–22.

Kulkarni, P.H., Paranjape, P. (1990) Clinical assessment of Ayurvedic anti-obesity drugs. A double blind placebo controlled trial. *Journal of the National Integrated Medical Association*, 32, 7–11.

Kuppurajan, K., Rajagopalan, S.S., Koteswara, Rao, Vijayalakshmi, A.N., Dwarkananth, C. (1973) Effect of Guggulu (*Commiphora mukul* Engl.) on serum lipids in obese subjects. *Journal of Research in Indian Medicine*, 8, 1–8.

Majumdar, A. (1979) Clinical studies of drugs (Bhallatak, Gourakh & Guggulu) in rheumatoid arthiritis. *Rheumatism*, 14, 118–130.

Majumdar, K.A. (1984) Role of gum guggulu with gold in rheumatic and other allied diseases. *Rheumatism*, 20, 9–15.

Malhotra, C.L., Agarwal, Y.K., Mehta, V.L., Prasad, S. (1970) The effect of various fractions of gum guggal on experimentally produced hypercholesterolemia in chicks. *Indian Journal of Medical Research*, 58, 394.

Mehra, B.L., Gurdip Singh (1986) A comparative study on the effect of Nirgundi Pak, Pinda Sneha and Suddh Guggal (controlled temperature) on the patients of Griva Hundanam (cervical spondylosis). *Rheumatism*, 21, 88.

Nair, P.R.C., Vijayan, N.P., Pillai, B.K.R., Venkatraghavan, S. (1978) The effect of Nirgundi Panchang and Guggal in sodhna cum samana and samana treatment of Gridhrasi (sciatica). *Journal of Research in Indian Medicine, Yoga and Homeopathy*, 13, 13–18.

Nandkarni, K.M. (1954) *Indian Materia Medica*. Part I. Popular Prakashan, Bombay.

Panda, M. (1990) The effect of Laksha Guggulu in the clinical management of fracture. *Journal of Research in Ayurveda and Siddha*, 11, 13–18.

Pandey, V.K., Sharma, A.K. (1986) Evaluation of *Vatahari* Guggal and Nadivaspa sweda in the management of rheumatic diseases. *Rheumatism*, 22, 1–6.

Pandit, M.M., Shukla, C.P. (1981) Study of shuddha guggulu on rheumatoid arthritis. *Rheumatism*, 16, 54–67.

Patil, N.D., Dewoolkar, Chheda, M.S. (1995) Effect of guggal on lipid profile and glycosylated HB in obese subjects, Project report. *Biorhythm*, 57–59.

Purushottam Dev (1979) Assessment of the ability of *Vatari Guggulu* to modify inflammatory pain. *Rheumatism*, 14, 39–44.

Rao, T.S., Kusuma Kumari, Netaji, B., Subhakta, P.K.J.P. (1985) A pilot study of svetpradra (leucorrhoea) with Amalaka guggulu. *Journal of Research in Ayurveda and Siddha*, 6, 213–237.

Sannd, B.N., Kumari, K. (1994) Preliminary clinical trial of Trikushtha guggulu in the treatment of sandhigatavata (osteoarthritis). *Sachitra Ayurveda*, 46, 765–771.

Satyavati, G.V. (1988) Gum guggal (*Commiphora mukul*) – The success story of an ancient insight leading to a modern discovery. *Indian Journal of Medical Research*, 87, 327–335.

Satyavati, G.V., Dwarkantah, C., Tripathi, S.N. (1969) Experimental studies on the hypocholesterolemic effect of *Commiphora mukul* Engl (Guggal). *Indian Journal of Medical Research*, 57, 1950–1962.

Saukhala, A., Mathur, P.N., Saukhala, A.K., Dashora, P.K. (1992) Comparative efficiency of Shilajeet and gum guggal (Commiphora mukul) in preventing diet-induced hypercholesterolemia in Wistar rats. *Indian Journal of Clinical Biochemistry*, 7, 45–48.

Shanavaskhan, A.E., Binu, S., Unnithan, M.D., Santoshkumar, E.S., Pushpangadan, P. (1997) Detoxification techniques of traditional physicians of Kerala, India on some toxic herbal drugs. *Fitoterapia*, 68, 69–74.

Sharma, J.N., Rajpal, M.N., Rao, T.S., Gupta, S.K. (1988) Some pharmacological investigations on the alcoholic extract of Triphala alone and in combination with petroleum ether extract of oleo-gum resin of Commiphora mukul. *Indian Drugs*, 25, 220–223.

Sharma, K., Puri, A.S., Sharma, R., Prakash, S. (1976) Effect of gum guggal on serum lipids in obese subjects. *Journal of Research in Indian Medicine, Yoga and Homoeopathy*, 11, 132–134.

Shukla, K.P., Singh, S.P., Kishore, N., Singh, D.R., Srivastava, S. (1985) Evaluation of Rasanadi Guggulu compound in the treatment of rheumatoid arthritis. *Rheumatism*, 21, 16–15.

Singh, A.K., Tripathi, S.N., Prasad, G.C. (1983) Response of *Commiphora mukul* (Guggulu) on melatonin-induced hyperthyroidism. *Ancient Science of Life*, 3, 85–90.

Singh, A.K., Tripathi, S.N., Prasad, G.C. (1985) Hormonal response of thyroid gland to *Commiphora mukul* and LATS in tissue culture. *Bulletin Ethno-Botanical Research*, 6, 155–164.

Singh, K., Chander, R., Kapoor, N.K. (1997) Guggulsterone, a potent hypolipidemic, prevents oxidation of low density lipoprotein. *Phytotherapy Research*, 11, 291–294.

Singh, R., Singh, R.P., Batliwala, P.G., Upadhyaya, B.N., Tripathi, S.N. (1993) Puskara-Guggulu-an antianginal and hypolipidemic agent in coronary heart disease (CHD). *Journal of Research in Ayurveda and Siddha*, 12, 1–18.

Tripathi, S.N., Gupta, M., Dwivedi, L.D., Sen, S.P. (1975) Regression of hyperlipidemia with an active principle of *Commiphora mukul*. *Journal of Research in Indian Medicine, Yoga and Homoeopathy*, 10, 11–16.

Tripathi, Y.B., Malhotra, O.P., Tripathi, S.N. (1984) Thyroid stumulating action of z-guggulosteron obtained from *Commiphora mukul*. *Planta Medica*, 50, 78–80.

Tripathi, Y. B., Tripathi, A., Malhotra, O.P., Tripathi, S.N. (1988) Thyroid stimulating action of (z) guggalsterone. Mechanism of action. *Planta Medica*, 54, 271–277.

Tyagi, M.K., Prasad, R.D. Clinical evaluation of the effect of Trayodshang guggulu and Vistundak vati in the management of Gridhrasi. *Seminar on Research in Ayurveda and Siddha, CCRAS*, New Delhi (India), 20–22 March, 1995.

Upadhyaya, G.P., Singh, R.H. (1979) Clinical trials of popular indigenous compounds. Part II. Clinical and microbiological studies on the role of Goksuradi Guggulu in urinary tract infection with obstructive uropathy (Mutrakricchra). *Journal of Research in Indian Medicine, Yoga and Homoeopathy*, 14, 25–33.

Varadani, B.V. (1973) Obesity and it's treatment by an indigenous drug LIPIDEX. *Indian Medical Gazaette*, 13, 33–43.

Verma, S.K., Barodia, A. (1988) Effect of *Commiphora mukul* (gum guggulu) in patients of hyperlipidemia with special reference to HDL cholesterol. *Indian Journal of Medical Research*, 87, 356–360.

Vyas, S.N., Shukla, C.P. (1987) A clinical study on the effect of Shuddha guggulu in rheumatic arthritis. *Rheumatism*, 23, 15–26.

23 Haritaki

Terminalia chebula Retz.
Family: Combretaceae

THE TREE AND ITS DISTRIBUTION

It is a medium-sized tree with dark brown bark and elliptic oblong, broad leaves (Fig. 14). The mature fruit is more or less a five angled drupe, 2.5 to 4 cm long, usually obovoid and glabrous. The tree grows in the sub-Himalayan tract and in the deciduous forests of India. It is commonly known by the name *harar*.

As per Hindu mythology, the tree originated from a few drops of nectar, which fell from heaven on the ground. Because of this divine origin, it has been given various names showing its virtues, such as *Haritaki* – born in the abode of *Hara* (Lord *Shiva*) on Himalayas, *Vijaya* – victorious or conquers all the diseases, *Rohini* – heals the wounds, ulcers, *Amrita* – nectar, *Shakla sreshta* – the best of all, *Abhya* – not fearful of any diseases, *Airytha* – cures all diseases, *Pramatha* – eradicates the disease from the source, *Amogh* – always beneficial, *Kayastha* – sustains the body, *Pratpathya* – extremely whole some, *Divya* – divine in nature, *Prananda* – offering life, *Jiva, Jivanti, Jivanika* – life promoting, *Putana*- sanctifying, *Shreyasi* – conferring prosperity, *Chataki* – increasing vitality, *Balyi* – gives strength, *Jivya priya* – liked by all, *Bhisak priya* – loved by physicians, *Pachoni* – digestive.

It has been considered a *Rasayana* since ancient times. Lord Budha and Guru Padmasambhav, the great Budhist sage who was instrumental in spreading Budhism beyond Himalayas, kept this fruit in their laps (Fig. 15). In ancient times the reputation of this fruit spread from India to the Middle East, and from there to Greece. Kabul (Afghanistan) became the biggest centre of its trade.

In earlier Ayurvedic texts, seven types of *haritaki* are mentioned, but now in India following three types are well known:

1 *Harar Jangi* or *Haleileh e Jung* or *Bal haritaki:* It is the immature fruit, black in colour and smaller in size.
2 *Harar:* It is available in different shapes and sizes. It is lustrous brown to greyish brown in colour. It may be sold as such, but very often the seed (stone) is separated from the pulp and the dry pulp is sold as *chilka* (cover) *harar.*

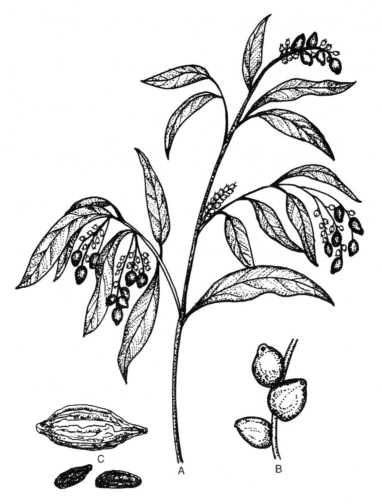

Figure 14 Terminalia chebula **A** twig, **B** young fruit, **C** dry fruit, **D** young dried fruit.

3   *Harar Kabuli:* It is about double the size of common *haritaki* fruit and is preferred
for *Rasayana* treatment. It is so heavy that it sinks in water. The name *Kabuli*
means from Kabul, the capital of Afghanistan, which at one time was a big centre
for the trade of this fruit. It is very expensive (more than ten times the price of the
common variety), so it is sometimes adulterated with moulded fruits made from
haritaki powder. Tuber of *Exogonium purga* Benth. (*Ipomoea jalap*) which is called
Jalap Harar is a common substitute for this fruit. *Jalap* tuber not only superficially resembles *Kabuli Harada* in shape but also in its laxative action. It is a
strong purgative. *Jalap Harar* is a tuber without a stone so it can be differentiated from *Kabuli Harar* on the basis of morphological characteristics. It has
striations on the outer surface and its powder causes a strong burning sensation in
the mouth.

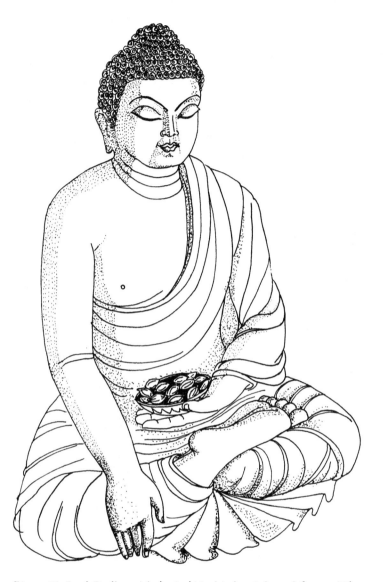

Figure 15 Lord Budha with *haritaki* in his lap (adopted from a Tibetan painting).

USES IN FOLKLORE AND AYURVEDA

As a good *Rasayana* it provides nutrition to the body in the same way that a mother provides to a foetus. The major uses of this fruit are:

As a laxative

In constipation, half a teaspoon of powdered immature fruit with cold water is given at bedtime. It is not only a good laxative but also regulates bowel movements. It operates rapidly without irritation or heat and can be used for a long time. It has a beneficial effect on the enlargement of the spleen. If as a result of its administration the faeces become watery, then the dose is reduced, but if hard, then the dose is increased. If dry powder is not easy to administer, it is mixed with an equal quantity of *ghee* and is given with water or 250 ml of milk. These fluids avoid astringency and lubricate the alimentary canal. *T. chebula* is an ingredient of a well-known household laxative *Triphala* (p. 28). A preserve called Muraba Harar made by an infiltration of sugar syrup in *haritaki* is also used as a laxative.

As a Rasayana

Haritaki provides strength to the body and delays the effects of old age. As a *Rasayana*, use three grams of *harar kabuli* powder in the morning when the stomach is empty. In the first half of winter ginger juice is added to *haritaki*, whilst in the second half long pepper is used. In the rainy season it is used with salt, in autumn with sugar and in spring with honey.

As an astringent

Through this activity, it cures spongy gums, ulcers, dysentery and chronic diarrhoea.

Contraindications

It should not be used by lean and thin people, in the case of extreme weakness, by people with poor digestion, in pregnancy or if there is haemorrhaging in any part of the body.

THERAPEUTIC INDICATIONS AND PHARMACOLOGICAL STUDIES

As an anti-spasmodic

Chebulin isolated from the fruit, possesses anti-spasmodic activity resembling that of papaverine (Thakur *et al.* 1989).

Hypolipidaemic activity

The feeding of a fraction of fruit extract to rats lowered their levels of low density lipoprotein lipids and increased the level of high density lipoprotein cholesterol, whilst reducing hepatic triglyceride (Khanna *et al.* 1993).

In liver problems

Sohni and Bhatt (1996) tried a compound herbal formulation containing this fruit in hepatic amoebiasis.

As a laxative

Tripathi and Tewari (1983) prescribed *haritaki* for simple constipation. The results were excellent in 20 per cent of the patients, and good in the rest. No side effects were observed in any case. Tamhana and Throat (1994) observed that the fruit affected gastric motility.

As an immunomodulator

The alcohol extract effectively scavenged the oxygen free radicals. It significantly inhibited chemiluminescence of human leucocyte and the bad effects of cigarette smoke (Fu Naiwu *et al.* 1992, Sohni and Bhatt 1996).

Cardiotonic property

Awsathi and Nath (1968) isolated a cardiac glycoside and Reddy *et al.* (1990) a phenolic compound responsible for cardiotonic activity. These compounds increased the force of contraction and cardiac output without altering the heart rate. Chebulinic acid – a major phenolic glycoside had a pronounced cardiotonic property. Its effect was greater on a hypodynamic heart than on a normal one. Various extracts from the fruit rind showed inhibition of Na^+, K^+, Mg^{2+} ATPase of frog heart muscle, which were dose dependent (Azeem *et al.* 1992). Srivastava *et al.* (1992), Reddy *et al.* (1994) also observed a cardiotonic effect of the fruit.

Cytoprotective effect

It had a cytoprotective effect when used with *Asparagus racemosus* (Dahanukar *et al.* 1983). The water extract of the fruit exhibited an anti-mutagenic activity when tested on *Salmonella typhimurium* (Grover and Saroj Bala, 1992). Hydrolyzable tannins and related compounds from the fruit had cytotoxic activity (Lee SeungHo, 1995).

Antimicrobial property

Sato *et al.* (1997) isolated gallic acid and its ester, which were effective against methicillin resistant *Staphylococcus aureus*. The aqueous extract of the fruit exhibited very strong anti-viral activity against duck hepatitis B virus and against HIV-1 protease (Xu Hong Xi *et al.* 1996, Chung *et al.* 1997).

In Uraemia

It is rich in tannins and thus has a uraemic toxin decreasing action (Yokozawa *et al.* 1995).

Chemical studies

The fruit has 30 to 32 per cent tannins and 13.9 to 16.9 per cent non-tannins. The tannins are of the pyrogallol type, rich in gallic acid, ellagic acid and a glycoside similar to sennoside. Chebulin and chebulinic acid have also been reported (Thakur *et al.* 1989).

References

Awasthi, L., Nath, B. (1968) Chemical examination of *Terminalia chebula* Roxb. Part I. A new cardiac glycoside. *Journal of Indian Chemical Society*, 45, 913.

Azeem, M.A., Reddy, B.M., Appa Rao, A.V.N., Prabhkar, M.C., Prasad, M.S.K. (1992) Effect of *Terminalia chebula* extracts on frog heart muscle (Na$^+$, K$^+$, Mg^{2+}) ATPase activity. *Fitoterapia*, 63, 300–303.

Chung, T.H., Kim, J.C., Lee, C.Y., Moon, M.K., Chae, S.C., Lee, I.S., Kim, S.H. Hahn, K.S., Lee, I.P. (1997) Potential antiviral effects of *Terminalia chebula, Sanguisorba officinalis, Rubus coreanus* and *Rheum palmatum* against duck hepatitis B virus (DHBV). *Phytotherapy Research*, 11, 179–182.

Dahanukar, S.A., Date, S.G., Karandikar, S.M. (1983) Cyptoprotective effect of *Terminalia chebula* and *Asparagus racemosus* on gastric mucosa. *Indian Drugs*, 20, 442–445.

Fu Naiwu, Quan Lanping, Huang Lei, Zhang Ruyi, Chen Yayan (1992) Antioxidant action of extract of *Terminalia chebula* and its preventive effect on DNA breaks in human white cells induced by TPA. *Chinese Traditional and Herbal Drugs* (in Chinese), 23, 26–29.

Grover, I.S., Saroj Bala (1992) Antimutagenic activity of *Terminalia chebula* (myroblan) in *Salmonella typhimurium. Indian Journal of Experimental Biology*, 30, 339–341.

Khanna, A.K., Chander, R., Kapoor, N.K., Singh, C., Srivastava, A.K. (1993) Hypolipidemic activity of *Terminalia chebula* in rats. *Fitoterapia*, 64, 351–356.

Lee Seung Ho, Ryu ShiYong, Choi SangUn, Lee ChongOck, No ZaeSung, Kim SeongKie, Ahn JongWoong (1995) Hydrolysable tannins and related compound having cytotoxic activity from the fruits of *Terminalia chebula*. *Archives of Pharmacal Research*, 18, 118–120.

Reddy, B.M., Ramesh, M., Appa Rao, A.V.N., Prabhakar, M.C. Isolation and studies on cardiotonic activity of active principles from the fruits Terminalia chebula. *Proceedings of 46th Annual Indian Pharmaceutical Congress*, Chandigarh, 28–30 December, 1994.

Reddy, V.R.C., Ramana Kumari, S.V., Reddy, B.M., Anzeem, M.A., Prabhakar, M.C., Appa Rao, A.V.N. (1990) Cardiotonic activity of the fruit of *Terminalia chebula*. *Fitoterapia*, 61, 517–525.

Sato, Y., Oketani, H., Singyouchi, K., Ohtsubo, T., Kihara, M., Shibata, H., Higuti, T. (1997) Extraction and purification of effective antimicrobial constituents of *Terminalia chebula* Rets. against methicillin resistant *Staphylococcus aureus*. *Biological and Pharmaceutical Bulletin*, 20, 401–404.

Sohni, Y.R., Bhatt, R.M. (1996) Activity of a crude extract formulation in experimental hepatic amoebiasis and in immunomodulation studies. *Journal of Ethnopharmacology*, 54, 119–124.

Srivastava, R.D., Dwivedi, S., Sreenivasan, K.K., Chandra Shekhar (1992) Cardiovascular effects of *Terminalia* species of plants. *Indian Drugs*, 29, 144–149.

Tamhana, M.D., Thorat, S.P. Alternations in gastric motility-induced by Ayurvedic agents. *Update Ayurveda-94*, Bombay (India) 24–26 Feb. 1994.

Thakur, R.S., Puri, H.S., Akhtar Hussain *Major Medicinal Plants of India*. Central Institute of Medicinal and Aromatic Plants, Lucknow, India 1989.

Tripathi, V.N., Tewari, S.K. (1983) Clinical trials of Haritaki (*Terminalia chebula*) treatment of simple constipation. *Sachittar Ayurveda*, 35, 733–740.

Xu HongXi, Wan Min, Loh BoonNee, Kon Oilian, Chow Pengwai, Sim KengYeow (1996) Screening of traditional medicines for their inhibitory activity against HIV-1 protease. *Phytotherapy Research*, 10, 207–210.

Yokozawa, T., Fujioka, K., Oura, H., Tanaka, T. (1995) Confirmation that tannin containing crude drugs have a uraemic toxin decreasing action. *Phytotherapy Research*, 9, 1–5.

24 Hing

Ferula foetida Regel
Syn. *F. foetida* (Bunge) Regel
F. asafoetida L.
F. rubricaulis Boiss
Family: Umbelliferae

THE PLANT AND ITS DISTRIBUTION

It is a large perennial herb, with a stem 1.5 to 3 m high, 2.5 to 7.5 cm thick, greenish
and furrowed. The leaves are few, radical and cauline, near the stem base (Fig. 16),
imparipinnate, 45 cm long and 10 to 15 cm broad. Flowers are small, monoecious and
yellow. Oleo-gum resin is obtained from *F. foetida* and other allied species. These
plants grow in western Afghanistan, Iran and adjoining Turkey in mountain slopes,
desolate wastes and sandy deserts.

Collection of oleoresin

The gum resin consists of milky sap, obtained from an incision of the green matured
root. The oldest plants are most productive and a plant less than four years old is
considered virtually worthless. From March to April, just before flowering, the upper
part of the carrot-shaped root is laid bare and the stem is cut off close to the crown.
The exposed surface is covered by a dome-shaped structure made from twigs and earth.
After a few days the exudative is scraped off and a fresh slice of the root is cut to
gather more latex. This process is continued for up to three months until there is no
more exudate. About 1 kg of gum may be obtained from each plant by this process.

The oleoresin

After collection and drying, the dry latex comes in various forms, such as light to dark
brown lumps or a thick paste and is graded for commercial purposes. It has a garlic-
like smell. It may be powdered either when excessively cold or by drying over freshly
burnt lime or exposure to a current of warm air, then reducing to a low temperature
or diluting with starch or magnesium carbonate (Culbreth, 1927).

In raw form asafoetida is nauseating so it is often fried in *ghee* before use. In India,
a compound of asafoetida diluted with starch is often used. It is prepared by boiling

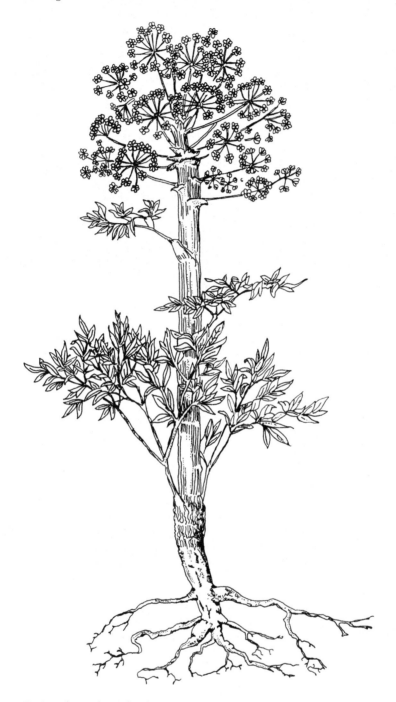

Figure 16 Ferula asafoetida the plant (diagrammatic).

asafoetida, starch and water to obtain a gelatinized mass. On cooling small lumps from this mixture are made and dried. It is sold under the name of *Bandhani Hing* or may be powdered. It is a household name in India and is a constituent of most of spice mixtures used for cooking. Earlier, in some parts of India, for honouring a guest it was common practice to smear the plate with a paste of asafoetida before serving dinner.

USES IN FOLKLORE AND AYURVEDA

Asafoetida is considered anti-spasmodic and hot in effect. It counteracts convulsions, paralytic attack, cough spasms and breathing obstructions, nervous irritability, depression and apathy. Because of a strong stimulant effect on the nervous system, it works as an excellent aphrodisiac. In hysteria it is prescribed with valerian. It is mainly an ingredient of an Ayurvedic digestive powder *Hingvastika churn*, used as carminative.

Uses in old western medicine

It was used for hysteria, hypochondriasis, convulsions, spasms, nervous apoplexy, whooping cough and flatulent constipation. Cerebral excitants were considered synergistic with it, whilst cerebral and arterial depressants were incompatible (Culbreth, 1927). It was commonly used in the form of tincture or as an emulsion, which was prepared by gradually triturating 4 g of asafoetida with 90 ml of water. The dose was 15–30 ml. A pill, made from equal parts of aloe extract and asafoetida, was also very popular for hyperacidity. With valerian, tincture asafoetida was commonly prescribed as a remedy for enuresis, hypochondria and hysteria, as it stimulated the general nervous system and circulation by raising arterial tension. It stimulated secretions and excretions and increased libido.

Toxicological studies

The raw asafoetida is nauseating due to essential oils, so it is heated before use.

Reference

Culbreth, D.M.R. *A Manual of Materia Medica and Pharmacology*. Lea & Febiger, Philadelphia, USA 1927.

25 Jaiphal and Javitri

Myristica fragrans Houtt.
Family: Myristicaceae

THE PLANT AND ITS DISTRIBUTION

It is indigenous to Moluccas Island, but grows in Java and Sumatra (Indonesia), Malaysia and is cultivated to a limited extent in Brazil, Granada, South India and Sri Lanka at an elevation of 300 m, along the sea coast in the tropical climate (Farrel, 1985). The name nutmeg is misleading as the seed is not a nut. It is a small evergreen tree, with alternate, oblong ovate, acute, entire, smooth dark green leaves (Fig. 17A). The flowers are small and pale yellow. The fruit is oval, smooth, lustrous and when the kernel is cut, dark veins are clearly visible due to the presence of aromatic oils.

The fruit cover is hard, about 2 cm long, oval to ovoid, enclosing mace, which is an outer covering on the nutmeg seed (Fig. 17B, C, D). On drying it separates from the seed as an orange-yellow papery material. It is used along with nutmeg in most cases. The mace is also sold under the name *flower of the nutmeg tree* (Ratsch, 1997).

Nutmeg has been used in most of the world for its stimulating effect, for its love-inciting property and as an aphrodisiac due to myristicin in its essential oil. The bigger fruits are preferred for medicinal purposes. Ingestion of several teaspoons of nutmeg can give mild hallucinogenic experiences, perceptual distortions, euphoria, mild visual hallucinations and a feeling of unreality. The active compounds myristicin and elimicin are somewhat like mescaline in action. Myristicin was the starting point for the love drug MDA or ecstasy. It appears to be transformed *in vivo* into highly active amphetamine derivatives (Ratsch, 1997).

USES IN FOLKLORE AND AYURVEDA

The tree is not a native of India but both mace and nutmeg are frequently mentioned in Ayurvedic literature. It is said to have saffron-like activity. According to Ayurveda, nutmeg is bitter, pungent, hot in effect, pleasant, light, digestant, anti-*kaph* and anti-*vata*. It helps bronchial troubles, nausea, vomiting and heart troubles. It is used in delirium tremens, insomnia and senile debility.

Being strong and hot in nature, it has a special effect on the nervous system and thus helps in sexual inadequacies. It has an irritating effect on the mucous membrane.

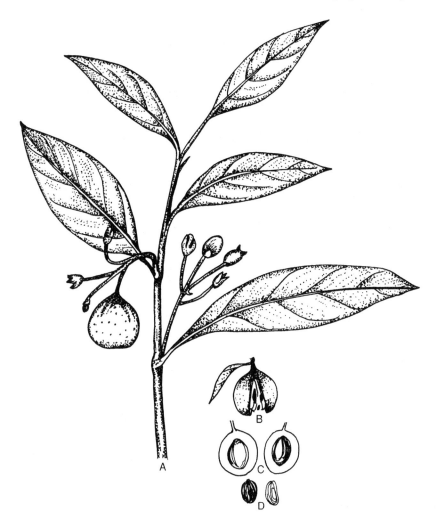

Figure 17 Myristica fragrans **A** twig, **B** fresh fruit cut open to show mace, **C** transection of the fruit, **D** nutmeg.

THERAPEUTIC INDICATIONS AND PHARMACOLOGICAL STUDIES

As a sedative

Bhagwat and Saifi (1980) studied the pharmacological action of volatile oils. It exhibited a sedative and skeletal muscle depressant effect. It produced a direct relaxant effect on the smooth muscles of the intestine, which was comparable to that produced by adrenaline. Shin *et al.* (1988) isolated a hepatic drug metabolism inhibitor from nutmeg. It significantly prolonged hexobarbital-induced sleeping time. Other tests confirmed CNS depressant properties in nutmeg.

Effects on digestive system

Rashid and Misra (1984) observed that the aqueous extract of the seed's paste had a marked inhibitory effect on the antienterotoxigenic effect produced by *Escherichia coli*. Shidore *et al.* (1985) found that the petroleum ether and water extract of nutmeg had anti-diarrhoeal activity, while the petroleum ether extract, when used alone, had anti-inflammatory properties. Chabra and Rao (1994) studied changes in the liver enzymatic system.

Hypolipidaemic effects

Hattori *et al.* (1993) found that mace had an inhibitory effect on lipids. Alpana Ram *et al.* (1996) studied the nutmeg extract for hypolipidaemic effect.

Chemical studies

Mace contains 11–15 per cent essential oil, while nutmeg has 16 per cent. Nutmeg also contains fixed oil 24–30 per cent of fatty oils, known as nutmeg butter (Farrell, 1985).

Toxicological studies

Hallstrom and Thuvander (1997) carried out a toxicological evaluation of myristicin, the major component of nutmeg.

Adulterants

M. malabarica is a large tree, growing in South India. It has fruits bigger than nutmeg but they are not aromatic. Nutmeg is often adulterated or substituted with these seeds.

References

Alpana Ram, Lauria, P., Rajeev Gupta, Sharma, V.N. (1996) Hypolipidemic effect of *Myristica fragrans* fruit extract in rabbits. *Journal of Ethnopharmacology*, 55, 49–53.

Chabra, S.K., Rao, A.R. (1994) Transmammary modulation of xenobiotic enzymes in liver of mouse pups by mace (*Myristica fragrans* Houtt.) *Journal of Ethnopharmacology*, 42, 167–177.

Bhagwat, A.W., Saifi, A.Q. (1980) Observations on the pharmaceutical actions of the volatile oil of *Myristica fragrans* (Houtt). *Journal of Scientific Research* (Bhopal), 20, 183–186.

Farrell, K.T. *Spices, Condiments and Seasoning*. Avi Publishing, Westport, Co., USA 1985.

Hallstrom, H., Thuvander, A. (1997) A toxicological evaluation of myristicin. *Natural Toxins*, 5, 186–192.

Hattori, M., Yang, X.W., Miyashiro, H., Namba, T. (1993) Inhibitory effects of monomeric and dimeric phenylpropanoids from mace on lipid peroxidation in vitro and vivo. *Phytotherapy Research*, 7, 395–401.

Rashid, A., Misra, D.S. (1984) Antienterotoxigenic effect of *Myristica fragrans* (nutmeg) on enterotoxigenic *Escherichia coli*. *Indian Journal of Medical Research*, 79, 694–696.

Ratsch, Christian *Plants of Love. The History of Aphrodisiacs and a Guide to their Identification and Uses*. Ten Speed Press, Berkeley CA, USA 1997.

Shidore, P.P., Majumdar, S.M., Shrotri, D.S., Majumdar, A.M. (1985) Antidiarrhoeal and antiinflammatory activity of nutmeg extracts. *Indian Journal of Pharmaceutical Sciences*, 47, 188–190.

Shin, K.H., Kim, O.N., Woo, W.S. (1988) Isolation of hepatic drug metabolism inhibitors from the seeds of *Myristica fragrans*. *Archives of Pharmacal Research*, 11, 240–243.

26 Kabab Chini

Piper cubeba L f.
Family: Piperaceae

It is also known as *sheetalchini* in commerce. The Sanskrit name is *kankol*.

THE PLANT AND ITS DISTRIBUTION

It grows wild in Borneo, and on the Indonesian islands of Java and Sumatra. It is cultivated in Sri Lanka and in some parts of Karnataka, in south India. It is a perennial, woody, evergreen creeper (Fig. 18A) with conspicuous nodes. The leaves are round to cordate, lanceolate, smooth, leathery, shining, glabrous, 15 cm long, with conspicuous vein islets. The flower is inconspicuous in 2.5 to 5 cm long bunches. The fruit is round like black pepper (Fig. 18B) 3–6 mm broad, with a brown to dark brown pericarp, coarsely reticulate. The fruit has a strong aroma, and characteristically pungent taste. The fruit is collected when fully developed but unripe.

USES IN FOLKLORE AND AYURVEDA

The drug of commerce is like black pepper. It is round, wrinkled, black with a small stalk at one end. When chewed it imparts an aroma and a cooling sensation like that of peppermint. Because of this characteristic it is called *sheetal*, which means cooling. It is bitter and pungent, sometimes used alone but often with *P. betle* leaves or other ingredients. It is said to increase the sex drive. Cubeba cigarettes are made by taking two parts *P. cubeba*, 1 part *Datura* leaves, 1 part peppermint leaves, and are used as a mild aphrodisiac and also in acute or chronic bronchitis. A medicated wine can also be prepared by immersing crushed seed in white wine (Ratsch, 1997).

In Ayurveda, it is considered a stimulant, digestive, diuretic and cardiotonic, having hot effect on the body. It has a strong antiseptic action, so it is used for venereal diseases. The seed's paste is applied to aches, pains, and inflammation. The oil distilled from the seed is applied as an antiseptic to wounds. It is particularly useful for mouth and throat infections.

In western medicine, it was earlier used for gonorrhoea, urethritis, vesical irritability, cystitis, prostate gland, abscesses, piles, chronic bronchitis and catarrh (Culbreth, 1927). The dose was 4–5 g powder and 5–20 drops oil.

It is also used as follows:

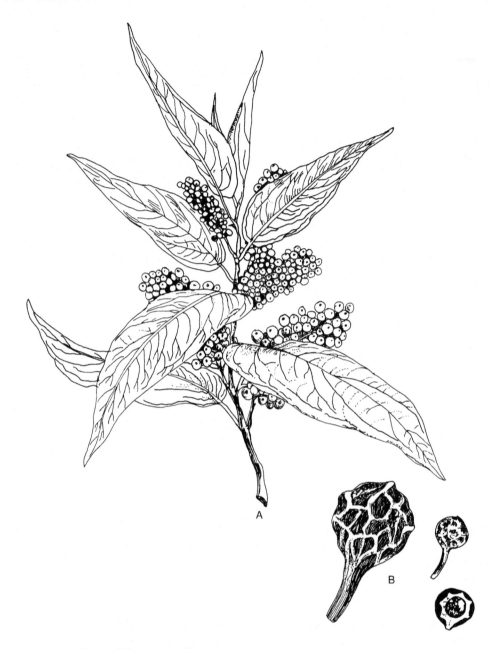

Figure 18 Piper cubeba **A** twig, **B** seed.

As an aphrodisiac

It is an ingredient of aphrodisiac preparations made with *Withania, Mucuna, Orchis* in the form of a candy.

For chronic syphilis

I. Mix powders of *kabab chini* (100 g), sodium bicarbonate (100 g) and alum (50 g). Take one teaspoonful twice daily with yogurt.

II. To one cup of boiling water, add one teaspoonful of *kabab chini* to make an infusion. When warm add 5 drops of *Santalum album* oil to this infusion. This preparation has a diuretic and an antiinflammatory effect.

For urethritis

Take 5 g of fine powder with sugar. Avoid fried, spicy food.

For piles

Take half a spoon of the herb twice daily with milk.

For chronic bronchitis

Mix a teaspoonful of fine powder of herb in honey.

For spermatorrhoea

Make a fine powder of 10 g each of *kabab chini*, cardamom seed, bamboo manna and long pepper. Add 40 g of sugar to it. Take half teaspoon twice daily with milk.

Ayurvedic preparation

Dhatu paushtik churn

Method   Make a fine powder of 10 g each of *kabab chini*, *shatawari*, *gokshru*, bamboo manna, *Sida cordifolia* seed, *Polygonum aviculare*, *Smilax chinesis*, processed *Mucuna* seed, long pepper, *vidarikand* and *Withania*. To this add 60 g of fine *Operculina turpethum* powder and 200 g sugar, and make a homogenous mixture.

Dose   One spoon twice daily with milk for 2–3 months. Avoid spicy and fried food.

Use   For making the body strong so as to have thick and viscous semen. It helps impotence, premature ejaculation, spermatorrhoea and in other sexual inadequacies.

Chemical studies

12–20 per cent essential oil, 6.4 to 8.5 per cent oleoresin, 3 to 4 per cent cubebin. Cubebol and cubic acid have been isolated from the seed.

Toxicological studies

It may cause headaches, giddiness, nausea, purging and paralysis. It is excreted by the bronchial mucous membrane, skin and kidneys and imparts a peculiar colour to urine.

References

Culbreth, D.M.R. *A Manual of Materia Medica and Pharmacology*. Lea and Febiger, Philadelphia, USA 1927.

Ratsch, Christian *Plants of Love. The History of Aphrodisiacs and a Guide to their Identification and Uses*. Ten Speed Press, Berkeley, CA, USA 1997.

27 Kalmegh

Andrographis paniculata (Burm. f.) Wall. ex Nees.
Family: Acanthaceae

THE PLANT AND ITS DISTRIBUTION

It grows wild as an under-shrub in tropical, moist deciduous forests of India.

It is an annual herb or small shrub, branches are sharply quadrangular, often narrowly winged towards the apical region. Leaves are petiolate, 5–8 cm long, lanceolate and acute. Flowers are small, solitary in panicle (Fig. 19). Fruits are 20 mm long, 3 mm wide, linear oblong acute at both ends. Seed are numerous, yellowish brown and glabrous.

USES IN FOLKLORE AND AYURVEDA

At one time many *Swertia* spp. (Indian name *chirayta*) were well esteemed as bitter tonics. These herbs grew in the temperate Himalayas, but because of over-exploitation these plants became scarce and hence expensive. *Andrographis* which has widespread distribution in India, was found to be a good substitute for *Swertia*, and it became popular as *Hara* (green) *chirayta*. It is well known as *kalmegh* in Ayurveda and sometimes as *kirayta*. It is sold as such in dry form; sometimes the leaves get separated, exposing the black twigs. Its main uses are as follows:

As a febrifuge

The herb is a bitter tonic and a febrifuge. It was included in the earlier editions of Indian pharmacopoeia. In Bengal (an Indian State), a preparation called *Alui* is prepared by taking powder of cumin and the seed of *Amomum subulatum* in the juice of this herb. *Alui* is prescribed for malaria.

For the digestive system

It encourages appetite and aids digestion. It is also used in dysentery, as an anthelmintic, stomachic, a liver stimulant, choleretic, cholagaogue, for jaundice, hepatotoxicity, etc. Decoction of the herb has been used for sluggish liver and in a certain form of

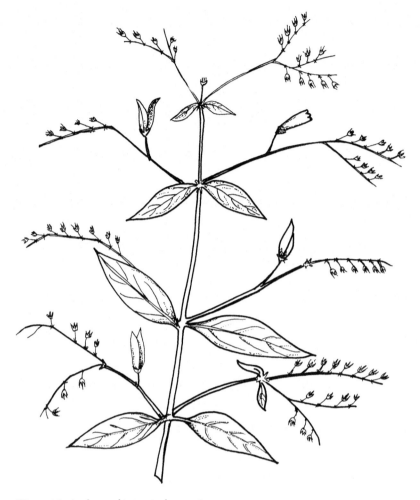

Figure 19 Andrographis paniculata twig.

dyspepsia, associated with gaseous distension. For children suffering from liver torpidity a dose of 5 g of the herb twice daily is adequate until cured

THERAPEUTIC INDICATIONS AND PHARMACOLOGICAL STUDIES

Anti-allergic activity

The bitter principles andrographolide and neoandrographolide showed significant anti-PCA (passive cutaneous anaphylaxis) and mast cell stabilizing activities. These activities were comparable to that of cromoglycate (Gupta *et al.* 1998). Madav *et al.* (1998) confirmed the anti-allergic activity of andrographolide. This compound significantly decreased degranulation of rat mast cells and reduced its liberation.

Effect on the liver

The action of the herb is entirely on gustatory nerves, resulting in increased flows of saliva and gastric juices. Handa and Sharma (1990a,b) showed hepatoprotective activity of andrographolides against galactosamine, paracetamol and carbon tetrachloride-induced intoxication in rats. Andrographolides brought about complete normalization of toxin-induced effects. Sarma and Tripathi (1992) found the herb effective in viral hepatitis. Andrographolides produced a significant dose dependent effect, as evidenced by increases in bile flow, bile salts and bile acids (Tripathi and Tripathi, 1991, Shukla *et al.* 1992). Visen *et al.* (1991, 1992) evaluated the hepatoprotective activity of andrographolide. These authors (Visen *et al.* 1992) carried out *in vitro* studies by using andrographolide on primary cultured rat hepatocytes. A curative effect against galactosamine toxicity was found. It protected rat hepatocytes against paracetamol-induced damage. It was more potent than silymarin, a standard hepatoprotective agent obtained from *Silybium marianum*. Pretreatment of rats with andrographolide significantly prevented the toxic effects of paracetamol, as judged by cell viability, certain biochemical markers and altered enzyme levels towards normal, which suggests it acts upon plasma membranes (Visen *et al.* 1993). The herb was effective against anti-human immunodeficiency virus type I (HIV-I) (Otake *et al.* 1995). Alcohol extract of the herb and two of its constituent diterpenes, andrographolide and neoandrographolide, showed significant antihepatotoxic action in *Plasmodium berghei*-induced hepatic damage in *Mastomys natalensis*. These preparations decreased the levels of liver peroxidation production and facilitated the recovery of superoxide dismutase and glycogen (Ramesh Chander *et al.* 1995).

Premila (1995), Bhatt and Bhatt (1996) have reviewed the literature on hepatoprotective effect of *Andrographis in vivo*, in animal studies, *in vitro* assays and in clinical trials.

Anti-ulcerogenic activity

The compound apigenin, isolated from the herb, exhibited dose-dependent anti-ulcer activity in Shay rats, histamine-induced ulcers in guinea pigs and aspirin-induced ulcers in rats (Vishwanathan *et al.* 1981).

Anti-inflammatory activity

In induced oedema, the herb gave a mean inhibition percentage of 65.35 per cent, compared with 76.50 per cent by butazone (Tajudin *et al.* 1983). Madav *et al.* (1995) found analgesic, anti-pyretic and anti-ulcerogenic activity in andrographolides. Madav *et al.* (1996), Shukla *et al.* (1992) noted that the herb had a good effect against all types of inflammatory agents. It also inhibited acetic acid-induced vascular permeability.

Effect on common cold

Hancke *et al.* (1995) observed this herb had a positive effect on common colds and sinusitis, with symptomatic relief and reduced duration of symptoms. There was a reduction in body temperature in 70 of 84 patients. In pharyngo-tonsilitis it was as effective as acetaminophen. It gave relief to all the patient's symptoms (Melchior, 1996/97).

Immunostimulant property

Water extract of the herb caused humoral immune response stimulation and cellular immune response suppression (Sutarjadi *et al.* 1991, Saxena, 1992). It caused significant stimulation of antibodies and delayed hypersensitivity responses to sheep red blood cells in mice. It also stimulated non-specific immune responses. It appears that compounds other than andrographolides in the herb are responsible for this activity (Puri *et al.* 1993).

In cardiac diseases

The herb was found to be an effective anti-thrombogenic agent in treating arterial thrombotic diseases. An anti-platelet aggregation effect on blood samples of volunteers was seen (Huo and Jinzhi, 1989). The flavone extract from the root prevented the formation of thrombi, as well as the development of myocardial infraction in dogs (Zhao and Fang, 1991). *Andrographis* prevented the atherosclerotic arterial stenosis and restenosis after angioplasty. Hypotensive properties in various fractions have been observed (Zhang and Tan, 1997; Wang and Zhao, 1997).

In leukaemia

The methanol extract of *A. paniculata* is reported to cause cell differentiation in mouse myeloid leukaemia cells. To confirm this Matsuda *et al.* (1994) isolated various compounds from this herb. Out of three diterpenoids isolated, two new compounds and andrographolides were found to be active.

CHEMICAL STUDIES

The diterpenoid and sesquiterpenoid compounds have been referred to as andrographolides.

Toxicological studies

When various concentrations of standardized extracts of herb were used for 60 days and evaluated using reproductive organ weight, testicular histology, ultra structural analysis of Leydig's cells and testosterone levels, no testicular toxicity was found (Burgos *et al.* 1997).

References

Bhatt, A.D., Bhatt, N.S. (1996) Indigenous drugs and liver diseases. *Indian Journal of Gastroenterology*, 15, 63–67.

Burgos, R.A., Caballero, E.E., Sanchez, N.S., Schroeder, R.A., Wikman, G.K., Hancke, J.L. (1997) Testicular toxicity assessment of *Andropgraphis paniculata* dried extract in rats. *Journal of Ethnopharmacology*, 58, 219–224.

Gupta, P.P., Tandon, J.S., Patnaik, G.K. (1998) Antiallergic activity of andrographolides isolated from *Andrographis paniculata* (Burm.f) Wall. *Pharmaceutical Biology*, 36, 172–174.

Hancke, J., Burgos, R., Caceres, D., Wikman, G. (1995) A double blind study with a new mono drug Kan Jang: decrease of symptoms and improvement in the recovery from common colds. *Phytotherapy Research*, 9, 559–562.

Handa, S.S., Sharma, A. (1990a) Hepatoprotective activity of andrographolide from *Andrographis paniculata* against carbon tetrachloride. *Indian Journal of Medical Research*, 92B, 276–283.

Handa, S.S., Sharma, A. (1990b) Hepatoprotective activity of andrographolide against galactosamine and paracetamol intoxication in rats. *Indian Journal of Medical Research*, 92B, 284–292.

Huo, T., Jinzhi, T. (1989) Study on antiplatelet aggregation effect of *Andrographis paniculata*. *Chinese Journal of Integrated Traditional and Western Medicine*, 9, 540–542.

Madav, S., Tandon, S.K., Lal, J., Tripathi, H.C. (1996) Anti-inflammatory activity of andrographolide. *Fitoterapia*, 67, 452–458.

Madav, S., Tripathi, H.C., Tandan, S.K., Dinesh Kumar, Lal, J. (1998) Antiallergic activity of andrographolide. *Indian Journal of Pharmaceutical Sciences*, 60, 176–178.

Madav, S., Tripathi, H.C., Tandon, S.K., Mishra, S.K. (1995) Analgesic, antipyretic and antiulcerogenic effects of andrographolide. *Indian Journal of Pharmaceutical Sciences*, 57, 121–125.

Matsuda, T., Kuroyanangi, M., Sugiyama, S., Umehara, K., Ueno, A., Nishi, K. (1994) Cell differentiation-inducing diterpenes from *Andrographis paniculata*. *Chemical and Pharmaceutical Bulletin*, 42, 1216–1225.

Melchior, J., Palm, S., Wikman, G. (1996) Controlled clinical study of standardised *Andrographis paniculata* extract in common cold: a pilot trial. *Phytomedicine*, 3, 314–318.

Otake, T., Mori, H., Morimoto, M., Ueba, N., Sutardjo, S., Kusumoto, I.T., Haitori, M., Namba, T. (1995) Screening of Indonesian plant extracts for anti-human immunodeficiency virus type I (HIV-1) activity. *Phytotherapy Research*, 9, 6–10.

Puri, A., Saxena, R., Saxena, R.P., Saxena, K.C., Srivastava, V. (1993) Immunostimulant agent from *Andrographis paniculata*. *Journal of Natural Products*, 56, 995–999.

Premila, M.S. (1995) Emerging frontier in the era of hepatoprotective herbal drugs. *Indian Journal of Natural Products*, 11, 7.

Ramesh Chander, Srivatava, V., Tandon, J.S., Kapoor, N.K. (1995) Antihepatotoxic activity of diterpenes of *Andrographis paniculata* (Kal-Megh) against *Plasmodium berghei*-induced hepatic damage in *Mastomys natalensis*. *International Journal of Pharmacognosy*, 33, 135–138.

Sarma, R.B.P., Tripathi, S.N. (1992) Effect of Kalamegh and amalkali compounds on viral hepatitis (Koshtha-Shakhashrita Kamala). *Aryavaidyan*, 5, 164–169.

Saxena, K.C. (1992) Immunomodulators from plants and their use in prophylaxis and therapy. *Proceedings 25th Indian Pharmacological Society Conference*, Muzzafarpur, 5–8, December, 1992.

Shukla, B., Visen, P.K.S., Patnaik, G.K., Dhawan, B.N. (1992) Choleretic effect of andrographolide in rats and guinea pigs. *Planta Medica*, 58, 146–149.

Sutarjadi, Santosa, M.H., Bendryman, Dyatmiko, W. (1991) Immunomodulatory activity of Piper betle, *Zingiber aromatica*, *Andrographis paniculata*, *Allium sativum* and *Oldenlandia corymbosa* grown in Indonesia. *Planta Medica*, 57 (supplement 2), p. A 136.

Tajuddin, Shahid, A., Tariq, M. (1983) Anti-inflammatory activity of *Andrographis paniculata* Nees (Chirayata). *Nagarjun*, 27, 13–14.

Tomar, G.S., Tiwari, S.K., Chaturvedi, G.N. (1982) Kalmegh (*Andrographis paniculata*) and its medicinal status. *Nagarjun*, 26, 76–78.

Tripathi, G.S., Tripathi, Y.B. (1991) Chloretic action of andrographolide obtained from *Andrographis paniculata* in rats. *Phytotherapy Research*, 5, 176–178.

Visen, P.K.S., Saraswat, B., Patnaik, G.K., Srimal, R.C., Dhawan, B.N. Curative effect of some hepatoprotective constituents isolated from plants against galactosamine toxicity: In vitro study on primary cultured rat hepatocytes. *Proceedings of 25th Indian Pharmacological Society Conference*, Muzaffarpur, 5–8 December, 1992.

Visen, P.K.S., Shukla, B., Patnaik, G.K., Dhawan, B.N. Evaluation of hepatoprotective activity of andrographolide isolated from the plant *Andrographis paniculata*. *Proceedings of 24th Indian Pharmacological Society Conference*, Ahmedabad, 29–31 December 1991.

Visen, P.K.S., Shukla, B., Patnaik, G.K., Dhawan, B.N. (1993) Andrographolide protects rat hepatocytes against paracetamol-induced damage. *Journal of Ethnopharmacology*, 40, 131–136.

Vishwanathan, S., Kulanthalvel, P., Nazimuddeen, S.K., Gopal Krishnan, V.T., Kameswaran, C. (1981) The effect of apigenin-7, 4'di-O-methyl ether of a flavone from *Andrographis paniculata* on experimentally induced ulcers. *Indian Journal of Pharmaceutical Sciences*, 43, 159.

Wang, D.W., Zhao, H. (1994) Prevention of atherosclerotic arterial stenosis and restenosis after angioplasty with *Andropgraphis paniculata* Nees and fish oil. *Chinese Medical Journal*, 107, 464–470.

Zhang, C.V., Tan, B.K.H. (1997) Mechanism of cardiovascular activity of *Andrographis paniculata* in the anaesthetised rat. *Journal of Ethnopharmacology*, 56, 97–101.

Zhao, H.Y., Fang, W.Y. (1991) Combined traditional Chinese and western medicine, Antithrombotic effects of *Andrographis paniculata* Nees in preventing myocardial infarction. *Chinese Medical Journal*, 104, 770–775.

28 Kawanch

Mucuna pruriens (L.) DC
Syn: *M. pruiens* Bakr.
M. prurita Hook.
Family: Leguminosae

THE PLANT AND ITS DISTRIBUTION

In India the plant's range is from the Himalayan foothills to sub-tropical forests. It is a liana with trifoliate leaves, which may be up to 12 cm long (Fig. 20A). The inflorescence (is) raceme with purple flowers and silky rachis. Pods vary in size and may be up to 7 cm long and 1 cm broad, curved at one end and covered with pale brown to steel grey bristles. These bristles cause intense irritation if touched. During seed collection great care is taken to avoid the pod touching the body. Some collectors burn the outer bristles to separate the seed from the pods, while others pluck the pods using a pair of tongs, store the pod in a thick bag, and separate the seed by beating the bag with a club. The seeds are picked by hand using a glove. Four distinct types of seed – variegated brown (big) (Fig. 20B), white (big) (Fig. 20C) dark brown (intermediate size), black (small) (Fig. 20D) – are available.

USES IN FOLKLORE AND AYURVEDA

As a component of the diet, the beans are soaked in water until they begin to sprout. They are washed in pure water, boiled or ground to form a paste for cooking.

For medicinal purposes, the seeds are not used as such but are mitigated before use, by boiling them in milk and removing the outer seed coat and embryo. The kernel which is obtained is dried and powdered. The milk in which these seeds are boiled is considered poisonous and is discarded. In south India (Shanavaskhan, 1997), seeds are first boiled in a solution of buffalo dung. On cooling, the seed coat and embryo is removed and the resulting kernel is stored in rice gruel, water, yogurt milk or lime juice for ten days. The seed kernels are washed after this treatment, with lime juice and dried in sunlight for three days. The common uses of these mitigated seeds are:

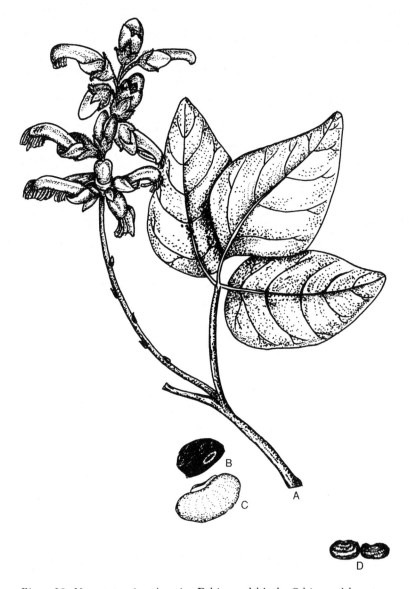

Figure 20 Mucuna pruriens **A** twig, **B** big seed black, **C** big seed brown,
× 3/4, **D** small seed black.

As a dietary supplement

These seeds are considered an aphrodisiac and a nervine tonic. A dietary supplement is
prepared by making small dough cakes of mitigated seeds and milk.

As an aphrodisiac

The seed is used in many aphrodisiac preparations. Some of these are:

1 Pulverize equal quantities of *Chlorophytum arundinaceum*, *Tinospora* starch, *Mucuna*, *Hygrophila*, *Salmalia* root, *Emblica* and sugar. The dose is 5 g, twice daily with milk, for three months.

2 Take 4 kg *Mucuna*, 20 litres cow's milk, 500 g *ghee*, 10 g each of nutmeg, mace, *Piper chaba*, clove, Indian thyme, *Anacyclus pyrethrum*, *Argyreia*, ginger, long pepper, black pepper, *Mesua ferea*, *Cinnamomum* spp. leaves, cinnamon, *Elettaria*, *Callicarpa macrophylla*, *Scindapsus officinalis* and 8 kg sugar. Make a fine powder of all the herbs and spices. Boil *Mucuna* seed in milk until it condenses to a solid mass. Roast this solid mass in *ghee* and add syrup prepared from 8 kg of sugar and mix all the herbs to it. Make candy balls of 20 g each from this mixture. Take one ball in the morning on an empty stomach and a second ball two hours after dinner. It is considered a supreme tonic.

A similar recipe without herbs and spices is called *Banar Gutika* (*Banar* is monkey and *gutika* pill). It is said that monkeys in jungles consume these seeds and remain physically and sexually active all the time.

3 Take 50 g of finely powdered *Asparagus*, *Mucuna*, *Hygrophila*, *Withania*, *Sida spinosa*, *Abutilon* root, 5 litres milk, 500 g *ghee*, with almonds, pistachios, pine nuts and dry grapes as per taste. Treat *Mucuna* seed with milk and *ghee* as above. Add the powdered herbs to the condensed milk and mix in the dry fruits. Make candy balls of 25–30 g each. Eat one ball at breakfast every day.

4 Take 50 g of finely powdered *Withania*, *Blepharis edulis*, *Mucuna*, *Argyreia*, *Tribulus*, *Hygrophila*, *Sida cordifolia* seed, *Abutilon* and mix it with 250 g sugar. This mixture is for middle-aged people, who may take a dose of 10 g mixed in *ghee*, followed by milk, twice daily in the morning before breakfast and two hours after lunch.

5 Pulverize 250 g *Mucuna*, 100 g *Hygrophila*, 350 g sugar and mix. The dose is one teaspoon, twice daily with milk.

6 Pulverize 250 g each of *Mucuna*, *Tribulus* and *Blepharis edulis* and add 400 g sugar. The dose is as above.

7 Pulverize 250 g each of *Mucuna* and *Phaseolus mungo* without their seed coats. Boil 2–3 teaspoons of this powder in 200 ml milk until condensed, cool and take twice daily.

8 Take 100 g each of *Withania*, *Argyreia*, *Cyperus scariosus*, *Mucuna*, *Tribulus*, *Asparagus*, *Triphala*, *Mimusops elengi*, poppy seed, 50 g of bamboo manna, nutmeg, cardamom and 500 g sugar. Make a fine powder of all these items. Use one teaspoon twice daily.

9 Pulverize *Chlorophytum arundinaceum*, *Salmalia* root, *Mucuna*, *Tribulus*, *Emblica* and starch from *Abrus precatorius*. Add the equivalent weight of sugar to that of the herbal powders. Dose: 15 g with 25 g *ghee*.

10 Pulverize 300 g *Mucuna*, 500 g *Tribulus*, 400 g *Piper cubeba*, 300 g *Hygrophila*, 200 g *Mesua ferrea*, 200 g *Chlorophytum*, 200 g *Salmalia* root, 200 g *Curculigo orchioides* and 300 g sugar. Dose: 15 g with milk twice daily.

11 Pulverize equal quantities of *Mucuna*, mace, camphor, *Argyreia*, *Calamus* powders with sugar. Dose: 1 g with milk.

Aphrodisiac for women:

Boil 500 g each of *Mucuna* and *Tribulus* in 4 litres of milk until the milk condenses. Add 1 kg sugar and make candy balls of 15 g each. Dry and steep these balls in honey. Use one ball per day for leucorrhoea, profuse menstruation and other gynaecological problems.

Antidote to *Mucuna* poisoning

If *kawanch* preparations show toxic symptoms, then a mixture of *ghee*, honey and sugar is a good antidote.

THERAPEUTIC INDICATIONS AND PHARMACOLOGICAL STUDIES

The consumption of improperly boiled seed increases body temperature and causes skin eruptions due to L-dopa (L 3,4 dihydroxyphenylalanine). Repeated boiling is known to reduce the L-dopa content and also that of anti-nutritional factors (Janardhanan and Lakshmanan, 1985). Mahajani *et al.* (1996) observed that L-dopa obtained from the seed or synthetic has the same activity. The major studies on the seed are:

In Parkinsonianism

L-dopa or the standardized seed extract can be used (Rajagopalan *et al.* 1978). The patient should start with a daily dose of 250 mg to 1 g of L-dopa, in five divided doses. If side effects occur then reduce the dose, otherwise increase it until intolerable. Improvement may take six months. This treatment controls speech, rigidity and helps swallowing of food. The therapeutic benefits in this disease cannot be ascribed to L-dopa alone. The residue of the seed left after the recovery of L-dopa is also effective.

In anorexia nervosa

Patients with anorexia nervosa improved and gained weight by using the seed.

For haircare

By stimulating hormones, L-dopa helps in the treatment of hyperseborrhoic cases. In patients with psoriasis, the results were excellent after four months' treatment. L-dopa helped in hair growth and development and may turn grey hair black. Hair pigmentation occurred in a white-bearded man after taking L-dopa for 8 months.

Effect on sexual behaviour

By acting on the hypothalamus, L-dopa may arouse sexual interest and cause excessive sexual behaviour. Sambasiva Rao *et al.* (1982) put forth the view that L-dopa facilitated sexual behaviour by increasing brain catecholamine. Saksena and Dikshit (1987) studied the effect of total alkaloids of the seed on spermatogenesis in rats. There was a noteworthy increase in numbers of spermatozoa, weight of testes, seminal vesicles and androgenic activity. Ahmad *et al.* (1991) noted that L-dopa had a stimulant effect at low doses but a depressant effect at high doses.

According to Elisabetsky *et al.* (1992) dopaminergic receptors are involved in male sexual arousal, including the sexual arousal caused by L-dopa. It increased a feeling of vigour, a sense of well-being and increased interest in oneself, family and surroundings. L-dopa stimulated the release of human growth hormones. In some cases, by administering levodopa, hypergrowth of the penis has also been observed. Sriniviasan *et al.* (1994) studied the aphrodisiac activity of the seed on rats. The treatment showed a significant increase in mounting and intermission frequency. Anantha Kumar *et al.* (1994) noted that seed powder, 75mg/kg body weight, increased the sexual activity of male rats considerably. Amin *et al.* (1993, 1993a, 1996) found that the seed improved sexual function, general mating behaviour, libido and potency in normal male rats. It produced a striking and sustained activity in depressed libido and helped in premature ejaculation. Uguru (1997) studied the effect of aqueous seed extract on the guinea pig ileum to determine the drug's mechanism of action. It was found to contain potent histamine receptor stimulants, which led to an influx of calcium and probably stimulated muscarinic receptors.

Ambekar and Khan (1991) tried a compound preparation of *Orchis, Mucuna* and *Alpinia* for its effect on castrated male rats. The compound increased the weight of sexual organs significantly, indicating an anabolic activity.

Anti-ageing effects

Studies on ageing have shown that in mice given near toxic levels of L-dopa, life expectancy increased considerably (personal communication).

Analgesic and anti-pyretic effects

Iauk *et al.* (1993) found that when L-dopa was administered to breast cancer patients, it reduced prolactin concentration to half, with complete relief of metastatic pain. Regression occurred on withdrawal of L-dopa.

It cured migraines but, when the drug was withdrawn, migraines reappeared.

As an anti-depressant

Singh *et al.* (1990) clinically tried this drug on cases of depressive sickness for two months. There was symptomatic improvement, with a decrease in the degree of anxiety and depression.

For healing fractures

Yang (1985) tried L-dopa as a promoter of fracture healing. A dose of 250–500 mg, thrice daily, was given orally for treatment of non-union, delayed union and fresh fractures.

Substitute

The seeds of *Mucuna utilis*, which are bigger than *M. pruriens*, are also used for the same purposes (Ghosh, 1982; Janardhanan and Lakshmanan, 1985).

Chemical studies

Seeds have about 5 per cent oil, 25.3 per cent protein and L-dopa. On boiling, L-dopa gets reduced but other constituents – glutathione, lecithin, alkaloids, gallic acid, seratonin – are heat stable.

Toxicological studies

It causes nausea, anorexia, vomiting and hypotensive palpitation. Involuntary movements are very common, along with abnormal limb movements. The seeds should be used with caution in glaucoma, cardiovascular, endocrine, hepatic, pulmonary, renal diseases, and in psychiatric disturbances. Expectant and nursing mothers should not use any preparations of these seed.

References

Ahmad, S., Taiyab, M., Amin, K.M.Y. Study of the activity of low and high doses of Tukhame-e-Konch (Mucuna pruriens) on CNS. *Conference of Pharmacology and Symposium on Herbal Drugs*, New Delhi, India, 15 March 1991.

Amin, K.M.Y., Khan, N.A., Rahman, S.Z. (1993) The sexual function improving effect of Tukhm-e-Konch (*Mucuna pruriens*) and its mechanism of action: An experimental study. *Proceedings of 1st National Seminar on Ilumal Advia*, Beenapara, India, 23–25 April 1993.

Amin, K.M.Y., Khan, N.A., Saleem, A.M. (1993a) The effect of Frah-E-Zilli, a herbal Unani drug, on male sexual function. *Proceedings of National Seminar on History of Unani Medicine in India*, New Delhi, India. 16–17 April 1993.

Amin, K.M.Y., Khan, M.N., Zilur-Rehman, S., Khan, N.A. (1996) Sexual function improving effect of *Mucuna pruriens* in sexually normal male rats. *Fitoterapia*, 67, 53–58.

Ambekar, M.S., Khan, N.A. (1991) Effect of a compound Unani drug on accessary reproductive organs of male rats. *Conference of Pharmacology and Symposium on Herbal Drugs*, New Delhi, India, 15 March 1991.

Anantha Kumar, K.V., Srinivasan, K.K., Shanbag, T., Rao, S.G. (1994) Aphrodisiac activity of the seeds of *Mucuna pruriens. Indian Drugs*, 31, 321–327.

Elisabetsky, E., Figueiredo, W., Oliveria, G, (1992) Traditional Amazonian nerve tonics as antidepressant agents: *Chaunochiton kappler*: a case study. *Journal of Herbs, Spices and Medicinal Plants*, 1, 125–162.

Ghosh, G. (1982) A note on pharmacognostic and chemical identification of *Mucuna utilis* seed, a substitute of *Mucuna pruriens. Indian Drugs*, 20, 24–25.

Iauk, I., Galati, E.M., Kirjavainen, S., Forestieri, A.M., Trovato, A., (1993) Analgesic and antipyretic effects of *Mucuna pruriens. International Journal of Pharmacognosy*, 31, 213–216.

Janardhanan, K., Lakshmanan, K.K. (1985) Studies on the pulse, *Mucuna utilis*: Chemical composition and antinutritional factors. *Journal of Food Science and Technology*, 22, 369–371.

Mahajani, S.S., Doshi, V.J., Parikh, K.M., Manyam, B. (1996) Bioavailability of L-Dopa from HP-200: a formulation of seed powder of *Mucuna pruriens* (Bak): a pharmacokinetics and pharmacodynamic study. *Phytotherapy Research*, 10, 245–256.

Rajagopalan, T.G., Antarkar, D.S., Purohit, A.V., Wadia, N.H. Treatment of Parkinson's disease with the cowhage plant: *Mucuna pruriens* Bak. *Symposium on Life and Health Science*, Bharat Vidya Bhawan, New Delhi, India 1978.

Saksena, S., Dixit, V.K. (1987) Role of total alkaloids of *Mucuna pruriens* Baker in spermatogenesis in albino rats. *Indian Journal of Natural Products*, 3, 3–7.

Sambasivarao, K., Tripathi, H.C., Jawahar, Lal, Gupta, P.K. (1982) Influence of drugs on male sex behaviour and its pharmacological aspects: A mini review. *Indian Drugs*, 19, 133–139.

Shanavaskhan, A.E., Binu, S., Unnithan, M.D., Santhoshkumar, E.S. Pushpangandan, P. (1997) Detoxification techniques of traditional physicians of Kerala, India on some toxic herbal drugs. *Fitoterapia*, 68, 69–74.

Singh, R.H., Nath, S.K., Behere, P.B. (1990) Depressive illness as a therapeutic evaluation with herbal drugs. *Journal of Research in Ayurveda and Siddha*, 11, 1–6.

Srinivasan, K.K., Anant Kumar, K.V., Gurumadhava Rao, S. Aphrodisiac activity of the seeds of *Mucuna pruriens* (abstract). *Proceedings of 46th Annual Indian Pharmaceutical Congress*, Chandigarh, 28–30 December, 1994.

Uguru, M.O., Aguiyi, J.C., Gosa, A.A. (1997) Mechanism of action of the aqueous seed extract of *Mucuna pruriens* on the guinea pig ileum. *Phytotherapy Research*, 11, 328–329.

Yang, H. (1985) L-dopa extracted from seeds of *Mucuna sempervirens* Hemsl., as a promoter of fracture healing. *Chinese Journal of Integrated Traditional and Western Medicine*, 5, 398–401.

29 Keshar

Crocus sativus L.
Family: Iridiaceae

THE PLANT AND ITS DISTRIBUTION

English "saffron" is derived from Persian *zafran*. It is mainly cultivated in Spain, France, Iran, Turkey and Italy. In India it is only grown in small areas near Srinagar in Kashmir and in Kishtwar of the Jammu region. Most saffron in India is imported from Europe, but that from Kashmir is considered the best.

In Kashmir, saffron cultivation starts in the late summer with the transplanting of the bulbs on the raised beds. The saffron flower (Fig. 21A) is purple in colour and blooms October–November. Three long styles (Fig. 21B), each with a distinct stigma, are picked from flowers by hand. Eighteen thousand flowers yield 28 g of saffron. The stigmas give the finest quality saffron which in Indian trade is called *Shahi Zafran*, the styles give the second grade and the saffron is called *Mongra Zafran*. The third grade is *Laccha Zafran* obtained from the remains of the flowers by cudgelling and winnowing them in water. By this process the petals float on the water while the other essential parts settle. This process is repeated three times to get *Laccha Zafran*. In the western countries saffron is also sold in powder form but this is considered inferior.

Saffron is the most expensive of all the spices. Commercial samples are thread-like, consisting of orange-red strands, trumpet in shape, 1–2 cm long. It is highly aromatic and bitter in taste. It is adulterated with the style, anther and corolla of saffron flowers, or with the floral parts of safflower (*Carthamus*) or marigold (*Tagetes* or *Calendula*), or with vegetable parts coloured with coal tar dyes. The stigma may be soaked in glycerin, sugar syrup or salt solution to give it a shine and to increase its weight. When a pinch of a genuine sample is placed on the surface of warm water, the stigma expands immediately and the colour spreads out slowly, whereas with artificially coloured materials it diffuses immediately (Madan *et al.* 1966). When dipped in ethanol, genuine saffron exudes colour without getting discoloured itself, whereas when using adulterated saffron the coloured materials are bleached after a while. The characteristic smell of saffron is produced on drying when picrocin, the bitter constituent, splits, releasing the volatile safranal.

For use in medicine dried saffron is required. Saffron is dried by placing it on a metallic plate. A metallic cup is heated and saffron from the plate is covered over with this hot cup. When the cup gets cold, the saffron is removed and is stored in airtight bottles.

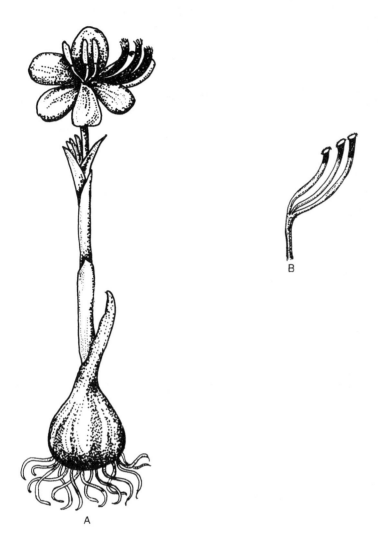

Figure 21   Crocus sativus **A** herb, **B** stigma (diagrammatic).

USES IN FOLKLORE AND AYURVEDA

In Ayurveda, saffron is considered bitter and anodyne. It vitiates the three *doshas* and helps diseases of the head. In the Greco-Arabic system (Unani medicine) saffron is used for slimming, enlarged livers, urinary, bladder and kidney infections, menstrual disorders, for strengthening the heart and cooling the brain. With *ghee*, it is said to help diabetes.

In traditional Chinese medicine it is used as an anodyne, sedative and emmenagogue (Sugiura *et al.*, 1995). It is said to make erogenous zones more sensitive and also has a hormone-like effect, which may be due to carotenoids (crocin and crocetin) contained in it. Other uses are:

In gynaecological practices

1 In painful menstruation and for regulating menstrual flow
   a A pellet of saffron kept in the uterus helps.
   b 250 mg saffron, triturated with half the amount of camphor, is prescribed three days before menstruation until the bleeding stops. Continue this treatment for six monthly periods.
2 In dysmenorrhoea, 4–5 pieces of saffron are given daily with goat's milk.
3 For pain in the uterus during pregnancy, 4–5 pieces with 20 g butter and 5 g sugar is given. The treatment is repeated every two hours until the pain subsides.

In paediatrics

For running noses of infants, give milk with one piece of saffron.

As a general tonic

Four to five stigmas of saffron are wrapped in a leaf of *Piper betle*. The leaf is then chewed. This is done every day throughout the winter.

In impotence

The essential oil contained in saffron produces an aphrodisiac effect due to slight stimulation of the central nervous system. In sexual debility, it is considered a sovereign remedy unsurpassed by the whole range of drugs in materia medica (Trivedi, 1997). It may be used as follows:

1. A mixture of 1 g saffron, 10 g mace and 10 g nutmeg is pulverized. Two grams of this mixture is taken daily for at least 60 days.
2. Boil 500 ml of milk with four dates, until the milk is reduced to half. Add 5–6 pieces of saffron and sugar to taste. Chew this milk for half an hour before retiring to bed every evening.

As a nerve tonic

It has an anti-inflammatory effect. It is also used for melancholia and neuralgia and rheumatic pains. For this, make a fine powder of 10 g each of saffron, senna, colchicum root and sugar. Take 125 mg of this mixture with water, twice daily.

Antidote to poisons

Used for both extraneous and internal toxins (Krishnamurthy, 1993).

Ayurvedic preparation

Ksheer pak

Ingredients   20 g saffron, 2 litres milk, 10 g of finely powdered *Orchis*, *Mucuna*, nutmeg, mace, *Argyreia*, long pepper, *Anacyclus*, processed iron and mica compounds, with 5 g *Makardhawaj* (red sulphide of mercury).

Method   Boil the saffron in milk, until the milk is concentrated into a semi-solid mass. Mix the fine powders of herbs and minerals in this concentrated milk and make the whole mass homogenous. Sprinkle very fine powdered *Makardhawaj* over this finished product and mix thoroughly.

Dose   Half teaspoonful twice daily for 60 days in winter.

THERAPEUTIC INDICATIONS AND PHARMACOLOGICAL STUDIES

Anti-cancerous activity

Nair *et al.* (1994) studied the effects of saffron on solid tumour growth in rats. Oral administration of 100 mg/kg of the saffron extract inhibited Dalton's lymphoma ascites (DLA) and S-180 solid tumours by 87 per cent and 41 per cent respectively. A dose of 150 mg delayed the onset of tumour formation and inhibited its further growth. Saffron also caused an increase in vitamin A and carotene levels in the serum of 180 tumour-bearing mice. The activity of saffron was due to crocin, which probably-induced the anti-tumour effect by its provitamin A activity and/or by antioxidant activity or by modulating the functional levels of the other antioxidants. Escribano *et al.* (1996) also observed that crocin, safranal and picrocrocin inhibited the growth of human cancer cells *in vitro*. Cells treated with crocin exhibited wide cytoplasmic vacuole-like areas, reduced cytoplasm, cell shrinkage and pyknotic nuclei. Saffron extract inhibited or prevented cancer and its pigments were used to treat papilloma, hypertension, spinal cord injury, cerebral oedema, arthritis and aflatoxin-induced hepatotoxic lesions (Dufresne *et al.* 1997). Konoshima *et al.* (1998) noted that crocin and crocetin derivatives and 50 per cent ethanol extract of saffron significantly inhibited Epstein-Barr virus early antigen activation, and mouse skin papilloma.

In heart problems

Due to crocetin, saffron indirectly reduced cholesterol levels in the blood (Baker and Negbi, 1983). Nishio (1987) noted that it showed a remarkable effect on blood coagulation and platelet aggregation. It accelerated the *in vitro* fibrinolysis activity of urikinase.

Immunomodulatory effect

Nair *et al.* (1991) observed that it had a modulatory effect on cisplatin-induced toxicity in mice. The saffron extract prevented the decrease in body weight, haemoglobin levels and leucocyte counts caused by 2 mg/kg of cisplatin. Saffron prolonged the life-span also.

Review

Rios (1996) has reviewed the literature on chemical composition and pharmacological properties of saffron between 1925–1994. The active constituents have shown anti-tumour, hypolipidaemic and tissue oxygenation enhancement properties.

Chemical studies

From saffron, 1.37 per cent essential oils, 13.45 per cent fixed oil, crocin (a natural carotenoid), picrocin and many other compounds have been reported. Genuine saffron has the colour of crocin, the aroma of safranal and the flavour of picrocrocin. The more intense the colouring, the better the saffron is.

Toxicological studies

In large doses it can be toxic, narcotic and even lethal, causing violet haemorrhages. Do not use saffron during pregnancy.

Substitute

In Italy, *C. longiflorus* also yields a saffron-like material. In this case the stigmas have a high dyeing power but less odour and bitterness (Casoria *et al.* 1996).

Ayurvedic substitutes

Nagkesar is the commonest substitute, obtained from the stamens of *Mesua ferrea*, *Ochrocarpus longifolius*, or *Calophyllum inophyllum*. Yellow *nagkesar* is obtained from buds or stamens of *Michelia champaca*.

The Ayurvedic scholars are also of the opinion that nutmeg has a saffron-like physiological effect and can be used in its place.

References

Baker, D., Negbi, M. (1983) Uses of saffron. *Economic Botany*, 37, 228–236.

Casoria, P., Laneri, U., Novella, N. (1996) A preliminary note on an interesting species of Crocus (*Crocus longiflorus*, Iridaceae) similar to saffron (*C. sativus*). *Economic Botany*, 50, 463–464.

Dufresne, C., Cormier, F., Dorion, S. (1997) In vitro formation of crocetin glucosyl esters by *Crocus sativus* callus extract. *Planta Medica*, 63, 150–153.

Escribano, J. Alonso, G.L., Coca-Prados, M., Fernandex, J.A. (1996) Crocin, safranal and picrocrocin from saffron (*Crocus sativus* L.) inhibit the growth of human cancer cell *in vitro*. *Cancer Letters*, 100 (1/2), 23–30.

Konoshima, T., Takasaki, M.M., Tokuda, H., Morimoto, S., Tanaka, H., Kwata, E., Xuan, L.J., Saito, H., Sugiura, M., Molnar, J., Shoyama, Y. (1998) Crocin and crocetin derivatives inhibit skin tumour promotion in mice. *Phytotherapy Research*, 12, 400–404.

Krishnamurthy, K.H. *Khas, Kesar, Nagkesar, Khaskhash*. Books for All, Delhi, India 1993.

Madan, C.L., Kapur, B.M., Gupta, U.S. (1966) Saffron. *Economic Botany*, 20, 377.

Nair, S.C., Salami, M.J., Panikkar, B., Panikkar, K.R. (1991) Modulatory effects of *Crocus sativus* and *Nigella sativa* extracts on cisplatin-induced toxicity in mice. *Journal of Ethnopharmacology*, 31, 75–83.

Nair, S.C., Varghese, C.D., Panikkar, K.R., Kurumboor, S.K., Parathod, R.K. (1994) Effects of saffron on vitamin A levels and its antitumour activity on the growth of solid tumours in mice. *International Journal of Pharmacognosy*, 32, 105–114.

Nishio, T., Okugawa, H., Kato, A., Hashimoto, Y., Matsumoto, K., Fujioka, A. (1987) Effect of Crocus (*Crocus sativus* Linn, Iridaceae) on blood coagulation and fibrinolysis. *Shoyakugaku Zasshi* (in Japanese), 41, 271–276.

Rios, J.L., Recio, M.C., Giner, R.M., Manez, S. (1996) An update of saffron and its active constituents. *Phytotherapy Research*, 10, 189–193.

Sugiura, M., Saito, H., Abe, K., Shoyma, Y. (1995) Ethanol extract of *Crocus sativus* L. antagonizes the inhibitory action of ethanol on hippocampl long term potentiation in vivo. *Phytotherapy Research*, 9, 100–104.

Trivedi, Madhuchandrika A best aphrodisiac, saffron. *Nirogadham* (in Hindi), October–December, 1997.

30 Kikar

Acacia nilotica (L.)Willd. ssp. *indica* (Benth.) Bre.
Syn: *A. arbica* Willd.
Family: Leguminosae

THE PLANT AND ITS DISTRIBUTION

The tree is common in arid zones of India. It can easily be identified by its dark coloured bark, bipinnate leaves and its spines, about 2 cm long at the base of the leaves (Fig. 22A). The inflorescence is yellow, globular and up to 2 cm in diameter. Pods are 15 cm long with 8–12 seeds. The tree yields a translucent gum, yellow to brown in colour, known as gum arabica, which resembles gum acacia obtained from *A. senegal* Willd. (Fig. 22B) in its physical properties.

USES IN FOLKLORE AND AYURVEDA

Gum arabica is a well known household item in the northwest part of India and is considered quite nutritive. It is mainly used after frying in *ghee*. The unripe pods are also well esteemed. They may be used as dry powder or in the form of a thick translucent sheet of dry juice extracted from the fresh pods.

As per Ayurveda, all parts of the tree provide energy to the body. *Kikar* is dry, heavy, astringent, cooling and helps in *kapha* and *pitta*. Gum is diuretic, astringent and helps ulcers of the buccal cavity, dry coughs, dryness and inflammation of the throat. Tender pods are astringent, used in various sexual deficiencies. They are anti-leprotic, anthelmintic, blood purifiers, healers of wound and vaso-constrictors. (All these properties may be due to tannins, which have an astringent effect.) The uses of the tree, some of which are as per Saxena Parvar (1998), are as follows:

As a general tonic

Fry the gum in *ghee* and dip it in the sugar syrup. Two to three teaspoons of this mixture, when taken daily, makes the body strong and healthy. It is also good for mental powers and virility. In another recipe, the legume *Phaseolus mungo* is soaked in water over night to remove the seed coat. The resulting seed kernel is ground to form a thick paste, which is then fried in *ghee*. When the paste turns brown, sugar syrup is

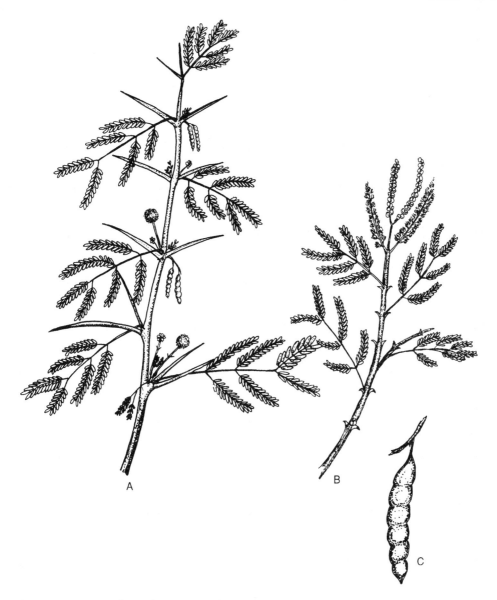

Figure 22 Acacia nilotica **A** twig, **C** pod, **B** *A. senegal* twig.

added and the whole mass is stirred until thick in consistency. To this mass, gum arabica and dry fruits are added as per taste and availability, and when hot, the whole mass is made into candy balls of 50–250 g each. The dose is as per the digestive power of the individual.

For bronchial troubles

The gum soothes the throat through its mucilaginous action, and coagulates any blood in the sputum.

For urinogenital diseases

1   Slightly heat 25 g each of gum arabica, gum tragacanth, gum kino (*Butea frondosa*), gum *mastagi roomi* (*Pistacia lentiscus*) and make a fine powder. One teaspoon of this powder with cold water may be taken twice daily for nocturnal emission.

2   When equal parts of dry leaves, bark, flowers and the gum of this tree are powdered and administered, it increases the viscosity of spermatic fluid and helps in other urinogenital diseases.

3   For venereal diseases, if pus and blood are passed through the urethra, make decoction of gum and tender leaves of acacia, sugar and black pepper. Drink 10 ml of this decoction, and douche the urethra with this solution.

4   For syphilis, steep 35 g of young tree buds in water for the night. In the morning macerate these buds by hand to form a thick infusion. Drink this infusion with 25 g of warm *ghee*. Repeat this treatment for 2–3 days or more, but for a week after that do not add *ghee* and drink the infusion only.

5   For urinary troubles, in summer, particularly in arid zones, the urine may become scanty because of lack of water in the body and may cause burning sensation during urination. In this situation gum arabica mucilage is prescribed for drinking, and the patient is advised to eat three to four dry acacia pods every day.

6   For scanty urine in the summer, 5 g of a fine powder made from equal quantities of dry, tender *kikar* and *Tribulus* fruit leaves is prescribed twice daily with milk. An infusion of tender pods may also be used.

For gynaecological problems

1   One dessertspoonful of finely powdered gum is fried in an equal quantity of *ghee*, and a cup of water and sugar are added as per taste, followed by a pinch of cardamom seed. This mixture is taken on an empty stomach in the morning. It is a tasty, nutritious preparation and, if consumed after menstruation, brings about contraction of uterus, vagina, and prevents leucorrhoea.

2   In leucorrhoea, a decoction of the bark with or with out alum is used for douching.

3   Two grams of equal quantities of powdered dry pod, gum and bark cures leucorrhoea and backache when given three times a day with milk or water.

4   A small piece of dry juice from the pods, if inserted in the vagina, acts as an anti-inflammatory agent. It also removes sluggishness of the muscles and brings about vaginal contractions.

5   Gum arabica fried in *ghee*, provides energy to both embryo and the mother when administered to an expectant mother.

6   A mixture of 3 g gum arabica with 3 g wheat flour helps excessive bleeding during menstruation.

For anal and vaginal prolapse

Boil acacia bark in water until reduced to one-fourth. Soak muslin in this decoction and insert it in the required place. The remaining decoction may be used for enema and douching.

For diarrhoea and dysentery

Soak small quantity of leaves and gum of *Acacia* tree in water and filter them after maceration. Prescribe two teaspoon of this filtrate every two hours. Gum alone may also be used. It provides nutrition to stomach and alimentary canal. The powder of tender leaves also helps gastroenteritis.

As an anabolic agent

Take 200 g almond kernel, 50 g gum arabica and 250 g raw sugar. Soak almond in water overnight, remove the seed coat in the morning, dry the kernel and make a fine powder. Fry gum arabica in a minimum quantity of *ghee* and make a fine powder. Mix the powders of almond, gum and sugar to the fried gum. Take 10 g of this mixture for 2–3 months with milk, twice daily, before breakfast and after dinner.

For eczema

Boil 25 g each of acacia and mango bark in 1 litre of water and foment the affected part with water vapours, followed by an application of *ghee*.

As a rejuvenator

Five grams of dry juice, when given with milk, helps the sexual power of weak, old and convalescent patients.

Ayurvedic preparations

Veerya shodhan churn

Method   Pulverize equal quantities of tender pods, tender leaves and gum arabica and mix them in an equal quantity of sugar.

Dose   10 g with milk, once or twice daily.

Use   Spermatogenic, increases the quantity and improves the quality of semen. Helps in all types of sexual inadequacy. Should be used for minimum of sixty days.

Rativallabh pak

Method   Take 500 g gum arabica, 100 g ginger, 100 g each of long pepper (fruit and root), 25 g clove, 25 g nutmeg, 25 g mace, 25 g *Bombax malabaricum* gum, 25 g *shilajit* (a herbomineral compound of natural origin), 10 g black pepper, 10 g cinnamon, 10 g *Cinnamomum* spp. leaves, 10 g *Mesua ferrea* flowers, 10 g cardamom seed, 10 g each of processed coral, iron, mica and tin, 5 g saffron, 250 g *ghee*, 2 kg sugar and dry fruits as per taste. Make a fine powder of gum and fry it in *ghee*. Pulverize all other herbs and spices but leave the saffron and minerals to be powdered separately.

Chop the dry fruits, almond, pistachio, dry dates, dry grapes and coconut, etc. Make a very fine powder of saffron and minerals and pass them through a sieve or muslin of mesh size 200. Make a syrup of sugar. To this syrup, when hot, add all the powdered herbs and spices, followed by saffron and minerals, and then dry fruits. Make candy balls of 25 g each from this mixture.

Dose In winter take 25–50 g as per the digestive power of the person. It should be chewed along with warm milk in the morning, when the stomach is empty.

Use A highly nutritious preparation, for the proper sexual life of both males and females. It is of immense use after childbirth; it imparts beauty and health both to the mother and the infant.

THERAPEUTIC INDICATIONS AND PHARMACOLOGICAL STUDIES

Both the bark and pod contain tannin and gallic acid, which help in the removal of catarrhal matter from the bronchi, arrest bleeding, sooth the inflamed pharynx, alimentary canal and urinogenital organs. Gum is useful in glycaemia and cholesterolaemia.

The bark has a hypoglycaemic property. It significantly reduced the blood glucose concentration, by peripheral utilization of glucose (Singhal, 1984).

Toxicological studies

Gum acacia from *A. senegal* was found quite safe as a food item (Anderson, 1986).

References

Anderson D.M.W. (1986) Evidence for the safety of gum arabic (*Acacia senegal.* Willd) as a food additive: a brief review. *Food Additives Contaminants*, 3, 225–230.

Saxena Pravar, S.R. *Herbal Treatment* (in Hindi). Rajasthan Patrika Parkashan, Jaipur, India 1998.

Singhal, P.C. (1984) Role of gum arabica and gum catechu in glycaemia and cholesterolemia. *Current Science*, 53, 91.

31 Kuchla

Strychnos nux vomica L.
Family: Loganiaceae

THE PLANT AND ITS DISTRIBUTION

The tree grows wild in tropical and semi-evergreen forests of central India.

It is a deciduous tree with short spines and thin, grey, smooth bark. Leaves are 7.5–15 cm long, 5–7.5 cm broad, elliptic (Fig. 23A), with numerous greenish white flowers. The fruit is globose, 2.5–7.5 cm and orange when ripe. The seed is (Fig. 23B) discoid concave on one side, convex on the other, up to 2.5 cm in diameter and covered with brown grey, silky hair, radiating from the centre. The seed is leathery and very difficult to powder.

USES IN FOLKLORE AND AYURVEDA

Mitigation of seed

The seed is very bitter and highly poisonous but some people get addicted to it and tolerate the lethal dose. For use in Ayurvedic preparations, it is partially detoxified by any of the following methods:

1 By boiling in equal quantities of milk and water, removing emerging cotyledons (said to be poisonous) when soft. The hot soft kernel turns hard on cooling, so these seed are boiled again until soft enough to pulverize.
2 Cow's urine is used in place of water and the seed is allowed to remain in it for a number of days until soft enough for crushing.
3 The seed is put in clean clay soil and allowed to remain in it until soft.
4 The easiest method for powdering the seed is to heat it in *ghee* in an iron pan over a mild heat until the outer skin of the seed turns red brown. Remove the outer skin and powder the kernel.
5 The seed is turned into dust-like powder using iron files.
6 In south India (Shanvaskhan, 1997) seed are boiled with rice and water for three hours. When they are cooked, after removal of seed coat, they are chopped into

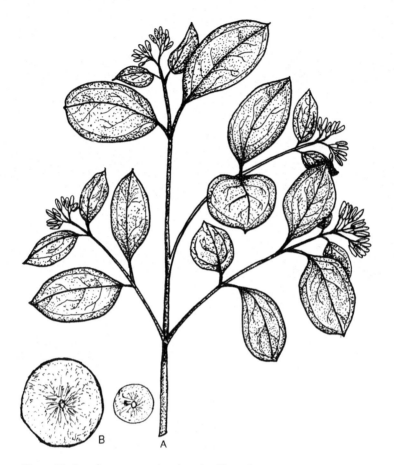

Figure 23 Strychnos nux vomica **A** twig, **B** seed.

small pieces and immersed in the juice of *Chenopodium ambrosiodes* for 3 hours and finally boiled in a decoction of *Semecarpus anacardium* seed.

These mitigation treatments deplete the alkaloid concentration (Agrawal and Joshi, 1977), without changing their composition (Bhanu and Vasudevan, 1977).

A dose of 30–60 mg of mitigated nux vomica is commonly given, sometimes it may be increased to 125 mg, but it may stimulate the heart at this dose and may be lethal.

The major uses of processed nux vomica are:

As an antidote to poisons

It is an antidote to lead poison, rabid dog bites, snakebites and opium overdose.

For wasting diseases

For wasting diseases in infants and children, mitigated nux vomica is given along with powder of dry liver and *kuchla* oil.

As a general stimulant

In Ayurveda, it is considered hot in effect and a stimulant for intellectuals and students, etc. It stimulates the respiratory system, neuromuscular system and makes the heart strong. It also helps lethargy of generative organs.

For the digestive system

For indigestion due to physiological weakness and for constipation, it is a drug of choice. It is used in obesity, as it burns fat from the liver. Nux vomica helps cases of acute gastric disturbance, when the patient's stools are watery, the patient has acute thirst, the stool is blood coloured (as in piles) or if the urge to pass stools and urine persists but regular movement is not there. It strengthens the stomach and digestive system by contractions of the alimentary canal.

For gynaecological problems

It relieves backache, delayed menstruation, dysmenorrhoea and leucorrhoea, when accompanied by yellow, foetid vaginal discharge.

Contraindications

It should be given in the minimum dose to people who live in solitude and get angry easily, and also to patients who have hyperacidity, acute flatulence, urinary incontinence, inflammation of the urethra, burning urination and nasal haemorrhages.

Toxicity

In the case of toxic symptoms, a leaf paste of *Abrus precatorius* along with gruel of arrow root (*Maranta arundinacea*) powder is given.

Ayurvedic preparations

Kuchla oil

Method   Heat 15 g nux vomica seed in 100 ml of sesame oil until seed turns brown, filter and use the oil.

Use   For external application in paralysis and wasting diseases of children. For migraines, make a paste of this oil with equal quantities of cinnamon, or *Piper longum* root, add cow's urine and apply.

Navjovan rasa

Method   Macerate 25 g processed nux vomica, 25 g processed iron, 5 g each of *ras sindur* (red sulphide of mercury), black pepper, long pepper and ginger in ginger juice and make pills of 60 mg each.

Use It is said to rejuvenate the body. It increases gastric juices so food is digested properly and provides strength to the body, nervous system, and stomach. It helps gastric problems, memory, chronic constipation, migraines or pain in any part of the body.

Laxmivillas ras

Method Take 75 g processed nux vomica, 75 g borax, 75 g black pepper, 50 g processed iron, 25 g purified sulphur and 12 g purified mercury. Triturate mercury and sulphur, add the powders of all other ingredients along with juice of ginger, followed by the juices of *Asparagus, Phyllanthus niruri* and *Eclipta* to saturate the mixture. Dry, repeat this process three times and make pills of 60 mg each.

Use As a rejuvenator it helps convalescence, wasting diseases, loss of vitality and spermatic liquid. It is a spermatogenic, makes skin look young and healthy and cures indigestion.

THERAPEUTIC INDICATIONS AND PHARMACOLOGICAL STUDIES

Strychnine stimulates respiratory and vasomotor centres. It has selective action on the central nervous system (CNS), more particularly on bone marrow. Small doses produce vasodilation. By its action on the cerebral cortex and peripheral nerves, it exhibits marked hyperactivity. It remains in the alimentary tract for a long time and exerts its influence on digestive system by gradual absorption.

Furukawa *et al.* (1985) observed that strychnine has direct depressant effect on the heart and inhibits the release of acetylcholine.

Panda and Panda (1993) tested its anti-gastric and anti-ulcer activity and found its effect equivalent to that of cimetidine.

Chemical studies

The seed has 1.8 to 2 per cent of total alkaloids, 42 per cent fatty oil and α-amyrin. The seed ratio of strychnine to brucine varies from 2 : 1 to 1 : 1. It is said that during germination or during treatments with aqueous fluids (mitigation), strychnine disappears whilst brucine, which occurs in the outer cells of the endosperm, is gradually converted into strychnine.

Toxicological studies

Large doses of nux vomica cause tetanic convulsions and eventually death results. Even with safe doses there may be some mental derangement.

References

Agrawal, V.K., Joshi, D. (1977) Effect of purification (Shodhna) on the alkaloidal concentration of kuchla seeds (*Strychnos nux-vomica* Linn). *Journal of Research in Indian Medicine Yoga and Homoeopathy*, 12, 43–45.

Bhanu, M.N., Vasudevan, T.N. (1989) Studies on sodhna of nux-vomica, *Indian Drugs*, 26, 150–152.

Furukawa, Y., Saegusa, K., Chiba, S. (1985) Suppression of strychnine on the two chronotropic and inotropic effects in the isolated blood perfused canine atrium. *Japanese Journal of Pharmacology*, 38, 439–441.

Panda, P.K., Panda, D.P. (1993) Anti-ulcer activity of nux vomica and its comparison with cimetidine in Shay rat. *Indian Drugs*, 30, 53–56.

Shanavaskhan, A.E., Binu, S., Unnithan, M.D., Santhoshkumar, E.S., Pushpagandan, P. (1997) Detoxification techniques of traditional physicians of Kerala, India on some toxic herbal drugs. *Fitoterapia*, 68, 69–74.

32 Kulanjan

Alpinia galanga Willd.
Family: Scitamineae

THE PLANT AND ITS DISTRIBUTION

It is a herb (Fig. 24A) growing in the tropical and sub-tropical areas of south and east India. The rhizome (Fig. 24B), sometimes imported from the Java islands of Indonesia, is reddish brown, cylindrical, about 3 cm in diameter and 4–8 cm long, with raised rings and scars on the leaf bases. Its fracture is hard, taste pungent and odour spicy. In India, it is known as *kulanjan* or *khuljanjan* or as a source of a controversial herb *rasna*. In Europe it is known as greater *galanga*. A closely allied species *A. officinarum* Hance, imported from southeast China, is called lesser *galangal* (Wren, 1975) or *galangol* (Ratsch, 1997).

USES IN FOLKLORE AND AYURVEDA

The Arabian physician Ibn Al-Baytar attributed a love promoting property to the root. It has been used as an aphrodisiac and as an additive to stimulating liquors since the 8th century. In German folk medicine it is also considered a tonic for sexual activities (Ratsch, 1997).

It is an aromatic, stimulant, carminative and expectorant. It is mainly used for bronchial troubles, where small pieces may be chewed, under the name *Pan ki Jar*. (It means root of *pan*, *Piper betle* is a wrong identification, galangal root has no relation with *P. betle*.) Sometimes it is prescribed for impotence and nervous debility, probably because of its vasodilator effect. In Ayurveda it is used in the treatment of various inflammatory diseases, diabetes mellitus and obesity (Achuthan and Padikkala, 1995).

THERAPEUTIC INDICATIONS AND PHARMACOLOGICAL STUDIES

Anti-microbial property

Janssen and Scheiffer (1985) showed that an essential oil from *A. galanga* has activity against gram positive bacteria, yeast and some dermatophytes.

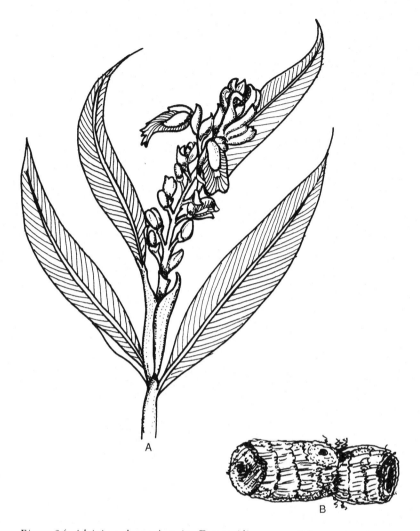

Figure 24 Alpinia galanga **A** twig, **B** root (diagrammatic).

Anti-tumour activity

Itokawa *et al.* (1987) isolated anti-tumour principles from it against Sarcoma 180 ascites in mice. Zheng *et al.* (1993) found two potential anticarcinogens in essential oils. These two isolated compounds exhibited carcinogen detoxification. A new potential chemopreventive agent was also detected.

Anti-ulcer activity

Al-Yahya (1990) observed gastric, anti-secretory, anti-ulcer and cytoprotective properties in the ethanol extract of the root. The extract significantly reduced the intensity of gastric mucosal damage and decreased gastric secretion. It had cytoprotective effect against sodium chloride-induced damage.

Anabolic effects

Weight gain in *A. galanga* treated animals was significantly higher compared with the control. Haematological studies revealed a significant rise in red blood cells and a significant drop in white blood cells. A significant gain in the weight of sexual organs and an increase in sperm motility and sperm count were observed (Quershi *et al.* 1992). Two groups of compounds, identified as gingerols and diarylhepatanoids, were effective against prostaglandin biosynthesizing enzymes (Kiuchi *et al.* 1992).

Anti-hepatotoxic effect

The ethanol extract of this root reversed the cytological and biochemical changes induced by cyclophosphamide in mice liver (Quershi *et al.* 1994). Jung *et al.* (1996) isolated a compound galangin from it, which was effective in induced hepatotoxicity.

In atherosclerosis

Achuthan and Padikkala (1995) studied the ethanol extract for hypolipidaemic activity and following the studies concluded that it might be useful in various lipid disorders especially atherosclerosis.

Chemical studies

The root contains an essential oil, which has 48 per cent methyl cinnamate, 20–30 per cent cineole, camphor and probably d-pinene (Nadkarni, 1976). A flavonoid glangin has also been reported (Jung *et al.* 1996).

Toxicological studies

Quershi *et al.* (1992) did not find any spermatotoxic effects in the root.

Substitutes

Kaempferia galangal is known as *galangal* in Europe. It may be *Kapur kachri* of India (*Hedychium spicatum* is also known by this name). It is an important ingredient of Indonesian *jamu* preparations. These preparations have aphrodisiac, stimulating and psychedelic properties (Ratsch, 1997).

References

Achuthan, C.R., Padikkala, J. (1995) Hypolipidemic effect of *Alpinia galanga* (Rasna) and *Kaempferia galanga* (Kachoor). *Amala Research Bulletin*, 15, 53–56.

Al Yahya, M.A., Rafatutlah, S., Mossa, J.S., Ageel, A.M., Al-Said, M.S., Tariq, M. (1990) Gastric, anti-secretory, anti-ulcer and cytoprotective properties of ethanolic extract of *Alpinia galanga* Wild in rats. *Phytotherapy Research*, 4, 112–114.

Itokawa, H., Morita, H., Sumitomo, T., Totsuka, N., Takeya, K. (1987) Antitumour principles from *Alpinia galanga*. *Planta Medica*, 53, 32–33.

Janssen, A.M., Scheiffer, J.J.C. (1985) Acetoxychavicol acetate, an antifungal component of *Alpinia galanga*. *Planta Medica*, 51, 507–511.

Jung, B.D., Kim, C.H., Kim, J.H., Heo, M.Y. (1996) Protective effect of galangin on carbon tetrachloride-induced hepatotoxicity. *Yakhak Hoeji*, 40, 320–325.

Kiuchi, F., Iwakami, S., Shibuya, M., Hanaoka, F., Sankawa, U. (1992) Inhibition of prostaglandin and leukotriene biosysnthesis by gingerols and diarylheptaniods. *Chemical and Pharmaceutical Bulletin*, 40, 387–391.

Nadkarni, A.K. *Indian Materia Medica*. Vol. I, Popular Prakshan, Bombay, India 1956.

Quershi, S., Shah, A.H., Ageel, A.M. (1992) Toxicity studies on *Alpinia galanga* and *Curcuma longa*. *Planta Medica*, 58, 124–127.

Quershi, S., Shah, A.H., Ahmed, M.M., Rafatullah, S., Bibi, F., Al-Bekairi, A.M. (1994) Effect of *Alpinia galanga* treatment on cytological and biochemical changes induced by cyclophosphamide in mice. *International Journal of Pharmacognosy*, 32, 171–177.

Ratsch, Christian *Plants of Love. The History of Aphrodisiacs and a Guide to their Identification and Use*. Ten Speed Press, Berkeley CA, USA 1997.

Wren, R.C. *Potter's New Cyclopaedia of Botanical Drugs and Preparations*. C.W. Daniel, Essex, England 1975.

Zheng, G.Q., Kenney, P.M., Lam, L.K.T. (1993) Potential anticarcinogenic natural products isolated from lemongrass oil and galanga root oil. *Journal of Agriculture and Food Chemistry*, 41, 153–156.

33 Kutaki

Picrorhiza kurrooa
Syn. *P. kurrooa* Royle ex Benth.
P. scrophulariaeflora
Family: Scrophulariaceae

In Indian literature, the name of this herb is commonly given as *Picrorhiza kurroa* Royle ex Benth. so in the present book this name has been used in place of the valid one, given above.

THE PLANT AND ITS DISTRIBUTION

P. kurrooa grows in the alpine Himalayas of North India, and *P. scrophulariaeflora* in the Eastern Himalayas and Tibet, at an altitude of 3,000–5,000 m. However these species are getting increasingly scarce by the day. The local name of the herb in north India is *kaur*, which means bitter. It is a small hairy herb, with rope-like rootstock, up to 0.5 cm thick, covered with the basis of withered leaves (Fig. 25A,B). Leaves are 5–10 cm long with a rounded tip and may be arranged in a rosette form. The flowering spike, with many flowers, is longer than the leaves.

USES IN FOLKLORE AND AYURVEDA

In Ayurveda, *kutaki* is considered a nutritive in the sense that it increases the appetite by stimulating gastric secretion. Because of its non-nauseating smell and taste, it is an ingredient of many preparations used as liver tonics and appetizers. It is not an astringent so it does not cause constipation. It helps in dyspepsia. It is a laxative in small doses, but cathartic in larger ones. It is commonly prescribed against fevers (*pitta jawar virodhi*), particularly for those patients who have a high temperature, burning sensation all over the body including the eyes, dry mouths with a frequent urge for water, and red eruptions on the skin.

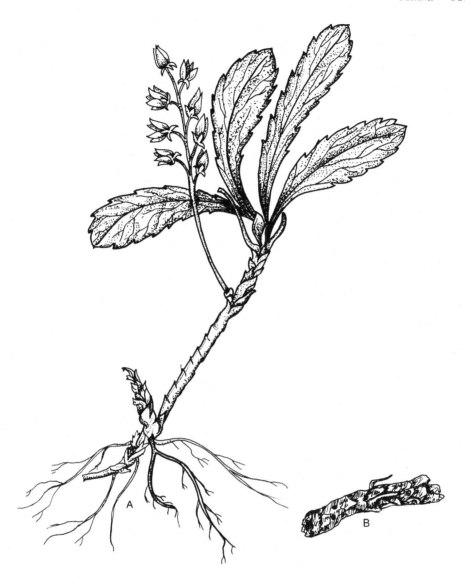

F*igure* 25 *Picrorhiza kurrooa* **A** twig, **B** root.

THERAPEUTIC INDICATIONS AND PHARMACOLOGICAL STUDIES

Both the whole root and Picroliv, as an isolated standardized preparation, containing two iridoid glycosides (picroside I and kutkoside) have been studied.

Antihepatotoxic activity

Some of the earlier studies on this herb indicated hepatoprotective and chloretic activity against carbon tetrachloride-induced hepatic damage. Later studies demonstrated that the various constituents of the root powder, its alcoholic extract, kutkin, picroside I and kutkoside had anti-inflammatory activity. Dass *et al.* (1976) confirmed that the bitter glucosides and its constituent, organic acids, cinnamic acid and vanillic acid have a significant chloretic and laxative effect. Hepatoprotective, chloretic and immunostimulant activity was seen in the alcoholic extract of the herb by Ansari *et al.* (1988). It stimulated both cell-mediated and humoral activity. Active principle kutkin showed significant activity in hepatic damage induced by galactosamine in rats and by *Plasmodium berghei* in *Mastomys*. Singh *et al.* (1982) observed anti-viral activity in the root against live vaccine virus, by the oral administration of *P. kurrooa* before and after the rise in temperature. It induced non-specific resistance in animals and thus was effective in viral hepatitis.

Picroliv provided significant protection to liver against carbon tetrachloride. The degree of protection was similar before and after the treatment (Dwivedi *et al.* 1990). Shukla *et al.* (1991) evaluated it for chloretic and anti-cholestatic activity. It showed a potent effect with significant reversal of enzymatic parameters. It also reversed thioacetamide-induced cholestasis. A significant reversal of these effects was achieved by treatment in a dose-dependent manner. It was more active than a known hepatoprotective compound, silymarin (Shukla *et al.* 1992). Picroliv provided protection against hepatitis B virus. It had oxygen-free radical scavenging property comparable with that of α-tocopherol. Rastogi *et al.* (1991) reported that it reversed enzymatic changes in liver toxicated with D-galactosomine or thioactamide. When studied for its effect on mice chromosomes in bone marrow cells, it was devoid of clastigenic activity (Jain and Sethi, 1992). Visen *et al.* (1994) studied the effect of Picroliv in combination with other bitters and hepatoprotectants, suh as andrographolide, obtained from *Andrographis paniculata*. One of these combinations showed hepatoprotection in 90–95 per cent of cases. Chander *et al.* (1994) administered Picroliv orally to *Mastomys natalensis* infected with *Plasmodium berghei*. It provided significant protection to *M. natalensis* by helping against the depletion of glutathione levels in the liver and brain. Srivastava *et al.* (1996) reported the effect of Picroliv on liver regeneration by administering 6 mg/kg of it to rats before hepatectomy. It enhanced liver DNA, RNA, protein and cholesterol levels compared with hepatectomized untreated rats. In patients with mycobacterial infection, where rifampicin was used and Picroliv administered along with it, the pharmacokinetics of the antibiotic were not modified but patients were protected against liver damage (Dwivedi *et al.* 1996). It also protected against alcohol-induced chronic hepatotoxicity.

Immunostimulant activity

Picrorhiza kurroa is a potent immunostimulant, inducing both cell mediated and humoral immunity, specific and non-specific (Singh *et al.* 1982). This characteristic is believed to impart positive health and it maintains organic resistance against infection by reestablishing body equilibrium and conditioning body tissues. It had a restorative, rejuvenator, protective effect and saved organisms from extraneous substances, maintaining homeostasis. Simons *et al.* (1989, 1990) found that this immunomodulating effect was due to two anti-complementary polymeric fractions from the aqueous extract of the root. These were dose dependent. Puri *et al.* (1992) studied the immunostimulant activity of Picroliv, it enhanced the non-specific immunoresponse characterized by an increase in macrophage migration index.

In vitiligo

Bedi *et al.* (1989) observed that the herb potentiated photochemotherapy in vitiligo.

Anti-cancerous property

The effect of *P. kurrooa* on the functions of macrophages obtained from mice treated with carcinogen ochratoxin A was investigated by Dhuley (1997). The chemotactic activity of murine macrophages was significantly decreased.

Anti-microbial property

The aqueous alcoholic extract displayed inhibitory action on virulent strains of *Salmonella typhi* septicemia. When a traditional polyherbal preparation containing *P. kurrooa* and the only roots of. *P. kurrooa* were studied, both had an inhibitory effect on *S. typhi*. It protected in cases of both pre- and post-infection, in single and multiple dose schedules (Sohni *et al.* 1995).

Hypolipidaemic activity

Khanna *et al.* (1994) found Picroliv was a hypolipidaemic agent, which acted through lowering protein and lipid levels by inhibiting cholesterol biosynthesis in liver, by bile acid excretion and by enhanced plasma lecithin.

Anti-ulcer activity

Biswas *et al.* (1992) found a *kutaki* effective in duodenitis, a pre-ulcerogenic condition, in duodenal ulcer. Singh *et al.* (1993) reported anti-inflammatory activity in its fractions. There was no effect on the spleen, thymus, adrenal gland or evidence of gastric mucosal damage through the use of this herb. Bandyopadhyay and Bandyopadhyay (1995) observed that it showed anti-ulcer activity by protecting gastric mucosa. It had a cytoprotective effect and it lowered gastric volume.

Antioxidant activity

Chander *et al.* (1991) observed antioxidant activity in Picroliv. Rastogi (1995) studied this activity in liver after partial hepatectomy.

Adulterants and substitutes

The common admixture is *Gentiana kurroo* (Family: Gentianaceae), but adulteration with *Helleborus niger*, called *khurasani kutaki* (Khurasan is a town in central Asia) has been recorded earlier. The root of *khurasani kutaki* is bigger, toxic and a high dose of it may induce purging and vomiting, leading to death.

References

Ansari, R.A., Aswal, B.S., Chander, R., Dhawan, B.N., Garg, N.K., Kapoor, N.K., Kulshreshtha, D.K., Mehdi, H., Mehrotra, B.N., Patnaik, G.K., Sharma, S.K. (1988) Hepatoprotective activity of kutkin-the iridoid glycoside mixture of *Picrorhiza kurrooa*. *Indian Journal of Medical Research*, April 1988, 401–404.

Bandyopadhyay, B., Bandyopadhyay, S.K. Evaluation of anti ulcer drug from an Indian origin plant *Picrorhiza kurrooa* (Katuki). *International Conference on Current Progress in Medicinal and Aromatic Plant Research*, Calcutta, India, 30 December 1994–1 January 1995.

Bedi, K.L., Zutschi, U., Chopra, C.L., Amla, V. (1989) *Picrorrhiza kurrooa*, an Ayurvedic herb may potentiate photochemotherapy in vitiligo. *Journal of Ethnopharmacology*, 27, 347–352.

Biswas, T.K., Mukherjee, B., Maity, L.N., Marji, B. Duodenitis: Effect of Kutaki in comparison with famotidine. *International Seminar-Traditional Medicine*, Calcutta, 7–9 November, 1992.

Chander, R., Kapoor, N.K., Dhawan, B.N. Picroliv: a biological antioxidant. *Proceedings 24th Indian Pharmacological Society Conference*, Ahmedabad, India, 29–31 December 1991.

Chander, R., Kapoor, N.K., Dhawan, B.N. (1994) Picroliv affects gamma-glutamyl cycle in liver and brain of *Mastomys natalensis* infected with *Plasmodium berghei*. *Indian Journal of Experimental Biology*, 32, 324–327.

Dass, P.K., Tripathi, R.M., Agarwal, V.K., Sanyal, A.K. (1976) Pharmacology of kutkin and two organic acid constituents, cinnamic acid and vanillic acid. *Indian Journal of Experimental Biology*, 14, 456–458.

Dhuley, J.N. (1997) Effect of some Indian herbs on macrophage functions in ochratoxin A treated mice. *Journal of Ethnopharmacology*, 58, 15–20.

Dwivedi, A.K., Rastogi, R., Singh, S., Dhawan, B.N. (1996) Effect of Picroliv on the pharmacokinetics of rifampicin in rats. *Indian Journal of Pharmaceutical Sciences*, 58, 28–31.

Dwivedi, Y., Rastogi, R., Ramesh Chander, Sharma, S.K., Kapoor, N.K., Garg, M.K., Dhawan, B.N. (1990) Hepatoprotactive activity of Picroliv against carbon tetrachloride-induced liver damage in rats. *Indian Journal of Medical Research*, 92B, 195–200.

Jain, A.K., Sethi, N. (1992) Effect of Picroliv, a hepatoprotective agent prepared from *Picrorhiza kurrooa* on mice chromosomes. *Fitoterapia*, 63, 255–257.

Khanna, A.K., Chander, R., Kapoor, N.K., Dhawan, B.N. (1994) Hypolipidaemic activity of Picroliv in albino rats. *Phytotherapy Research*, 8, 403–407.

Puri, A., Saxena, R.P., Sumati, Guru, P.Y., Kulshreshtha, D.K., Saxena, K.C., Dhawan, B.N. (1992) Immunostimulant activity of picroliv, the iridoid glycoside fraction of Picrorhiza kurrooa and its protective action against *Leishmania donovani* infection in hamsters. *Planta Medica*, 58, 528–532.

Rastogi, R., Dwivedi, Y., Garg, N.K., Dhawan, B.N. (1991) Perfusion of rat liver with picroliv reverse enzyme changes induced by D-galactosamine or thioacetamide. *Proceedings 24th Indian Pharmacological Society Conference*, Ahmedabad, India, 29–31 December 1991.

Rastogi, R., Seema, S., Garg, N.K., Dhawan, B.N. (1995) Effect of Picroliv on antioxidant system in liver of rats, after partial hepatectomy. *Phytotherapy Research*, 9, 364–367.

Shukla, B., Visen, P.K.S., Patnaik, G.K., Dhawn, B.N. Prevention of carbon tetrachloride-induced hepatic damage by picroliv. *Proceedings 24th Indian Pharmacological Society Conference*, Ahmedabad, India, 29–31 December 1991.

Shukla, B., Visen, P.K.S., Patnaik, G.K., Dhawan, B.N. (1992) Reversal of thioacetamide-induced cholestasis by picroliv in rodents. *Phytotherapy Research*, 6, 53–55.

Simons, J.M., t'Hart, L.A., Labadie, R.P., van Dijk, H., de Silva, K.T.D. (1990) Modulation of human complement activation and the human neutrophil oxidative burst by different root extracts of *Picrorhiza kurrooa*. *Phytotherapy Research*, 4, 207–211.

Simons, J.M., t'Hart, L.A., van Dijk, H., Fischer, F.C., de Silva, K.T.D., Labadie, R.P. (1989) Immunomodulatatory compounds from *Picrorhiza kurrooa*: Isolation and characterisation of two anti-complementary polymeric fraction from an aqueous root extract. *Journal of Ethnopharmacology*, 26, 169–182.

Singh, G.B., Sarang Bani, Surjeet Singh, Khujuria, A., Sharma, M.L., Gupta, B.D., Banerjee, S.K. (1993) Antiinflammatory activity of iridoids kutkin, picroside-1 and kutkoside from *Picrorhiza kurrooa*. *Phytotherapy Research*, 7, 402–407.

Singh, N., Mishra, N., Singh, S.P., Kohli, R.P., Bhargava, K.P. (1982) Protective effect of *Picrorhiza kurrooa* against cutaneous vaccinial (viral) infection in Guinea pigs. *Journal of Research in Ayurveda and Siddha*, 3, 162–171.

Sohni, Y.R., Padmaja Kaimal, Bhatt, R.M. (1995) Prophylactic therapy of *Salmonella typhi* septicemia in mice with traditionally prescribed crude drug formulation. *Journal of Ethnopharmacology*, 45, 141–147.

Srivastava, S., Srivastava, A.K., Patnaik, G.K., Dhawan, B.M. (1996) Effect of picroliv on liver regeneration in rats. *Fitoterapia*, 67, 252–256.

Visen, P.K.S., Saraswat, B., Patnaik, G.K., Dhawan, B.N. Hepatotprotective activity of combination of active material isolated from medicinal plants. *Fourth International Congress of Ethnobiology*, NBRI, Lucknow (India), 17–21 November 1994.

34 Kuth

Saussurea costus (Falc.) Lipsch.
Syn. *S. lappa* (Decne) Sch.-Bip
(Sometimes an old name *Aplotaxis auriculata* is used)
Family: Compositae (Asteraceae)

THE PLANT AND ITS DISTRIBUTION

It is cultivated in the alpine zone of the western Himalayas (Lahaul and Spiti, and along the Indo-Tibetan border). Earlier it was collected from these areas and cultivated in some parts of alpine Kashmir. In the last century, it was a precious commodity in the Indo-Chinese trade and was one of the few medicinal plants which were cultivated in Kashmir. Chinese merchants at that time would pay the equivalent weight of the roots in silver, so at that time the *kuth* plantations in Khilanmarg (Kashmir) were guarded day and night by security men to ensure the roots were not stolen. Recently the trend has changed. This herb is now being cultivated on a large scale in China and is being smuggled from China into India through the eastern Himalayas. In Chinese medicine it is used under the name *Saussureae Radix*.

The plant (Fig. 26A) may grow up to 2 m in length. The radical leaves have a long stalk. The flower head is sessile, hard, round and 3–5 cm in diameter, with dark purple to black flowers. The seeds are achene, about 3 mm long, curved and compressed. The aromatic root (Fig. 26B) is horn-like, rough from outside, up to 10 cm thick and may be 20 cm or more long, but in trade broken pieces are often available. When cut, the root depicts a dark brown cylindrical centre.

The Sanskrit name of the root is *kushta*, but the trade name *kuth* or bitter *kuth*, is well known in the Indian subcontinent. Sometimes, because of the root's close resemblance with *Inula racemosa*, it is identified as *pushkarmul*, with which it is often confused. A number of aromatic, tuberous, tapering roots obtained from various species of *Inula*, *Costus*, *Iris* or of wild *Withania* are known as *meetha kuth* (*meetha* means sweet) to differentiate them from the genuine herb, which is called bitter *kuth*.

USES IN FOLKLORE AND AYURVEDA

As per Ayurveda it is hot, aromatic, carminative, stimulant, diuretic and alterative. The major uses of the root are:

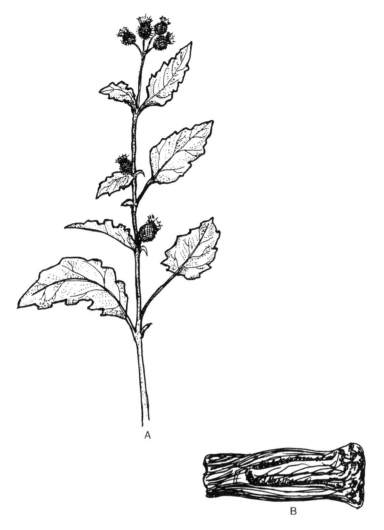

Figure 26 Saussurea lappa **A** twig, **B** root.

As a tonic

It has a good effect on the central nervous system. As a *Rasayana* fine powder of the herb with *ghee* and honey is licked twice daily. It keeps all infections away and imparts longevity.

For bronchial problems

In asthma, fine powder of the root, 3–4 times a day, is a prophylactic before an attack. It does not have side effects like those of adrenaline or of anti-asthmatic cigarettes. After prescribing for 10–15 days, the medication should be stopped to see the effects. If required, the treatment may be repeated again. It has not got a cumulative or intolerance effect. When smoked in small quantities, it reduces the swelling and clears a sore throat.

As an anti-inflammatory agent

In arthritis, powder of *kuth* with castor oil is administered internally and applied externally. As an anti-inflammatory agent, it gives relief from headache and other body aches and pains. For external purposes, it is mixed with rose water and applied.

As a hair darkner

In China, hair is fumigated with the smoke from the root for darkening grey hair.

For healing ulcers

In skin diseases, root powder mixed in ointment is applied on ulcers.

THERAPEUTICAL INDICATIONS AND PHARMACOLOGICAL STUDIES

Anti-microbial properties

Essential oils are strongly antiseptic and disinfectant, especially against *Streptococcus* and *Staphylococcus* bacteria (Nadkarni, 1954). Chen *et al.* (1995) examined the anti-viral activities of the crude extract. Two active constituents, costunolide and dehydrocostus lactone, showed a strong suppressive effect on the component of the hepatitis B surface antigen (HBsAg) in human hepatoma Hep3B cells.

Anti-inflammatory activity

It suppressed chemokines, which are involved in the migration of leucocytes from circulation to accumulated inflamed sites, and thus has an important role in rheumatoid arthritis and psoriasis (Jung *et al.* 1998).

As a cardio-stimulant

It relaxed involuntary muscles and acted as a cardiostimulant (Nadkarni, 1954). Dwivedi *et al.* (1987, 1989) observed the root's prostaglandin E2-like activity in the ischaemic aorta. The crude powder reduced the frequency of angina.

As a bronchodilator

An alkaloid saussurine obtained from the root had a depressant effect on the vagus nerves in the medulla, on bronchioles and on involuntary muscles, which relaxed the respiratory tubules (Nadkarni, 1954).

Anti-tumour effect

The root resolved tumours (Nadkarni, 1954). Lee *et al.* (1995) observed that various fractions of the root had inhibitory effects on IL-8 induction in lipopolysaccharide activated rat macrophages. Taniguchi *et al.* (1995) isolated costunolide and dehydrocostus lactone from the root, which acted as inhibitors of the killing function of cytotoxic T lymphocytes. Cho *et al.* (1998) reported that the total methanolic extract (sesquiterpenes) showed a potent inhibitory effect on the production of tumours.

Hypoglycaemic effect

Singh and Sharma (1990) reported anti-diabetic (diabetes mellitus) activity in the root. Chaturvedi *et al.* (1993) studied the effect of alcoholic extract of the root on glucose metabolism. It showed a significant hypoglycaemic response by stimulating the thyroid. Chaturvedi *et al.* (1995) compared this hypoglycaemic activity of the root with that of *Inula racemosa*. *Kuth* extract increased concentrations of liver glycogen but reduced that of plasma insulin (Upadhyay *et al.* 1996).

Inulin contained in the root may be playing a part in anti-diabetic activity. Inulin helps to stabilize blood glucose levels as it has a zero glycaemic index.

Aphrodisiac activity

Chopra *et al.* (1958) postulated that the essential oils contained in the root, when excreted, produce a certain amount of irritation in the urethra, giving rise to penile erection. Other studies showed that this activity might be due to alkaloid saussurine, which has an adrenalin-like effect.

Anti-ulcer effect

Yamahara *et al.* (1985, 1990) observed that costunolide from acetone extract had cholagogic, anti-ulcer and a gastrointestinal motility enhancing effect. Yoshikawa *et al.* (1993) isolated an anti-ulcer principle, saussureamine A, which exhibited inhibitory activity on stress-induced ulcer formation.

A herbal preparation containing *S. lappa* had a protective effect on gastric and duodenal ulcers induced by chemical and physical agents (Mitra *et al.* 1996).

Neuroleptic effect

A compound isolated from the benzene fraction had an effect similar to that of chlorpromazine (Okugawa *et al.* 1996).

In gynaecological practice

Saussurea polysaccharides had a stimulating effect on isolated rat uterus, which was dose dependent (Lin and Wang, 1986).

In digestive problems

Inulin present in the root is a non-digestible food ingredient, an appetite suppressant. It increases the faecal matter and improves the bacterial ecology in the colon. It stimulates the growth and activity of one or a limited number of bacteria in the colon (such as *bifidobacteria*) and cleanses the intestine by reducing the amount of harmful intestinal bacteria. It increases the *bifidobacterial* count 5–8 times and brings a significant reduction in *Bacteriosides fusobacteria* and *Clostridia* (Kleessen *et al.* 1997, Gibson *et al.* 1995, Bouhnik *et al.* 1996).

Chemical studies

The root contains 2–5 per cent essential oils, 0.5 per cent alkaloid saussurine, 18 per cent inulin, 6 per cent resin, potassium nitrate and valeric acid.

Toxicology

When smoked, it has an opium-like narcotic effect, but no toxic effect has been observed in alcohol extract (Chaturvedi *et al.* 1993).

Adulterants and substitutes

The root is sometimes substituted by *Echinops latifolia* in Russia (Batorova *et al.* 1980).

References

Batorova, S.M., Rakshain, K.V., Bogdanov, T.V., Shantanova, L.N. (1980) Pharmacological evaluation of the decoction of roots of *Echinops latifolia*. *Rastitelnye Resursy* (in Russian), 16, 134–136.

Bouhnik, Y., Flourie, B., Andrieux, C., Bissetti, N., Brief, F., Rambaud, J.C. (1996) Effects of bifidobacterium sp fermented milk ingested with or without inulin on colonic bifidobacteria and enzymatic activities in healthy humans. *European Journal of Clinical Nutrition*, 50, 269–273.

Chaturvedi, P., Shukla, S., Tripathi, P., Chaurasia, S, Singh, S.K., Tripathi, Y.B. (1995) Comparative study of Inula racemosa and Saussurea lappa on the glucose levels in albino rats. *Ancient Science of Life*, 15, 62–70.

Chaturvedi, P., Tripathi, P., Pandey, S., Singh, U., Tripathi, Y.B. (1993) Effect of *Saussurea lappa* alcoholic extract on different endocrine glands in relation to glucose metabolism in the rat. *Phytotherapy Research*, 7, 205–20.

Chen, H.C., Chou, C.K., Lee, S.D., Wang, J.C., Yeh, S.F. (1995) Active compounds from *Saussurea lappa* Clark that suppresses hepatitis B virus surface antigen gene expression in human hepatoma cells. *Antiviral Research*, 27, 99–109.

Cho, J.Y., Park, J., Yoo, E.S., Baik, K.U., Jee, H.J., Lee, J., Park, M.H. (1998) Inhibitory effect of sesquiterpene lactones from *Saussurea lappa* on tumour – production in murine macrophage like cells. *Planta Medica*, 64, 594–597.

Chopra, R.N., Chopra, I.C., Handa, K.L., Kapur, L.D. *Chopra's Indigenous Drugs of India*. 2nd Edition. U.N. Dhur & Sons, Calcutta, India 1958.

Dwivedi, S., Chansuria, J.P.N., Somani, P.N., Udupa, K.N. (1987) Influence of certain indigenous drugs on the prostaglandin E2 like activity in the ischaemic rabbit aorta. *Indian Drugs*, 24, 378–382.

Dwivedi, S., Somani, P.N., Udupa, K.N. (1989) Role of Inula racemosa and *Saussurea lappa* in management of angina pectoris. *International Journal of Crude Drug Research*, 27, 217–222.

Gibson, G.R., Beatty, E.R., Wang X., Cummings J.H. (1995) Selective stimulation of bifidbacteria in the human colon by oligofructose and inulin. *Gastroenterology*, 108, 975–982.

Jung, Jee, H., Ha, Joo Yong, Min, K.R., Shibata, F., Nagagawa, H., Kang, S.S., Chang, F.L., Moo, Kim Y. (1998) Reynosin from *Suasuurea lappa* as inhibitor on CINC-1 induction in LPS stimulated NRK 52 E cells. *Planta Medica*, 64, 454–455.

Kleessen, B., Sykura, B., Zunft, H.J., Blaut, M. (1997) Effects of inulin and lactose on fecal microflora, microbial activity and bowel habit in elderly constipated persons. *American Journal of Clinical Nutrition*, 65, 1397–1402.

Lee, G.I., Ha, J.Y., Min, K.R., Nakagawa, H., Tsurufuji, S., Chang, I.M., Kim, Y.S. (1995) Inhibitory effects of oriental herbal medicines on IL-8 induction in lipopolysaccharides-activated rat macrophages. *Planta Medica*, 61, 26–30.

Lin, X.Z., Wang, G.X. (1986) The effects of *Saussurea* polysaccharides on isolated rat uteri. *Acta Pharma Sinica*, 21, 220–222.

Mitra, S.K., Gopumadhavan, S., Hemavathi, T.S., Murlidhar, T.S., Venkataranganna, M.V. (1996) Protective effect of UL-409, a herbal formulation against physical and chemical factor-induced gastric and duodenal ulcers in experimental animals. *Journal of Ethnopharmacology*, 52, 168–169.

Nadkarni, K.M. *Indian Materia Medica*. Vol I Popular Book Depot, Bombay, India 1954.

Okugawa, H., Ueda, R., Matsumoto, K., Kawanishi, K., Kato, A. (1996) Effect of dehydrocostus lactones and costunolide from *Saussurea* root on the central nervous system in mice. *Phytomedicine*, 3, 147–153.

Singh, D.C., Sharma, B.P. (1990) Management of Madhumeha (diabetes mellitus) by indigenous drugs Bijaysar and Kushtha. *Aryavaidyan*, 4, 21–23.

Taniguchi, M., Kataoka, T., Suzuki, H., Uramoto, M., Arao, K., Magae, J., Nishimura, T., Stake, N., Nagai, K. (1995) Costunolide and dehydrocostus lactone as inhibitors of killing function of cytotoxic T lymphocytes. *Bioscience, Biotechnology and Biochemistry*, 59, 2064–2067.

Upadhyay, O.P., Singh, R.H., Dutta, S.K. (1996) Studies on antidiabetic plants used in Indian folk-lore. *Aryavaidyan*, 9, 159–167.

Yamahara, J., Chisaka, T., Hunag, Q., Kishi, K, Kobayashi, H., Kawahara, Y. (1990) Gastrointestinal motility enhancing effect of Saussureae Radix. *Phytotherapy Research*, 4, 160–161.

Yamahara, J., Kobayashi, M., Miki, K., Kozuka, M., Sawada, T., Fujimura, H. (1985) Cholagogic and antiulcer effect of Saussureae radix and its active components. *Chemical and Pharmaceutical Bulletin*, 33, 1285–1288.

Yoshikawa, M., Hatkeyama, S., Inoue, Y., Yamahara, J. (1993) Saussureamines A, B, C, D and E, new anti-ulcer principles from Chinese Saussureae Radix. *Chemical and Pharmaceutical Bulletin*, 41, 214–216.

35 Malakangani

Celastrus paniculatus Willd.
Family: Celastraceae

THE PLANT AND ITS DISTRIBUTION

It grows as a deciduous climber in the warm hilly areas of Himalayas up to 1,000 metres, in hotter parts of south and east India, and the middle and south of Andamans islands. The plant has white spots on young twigs. Leaves are 5–12 cm long in various rounded shapes (Fig. 27A). The flowers are greenish yellow and about 1 cm in diameter. The seed are black (Fig. 27B), pepper-like but with a yellow to red cover. On pressing between the fingers, the seed coat gets separated from the kernel and on further pressing changes into an oily mass.

USES IN FOLKLORE AND AYURVEDA

In Ayurveda, the seed is considered hot, dry and is either applied externally or administered internally, in the following forms:

1   When the seed alone is prescribed, the initial dose is one seed for the first day, increased by one seed each day until a maximum dose of fifty seeds is achieved.
2   Seeds are boiled in milk and used.
3   An oil is prepared by heating the seed in an inverted bottle. The pure oil which is obtained is pungent, scarlet or yellow in colour. Dose: 10–20 drops.
4   *Krishna tailam* or Black oil is prepared from a mixture of *malakangni* seed, benzoin, clove, nutmeg and mace. Dose: 10–30 drops
5   Triturate a mixture of 40 g each of *Celastrus* oil, honey and *ghee* for a few hours. The mixture is stored in a sealed container and is allowed to ferment for six months in a warm place. When ready, a dose of 125 mg is prescribed, three times daily for three months, as a brain tonic in winter.

The above preparations are used as nervine tonic in gout, paralysis, rheumatism, leprosy, in mental illness, to promote memory, to stimulate intellect and as an aphrodisiac. The oil has a powerful stimulant action in paralysis. In the Siddha system of medicine, the oil is given to build stamina. During the administration of this seed in any form, a strict diet of just milk, roasted meat and bread is given.

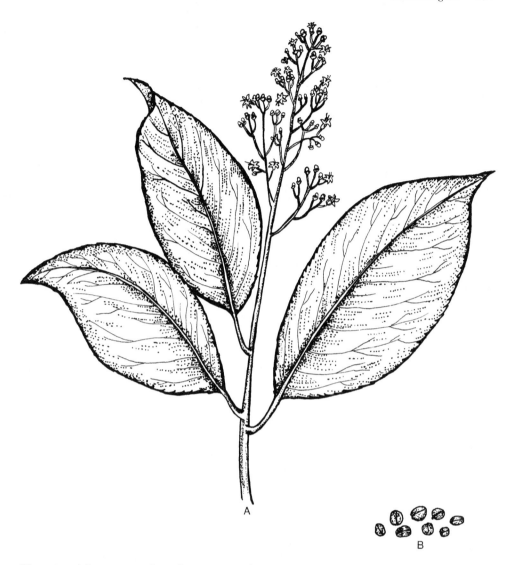

Figure 27 Celastrus paniculatus **A** twig, **B** seed.

In the Philippines, it is prescribed as an antidote to opium poisoning. It is also being used to reverse brain damage caused by organophosphate pesticides and similar toxins.

THERAPEUTIC INDICATIONS AND PHARMACOLOGICAL STUDIES

As a tranquillizer

The oil acted as a tranquillizer in low doses. At a dose of 50–100mg/kg, the oil produced a gradual fall in cardiac output, bradycardia and a marked increase in pulse pressure in isolated heart and lung preparations (Gaitonde *et al*. 1957, Seth *et al*.

1963). It was found to be a central nervous system active agent (Dandiya and Chopra, 1970, Singh *et al.* 1974, Ahumada *et al.* 1991). Further tests suggested that it had tranquillizing, anti-convulsant, muscle relaxant property, and anti-pyretic, analgesic and anti-ulcerogenic effects, which shows it is a good adaptogen. It was effective in psychiatric cases of depression and hysteria (Balaraman, 1971).

An Ayurvedic drug containing this oil, when tested by Kakrani *et al.* (1985), reduced depletion of liver glycogen, inhibited glycogenolysis in the muscle fibres of rats, indicating the protective effect in stress. There was a significant increase of the narcosis time in both male and female mice. Another Ayurvedic preparation containing *malkangani* was effective in residual schizophrenia (Tripathi and Singh 1994).

For enhancing memory

It hastened the learning process in rats, which was statistically significant and the results were comparable to that of vasopressin, a known agent for the learning process (Karnath *et al.* 1980, 1994). Through its use the three monoamines, norepinephrine, dopamine and serotonine and their metabolites, which are involved in the memory and learning process, decreased significantly in the brain. Nalini *et al.* (1995) found significant memory retention in rats treated with this drug.

In hemiplegia

Namboodiri *et al.* (1991) found an oil containing *Celastrus* to be effective in hemiplegia.

Hypolipidaemic effect

The 50 per cent alcohol extract of the seed showed hypolipidaemic and anti-arterosclerotic effects in rats. It reduced both serum cholesterol and LDL and prevented atherogenesis. It prevented the accumulation of cholesterol and triglycerides in liver and aorta, regressed atheromatous plaques of ascending thoracic and abdominal aorta. Faecal secretion of cholesterol was significantly increased, suggesting that the modulation of absorption was affected (Mathur *et al.* 1993).

Chemical studies

Two alkaloids, celastrine and paniculatine are reported.

Toxicological studies

At low doses, it is clinically safe, with low toxicity. Large doses cause burning of the skin. An oil fraction produced a transient fall in fatty degeneration in the liver and transient tubular damage in the kidney, but it was not found harmful in the long run. (Bidwai *et al.* 1990).

References

Ahumada, F., Trincado, M.A., Arellano, J.A., Hancke, J. Wikman. G. (1991) Effect of certain adaptogenic plant extracts on drug-induced narcosis in female and male mice. *Phytotherapy Research*, 5, 29–31.

Balaraman, S. (1971) Rapid screening of the behavioural effects of *Celastrus paniculatus* and sodium pentobarbital with fixed internal schedules of reinforcement. *Journal of Research in Indian Medicine*, 8, 61–68.

Bidawi, P.P., Wangoo, D., Sharma, V. (1990) Effect of polar and semipolar compounds from the seeds of *Celastrus paniculatus* on the liver and kidney in rats. *Fitoterapia*, 61, 417–424.

Dandiya, P.C., Chopra, Y.M. (1970) *Celastrus paniculatus* Willd, CNS active drugs from plants indigenous to India. *Indian Journal of Pharmacology*, 2, 69–70.

Gaitonde, B.B., Raikar, B.P., Shroff, F.N., Pateljal, R. (1957) Pharmacological studies with Malkangani: an indigenous tranquilizer drug. *Current Medical Practitioner*, 1, 619–621.

Kakrani, H.K., Nair Vijaynathan, G., Kalyani, G.A., Satyanaryana, D. (1985) Studies on Ayurvedic drug. I Evaluation of antifatigue effect of the Ayurvedic drug *Alert* in rats. *Fitoterapia*, 65, 293–295.

Karnath, K.S., Haridas, K.K., Gunasundri, S., Guruswami, M.N. (1980) Effect of *Celastrus paniculatus* on learning process. *Arogya – Journal of Health Science*, 6, 137–139.

Karnath, K.S., Padma, T.K., Guruswami, M.N. Preliminary report of *Celastrus paniculatus* on memory process (abstract). *Proceedings of the 46th Annual Congress of Indian Pharmaceutical Society*, Chandigarh, 28–30 December 1994.

Mathur, N.T., Varma, M., Dixit, V.P. (1993) Hypolipidaemic and antiatherosclerotic effect of *Celastrus paniculatus* seed extract (50 percent EtOH) in cholesterol fed rabbits. *Indian Drugs*, 30, 76–82.

Nalini, K., Karanth, K.S., Rao, A., Aroor, A.R. (1995) Effects of *Celastrus paniculatus* on passive avoidance performance and biogenic amine turnover in albino rats. *Journal of Ethnopharmacology*, 47, 101–108.

Namboodiri, P.K.N., Menon, T.V., Parbhakran, V.A., Vijayan, N.P., Pillai, N.G.K. Santhakumari, K. (1991) Comparative effect of J.J. tailam internal and external in Paksavadha (Hemiplegia). *Journal of Research in Ayurveda and Siddha*, 12, 41–46.

Seth, U.K., Vaz, A., Daliwala, C.V. Billore, R.A. (1963) Behavioural and pharmacologic studies of tranquilising fraction from the oil of *Celastrus paniculatus* (Malkanagani oil). *Archives International Pharmacodynamics*, 144, 35–50.

Singh, N., Chand, N., Kohli, R.P. (1974) Pharmacological studies on *Celastrus paniculatus* (Malkanagani). *Journal of Research in Indian Medicine*, 9, 1–8.

Tripathi, J.S., Singh, R.H. (1994) Clinical evaluation of Smrtisagar Ras in cases of residual schizophrenia. *Journal of Research in Ayurveda and Siddha*, 15, 8–16.

36 Mandukparni (*Gotu Kola*)

Centella asiatica (L.) Urban
Syn. *Hydrocotyle asiatica* L.
Family: Umbelliferae

The herb is known as *brahmi* in the Indian subcontinent and *gotu kola* in the western world.

THE PLANT AND ITS DISTRIBUTION

It is cosmopolitan in its natural distribution and grows along damp shady streams, in ponds, particularly on the marshy land, along the river banks and in irrigated fields up to 2,000 m high ((Bagchi and Puri, 1988) in India, Sri Lanka, Malaysia, Indonesia, Madagascar and South Africa. It is cultivated in east India, Kenya and Hawaii. The plant is a herb, a ground creeper (Fig. 28A) having orbicular-reniform, crenate leaves, up to 7 cm in diameter (Fig. 28B), which can be easily identified by epidermal peel in its dry form (Fig. 28C, D); 3–6 flowers are arranged in an umbel. The seeds are compressed.

USES IN FOLKLORE AND AYURVEDA

Mandukparni is considered cool, bitter, a brain tonic and a *Rasayana*. The major uses of this herb are:

As a *Rasayana*

An old proverb says that *Two leaves a day will keep old age away*.

In *Rasayana chikitsa* (rejuvenation treatment) the juice of the herb or a polyherbal preparation called *Brahmi ghrit* is prescribed for *kayakalp* (complete overhaul of body systems). It may be used during daily routines but *kuti praveshika* (confinement to an isolated hut for treatment) is said to give better results.

As a brain tonic

It is one of three major *Medhya Rasayana* (tonics for brain) herbs and is said to sharpen memory. In an earlier ethnobotanical study by a European, who lived in India in the nineteenth century, it was mentioned that consuming a few leaves of *Centella* strengthened and revitalized the mind to a remarkable degree, providing the body is exposed to sun.

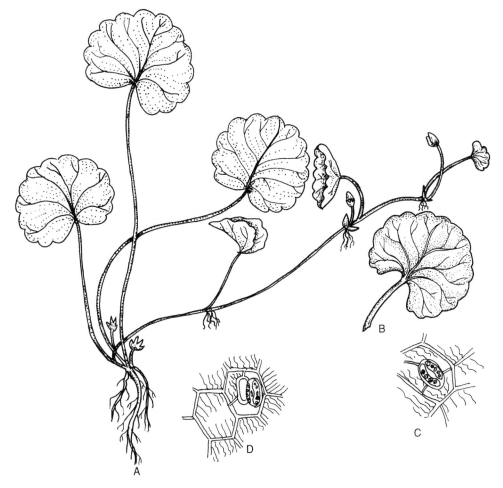

Figure 28 Centella asiatica **A** herb, **B** a leaf, C, D epidermal peel (diagrammatic).

It prevented brain fog and nervous breakdown. In 1914 an American tutor (Miss Mary E. Forbes) in a princely Himalayan state of Mandi, (now in Himachal Pradesh in India) began eating a few tender leaves of *Centella* in salad. After a few months she never knew what brain fatigue was! It gave relief in rheumatism, neuritis and nervous breakdown. The villagers in Sri Lanka asserted that the elephants kept their youth and strength for hundreds of years by regularly consuming this herb (Lucas, 1966).

In Chinese medicine this herb is said to be a brain food and an elixir of long life. It has ginseng-like rejuvenating and energizing effects on the brain cells and endocrine glands.

For nervous disorders

In nervous debility, 300–600 mg of powder is given thrice daily. A paste prepared from powders of 5 parts *Centella*, 4 parts *Saussurea* and honey is prescribed in a dose of 200–350 mg, three times daily, during speech therapy in children, in insanity and in hypochondriasis. If this mixture suppresses appetite, *calamus* is added as a carminative.

For sterility

When *Centella* was provided as a homoeopathic medicine, a special effect on female generative organs was observed, indicating its use for sterility. For this purpose equal quantities of this herb and *Trichodesma indicum* with half the quantity of sugar was mixed. Three grams of this mixture was prescribed, twice daily with milk for 3 days, after menstruation. It is not effective if the patients have obesity, leucorrhoea or dysmenorrhoea (Ghosh, 1930).

For skin diseases

It is said to bring about *kaya kalp* – complete rejuvenation of body. It makes the skin disease-free, lustrous and charming. The plant in the form of juice, pulp, dry powder, ointment or water extract, is used for various skin diseases, such as chronic and obstinate ulcers, eczema, psoriasis, sores, elephantiasis, leprosy, scrofula, etc. In scrofula, the powder of the herb is dusted all over. In leprosy it gives symptomatic relief. In syphilis, when prescribed in the second and third stage, healing of skin occurs. It is an ingredient of popular hair oil, along with *Eclipta alba*, *Emblica officinalis* and sesame oil. This oil is said to help hair growth and make it black and healthy.

For leprosy

The European physician Dymock in the nineteenth century (Ghosh, 1930) remarked, "The administration of this drug to lepers causes a sensation of warmth and pricking in the skin at first, especially of the hands and feet. This is followed by a few days of a general sensation of warmth, sometimes almost intolerable. The capillary circulation is accelerated and after about a week the appetite improves, the skin becomes softer, throws off the thickened epidermis and recovers its transpiratory faculties."

In gastroenteritis of infants

The juice of 2 to 4 leaves is prescribed and a paste of the leaves is applied on the naval region.

For various types of fevers

Equal parts of fresh sacred basil leaves (*Ocimum sanctum*), black pepper and *Centella* are ground to form a paste and on drying made into pills of 2 g each. These are prescribed three times a day.

Ayurvedic preparations

Brahmi ghrit

Ingredients   1 litre of *Centella asiatica* juice (if the juice is not available a decoction of herb is used), 500 g *ghee* and 30 g each of *Acorus calamus*, *Saussurea lappa* and *Convolvulus arvensis*.

Method   Make a paste by macerating the above powdered herbs in the juice of *Centella*, mix it in *ghee* and warm to a slow to moderate heat, until all the water evaporates.

Dose   5–10 g with sugar followed by sweet, warm milk.

Use   As a mental tonic, particularly useful for scholars and students, for mental and physical fatigue, and in forgetfulness.

Saraswat ghrit

Ingredients   3 litres *Centella* juice, 750 g *ghee* and 50 g each of turmeric, jasmine flower, *Saussurea lappa*, *Ipomaea turpethum*, *Terminalia chebula*, and 25 g each of *Embelia ribes*, salt, sugar and calamus.

Method   Mix the powdered herbs with *Centella* juice, *ghee*, and heat slowly until all the water evaporates, strain and preserve the fatty matter.

Dose   10–25 g depending on the digestion power. Use with milk.

Use   This *ghee* makes a person intelligent and virile so it is used to increase sexual power and memory. It is also considered useful in all types of skin diseases.

THERAPEUTIC INDICATIONS AND PHARMACOLOGICAL STUDIES

Bagchi and Puri (1988, 1989) reviewed the literature on various aspects of this herb's chemistry, pharmacology and toxicology. The salient features of these and the other studies are as follows:

As a sedative

Singh *et al.* (1981) tried the herb with patients suffering from anxiety neurosis. A six-week treatment not only provided significant relief but a quantitative reduction in the anxiety levels, leading to improved mental functions, studied in terms of mental fatigue and immediate memory span. Experimental studies on the psychotropic effect in rats showed a significant barbiturate hypnosis potentiation effect, besides producing significant alternations in the neurochemistry of the brain. The histamine and catecholamine contents in the brains of the treated group increased significantly.

Agrawal (1981) observed that the alcohol extract of the herb showed a varying degree of sedation. It prolonged the hypnotic effect of sodium phenobarbitone in rats. It decreased the acetylcholine and histamine content of the whole brain, while catecholamine was increased. Its effect on the central nervous system resembled that of chlorpromazine and reserpine. It also had an anti-amphetamine activity. It produced hypothermia, reduced the motor activity and was a potential neuroleptic. Shukla (1989) observed a barbiturate hypnosis potentiation effect in different fractions while Sakina and Dandiya (1990) detected a depressant property in this herb.

Kapoor (1986) found a polyherbal preparation containing *Centella* quite effective in insomnia. Kuppurajan *et al.* (1992) noted that a mixture of *Centella*, liquorice, *Nardostachys* in the ratio of 1:2:2 was more active in psychomotor performance, compared with a well-known tranquillizer, diazepam, and a placebo. The drug was effective in controlling somatic and psychic anxiety, preferably in old age. In another study (Kuppurajan, 1995) *Ksheerbala tailam* (see *bala*) a mixture of herbs was suspended in milk and oil emulsion, and dropped on the forehead to see its anxiolytic property. The preparation was effective in enhancing perceptual discrimination and psychomotor performance.

Effect on mentally retarded children

Appa Rao *et al.* (1973) observed that the herb increased the intelligent quotient and changed the behaviour of mentally retarded children. There was an overall general adjustment. With the administration of the herb, shy and withdrawn children or those who were restless became expressive, communicative and cooperative. The herb also increased concentration power and attention span. In further studies Appa Rao *et al.* (1977) observed a significant increase in the general mental ability of mentally retarded children after 3–6 months of administering this herb. Sharma *et al.* (1985) administered a powder of the herb for six to twelve months to educable, mentally retarded children within the age range of 8–12 years. These children were followed for one year. They showed significant improvement, with good performance in school. Nalini *et al.* (1992) studied the effect of aqueous extract of the herb on learning, memory and also on levels of norepinephrine (NE), dopamine (DA), 5-HT and their metabolites in the brain. By using this concentration all of these decreased significantly, which showed that all these compounds are involved in learning and memory. Anbuganapathi (1995) studied the effect of the syrup prepared from *Centella* and *Bacopa* on the learning ability of albino mice and school children and found it quite effective.

Immunopotentiating effect

When a powder of the herb (3 g/day) was given for three months to patients, it increased memory, sleep and appetite. It relieved anxiety and mental fatigue (personal communication). Plohmann *et al.* (1994) found an immunomodulatery effect in the triterpenoid saponins of *Centella*. Praveen Kumar (1996) noted that the oral administration of *Brahma Rasayana*, containing *Centella*, significantly increased white blood cell count, bone marrow cellularity, natural killer cells and antibody dependent cellular activity in mice exposed to gamma radiation. It reduced radiation-induced peroxidation in the liver.

Anabolic effect

When albino rats were fed on a low protein diet and *Centella*, it prevented mortality due to gross protein deficiency. It increased the blood protein nitrogen and prevented fatty acid infiltration of liver. The increase in haemoglobin content was quite high and statistically significant. It decreased the mean level of blood urea (personal communication).

Anti-cancer studies

Babbu and Padikkala (1993) found that a partial purified fraction of methanol extract of the herb inhibited the growth of tumour cells with no toxic effect against lymphocytes. Babu and Padikkala (1994) studied *C. asiatica*-induced apoptosis in Ehrlich Ascites tumour cells. Babu and Padikkala (1995) also studied the role of the extract of this herb on chemotherapeutic drug-induced toxicity. There was a reduction in myelosuppression. Babu *et al.* (1995) observed that the extract destroyed 100 per cent tumour of the cells in normal human lymphocytes. In follow-up action in animals, it doubled the lifespan of cancerous mice without any toxicity.

Anti-inflammatory effect

Jain *et al.* (1994) observed an anti-inflammatory activity in a polyherbal Ayurvedic preparation *Brahmi rasyana*, which contains *Centella* as well as other herbs.

For ulcers

Centella has been studied for its activity in connective tissue metabolism and endothelial integrity in various ulcers and venous hypertension. Shin *et al.* (1982) noted that the herb, in 93 per cent cases of duodenal and gastric ulcers, exhibited definite improvement. Grimaldi *et al.* (1990) also tested it on venous ulcers. Chatterjee *et al.* (1992) showed that extract of the herb significantly inhibited gastric ulcerations-induced by cold stress in rats. It increased GABA levels, which were dose dependent. Sarma *et al.* (1995) tried an ethanol extract of *T. cordifolia* and *Centella* at dose of 100 mg/kg daily. These had marked protective action against stress-induced ulceration due to the adaptogenic property of the mixture.

Effect on skin

Bonte *et al.* (1994, 1995) tested the effects of various compounds from *Centella* on collagens. It was seen that both asiaticoside and madecosside stimulated collagen secretion. Sunil Kumar *et al.* (1998) applied topically various formulations containing aqueous extract of *Centella* to open wounds. It increased cellular proliferation and collagen synthesis at the wound site. Treated wounds epithelized faster and the rate of wound contraction was higher, compared to the control.

Anti-filarial effect

A mixture of ethanol extract of *C. asiatica* and *Acacia auriculiformis* was administered to dogs naturally infected with *Dirofilaria immitis* by Sarkar *et al.* (1998). It resulted in a considerable decrease in filarial count.

Chemical studies

Three principle compounds reported from the herb are asiatic acid, madecassic acid and asiaticoside. In the body asiaticoside gets transformed into asiatic acid, which is the most active (Grimaldi *et al.* 1990). Two saponins are brahmoside and brahminoside

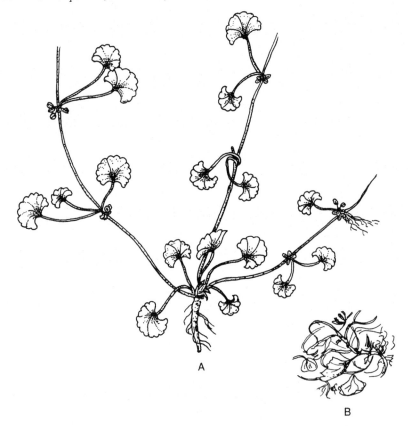

Figure 29 Hydrocotyle javanica, **A** herb, **B** dry herb.

and the two triterpenic acids are brahmic acid and isobrahmic acid (Thakur *et al.* 1989). It also contains essential oil.

Toxicological studies

In high doses it is a narcotic, causing heaviness of the head, headaches and vasodilation, which may lead to coma. Studies on the compound asiaticoside showed that it is not very toxic. At higher concentrations it affected the epidermis by keratinization. The herb caused 20 per cent mortality at a dose of 10 g/kg (Agrawal, 1981). *Centella* may cause contact dermatitis on external application (Danese *et al.* 1994).

Adulterants and substitutes

The Chinese herb *Fo-Ti tieng*, which means *elixir for long life*, is obtained from a closely allied plant, *Hydrocotyle asiatica minor*, and is sometimes supplied as *gotu kola*. A variety of *Centella* known as *thankuni* grows in east India. It is smaller than *C. asiatica* of Indo-gangetic plains and is less bitter. It is cooked and eaten as spinach. It is also sold as a genuine herb but is considered inferior.

Mandukparni is a herb with semi-lunar or orbicular leaves so other herbs or plants with the same types of leaves are sometimes substituted for it. Some of the known adulterants are: *Merremia emerginata* Hallier, Syn. *Ipomoea reniform* Choisy, *Evolvulus emarginatus* Burm., *Hydrocotyle javanica* Thunb. (Figs. 29A & B) and *H. rotundifolia* Roxb. (Bagchi and Puri, 1989). Recently a large-scale adulteration of the herb with *Malva rotundifolia* has been observed.

References

Agrawal, S.S. (1981) Some CNS effects of *Hydrocotyle asiatica* Linn. *Journal of Research in Ayurveda and Siddha*, 2, 144–149.

Anbuganapathi, G. (1995) The synergistic effect of Vallarai and Brahmi on learning ability of albino mice and school children. *International Seminar on Recent Trends in Pharmaceutiucal Sciences*, Ootacamund. (TN, India) 18–20 Feb. 1995.

Appa Rao, M.V.R., Srinivasan, K., Koteswara Rao, T. (1973) The effect of mandookparni (*Centella asiatica*) on the general mental ability (medhya) of mentally retarded children. *Journal for Research in Indian Medicine*, 8, 9–16.

Appa Rao, M.V.R., Srinivasan, K., Koteswara Rao, T. (1977) The effect of *Centella asiatica* on the general mental ability of mentally retarded children. *Indian Journal of Psychiatry*, 19, 54–59.

Babu, T.D., Kuttan, G., Padikkala, J. (1995) Cytotoxic and anti-tumour properties of certain taxa of Umbelliferae with special reference to *Centella asiatica* (L.) Urban. *Journal of Ethnopharmacology*, 48, 53–57.

Babu, T.D., Paddikkala, J. (1993) Anticancer activity of an active principle from *Centella asiatica*. *Amala Research Bulletin*, 13, 46–49.

Babu, T.D., Padikkala, J. (1994) DNA frgamentation in Ehrlich Ascites tumour cells by extract of herbal plant *Centella asiatica* (L.). *Amala Research Bulletin*, 14, 52–56.

Babu, T.D., Padikkala, J. (1995) The role of *Centella asiatica* extracts on chemotherapeutic drug-induced toxicity in mice. *Amala Research Bulletin*, 15, 41–45.

Bagchi, G.D., Puri, H.S. (1988) *Centella asiatica* I. *Herba Hungarica*, 27, 137–140.

Bagchi, G.D., Puri, H.S. (1989) *Centella asiatica* II. *Herba Hungarica*, 28, 127–134.

Bonte, F., Dumas, M., Chaudagne, C., Meybeck, A. (1994) Influence of asiatic acid, madecassic acid and asiaticoside on human collagen I synthesis. *Planta Medica*, 60, 133–135.

Bonte, F., Dumas, M., Chaudagne, C., Meybeck, A. (1995) Asiaticoside and madecassoside activity on human fibroblast type I and II collagen secretion. *Annales Pharmaceutiques Francaises*, 53, 38–42.

Chatterjee, T.K., Chakraborty, A., Pathak, M. (1992) Effect of plant extract *Centella asiatica* (Linn.) on cold restraint stress ulcer in rats. *Indian Journal of Experimental Biology*, 30, 889–891.

Danese, P., Carnevali, C., Bertazzoni, M.G. (1994) Allergic contact dermatitis due to *Centella asiatica* extract. *Contact Dermatitis*, 31, 201.

Ghosh, S.T. *Drugs of Hindoostan*. Hahneman Publishing Co, Calcutta, India 1930.

Grimaldi, R., De Ponti, F., D'Angelo, L., Caravaggi, M., Guidi, G., Lecchini, S., Frigo, G.M., Crema, A. (1990) Pharmacokinetics of the total triterpenic fraction of *Centella asiatica* after single and multiple administration to healthy volunteers, a new assay for asiatic acid. *Journal of Ethnopharmacology*, 28, 235–241.

Jain, P., Khanna, N.K., Trehan, N. (1994) Antiinflammatory effects of an Ayurvedic preparation Brahmi Rasayan in rodents. *Indian Journal of Experimental Biology*, 32, 633–636.

Kapoor, K.B. (1986) Study of Yogi Rasayan (Brami jam) in insomnia. *Journal of Scientific Research on Plants and Medicine*, 7, 50–53.

Kuppurajan, K. Anti-anxiety effect of an ayurvedic compound preparation. A cross over trial. *Seminar on Research in Ayurveda and Siddha*, CCRAS, New Delhi, 20–22 March 1995.

Kuppurajan, K., Seshadri, C., Rajagopalan, V., Srinivasan, K., Sitaraman, R., Indurthi, J., Venkataraghavan, S. (1992) Anti-anxiety effect of an Ayurvedic compound drug – a cross over trial. *Journal of Research in Ayurveda and Siddha*, 13, 107–116.

Lucas, Richard *Natures's Medicine*. Park Publishing, UK 1966.

Nalini, K., Aroor, A.R., Karanth, K.S., Rao, A. (1992) Effect of *Centella asiatica* fresh leaf aqueous extract on learning and memory and biogenic amine turnover in albino rats. *Fitoterapia*, 63, 232–237.

Plohmann, B., Bader, G., Streich, S., Hiller, K., Franz, G. (1994) Immno-modulatory effects of triterpenoid saponins. *European Journal of Pharmaceutical Sciences*, 21, 120.

Praveen Kumar, Kuttan, V.R., Kuttan, G. (1996) Radioprotective effects of Rasayanas. *Indian Journal of Experimental Biology*, 34, 848–850.

Sarkar, P., Sinha Babu, S.P., Sukul, N.C. (1998) Antifilarial effect of a combination of botanicals from Acacia auriculiformis and *Centella asiatica* on canine dirofilariasis. *Pharmaceutical Biology*, 36, 107–110.

Sakina, M.R., Dandiya, P.C. (1990) A psycho-neuropharmacological profile of *Centella asiatica* extract. *Fitoterapia*, 61, 291–296.

Sarma, D.N.K., Khosa, R.L., Chansauria, J.P.N., Sahai, M. (1995) Antiulcer activity of Tinospora cordifolia Miers and *Centella asiatica* Linn extracts. *Phytotherapy Research*, 9, 589–590.

Sharma, R., Jaiswal, A.N., Suresh Kumar, Chaturvedi, C., Tewari, P.V. (1985) Role of Brahmi in educable mentally retarded children. *Journal of Research in Education of Indian Medicine*, 1, 55–77.

Singh R.H., Shukla, S.P., Mishra, B.K. (1981) The psychotropic effect of Medhya rasayana drug, Mandukparni (*Hydrocotyle asiatica*): an experimental study. Part II. *Journal of Research in Ayurveda and Siddha*, 2, 1–10.

Shin, H.S., Chou, I.C., Lee, M.H., Pack, K.N. (1982) Clinical trials of medecassol: *Centella asitica* on gastro-intestinal ulcer patients. *Korean Journal of Gastroenterology*, 14, 49–56.

Shukla, S.P. (1989) A study on barbiturate hypnosis potentiation effects of different fraction of indigenous plant drug Mandukparni (*Hydrocotyle asiatica* Linn). *Bulletin of Medico-Ethnobotanical Research*, 10, 119–123.

Sunilkumar, Parameshwaraiah, S., Shivakumar, H.G. (1998) Evaluation of topical formulations of aqueous extract of *Centella asiatica* on open wounds in rats. *Indian Journal of Experimental Biology*, 36, 569–572.

Thakur, R.S., Puri, H.S., Akhtar Hussain *Major Medicinal Plants of India*. CIMAP, Lucknow, India 1989.

37 Mundi

Sphaeranthus indicus L.
S. africanus L.
Family: Asteraceae (Compositae)

THE PLANT AND ITS DISTRIBUTION

These plants are hygrophytic weeds, growing in winter in the warmer part of the Indian subcontinent. The plant is aromatic, up to 30 cm long with spreading roots. The leaves are herbaceous, serrate and 2–5 cm long. The inflorescence is pink to light violet in colour and may be up to 2 cm long. The herb has a strong smell and, if ingested, its excretion can be perceived by the unpleasant smell of urine and sweat.

USES IN FOLKLORE AND AYURVEDA

As per Ayurveda it is light, dry, bitter, sweet, hot, a blood purifier, diuretic, and sudorific.

For urinary inflammation

In syphilis, when there is acute pain passing urine and the urethra is inflamed, a decoction of the herb is given orally, as well as injected into the urethra. Through this treatment inflammation, swelling and pain subside and urine flow becomes normal. This treatment also helps these symptoms in women. It relieves various skin diseases as well. It helps in polyurea, when used for 4–6 months.

For development of the breast

Make a paste of *mundi* and long pepper with oil, filter and use it as nasal drops and for massaging on the breast.

For migraines

Heat the juice of *mundi* until warm and add black pepper powder to it. Use it before meals for seven days.

As a *Rasayana*

A powder prepared from the whole plant or from flowers has a rejuvenating effect and keeps old age away (Vaidya, 1998). It may be used as follows:

1. For physical strength and as a mental tonic, use the herb with *ghee*.
2. Root juice of the herb or tea improves youthful vigour, prevents premature greying of hair and wrinkles on the skin. The same effects are achieved when this herb is used with an equal quantity of *Eclipta*.
3. For a spermatogenic effect, the herb is given with sugar.

Ayurvedic preparations

Arq mundi (aqua mundi) I

Method   Soak 1 kg flowers in 8 litres of water and distil to obtain 5 litres of distillate (Some people mix 1 kg of fresh rose petals to above, before distillation).

Dose   125 ml.

Use   Cepahalic tonic, cardiac stimulant and for improving eyesight.

Arq mundi (aqua mundi) II

Method   Mix the juice of the ground root. When the mixture is dry add a few drops of jasmine oil. Distil the whole mass and collect the distillate.

Dose   Smear this distillate on betel leaf and chew it with betel nut.

Use   For rejuvenation.

Mundi resinoid

Method   The whole herb is distilled and the resinoid, which floats on the top of the distillate, is separated. The distillate obtained is used for further distillation of the fresh herb and more resinoid is collected.

Dose   One drop of the resinoid in a teaspoon of sugar for 40 days.

Use   Elixir for vigour and vitality and for rejuvenating the whole system.

Halwa mundi

Method   Take equal quantities of wheat flour, sugar, *ghee* and the dried, powdered whole plant of *mundi*. Make a thick syrup of sugar. Roast wheat flour in *ghee*, add the sugar syrup followed by the herb. Mix thoroughly and let it cool.

Dose   30–50 g *Halwa* daily for 40 days.

Use   Keeps the body young, energetic and provides enough strength for day-to-day activities.

It is a preparation chosen by fugitives inhabiting forests in central India. It is said to provide them enough strength and energy to remain in the ravines without food and water for days.

THERAPEUTIC INDICATIONS AND PHARMACOLOGICAL STUDIES

Immunostimulant activity

This activity has been observed in sesquiterpene glycosides of the herb (Shekhani *et al.* 1990).

Anti-tumour property

An Ayurvedic preparation which contains *Curculigo, Gymnema, Sphaeranthus, Vanda, Glycyrrhiza*, etc. protected rats against induced mammary tumours (Sharma *et al.* 1991).

Chemical studies

Alkaloid sphaeranthine, 0.02 per cent essential oil and sesquiterpene glycoside.

Substitute

Sphaeranthus amaranthoides grows in the rice fields of south India. This herb is bigger than the two species mentioned above. In this case the leaves may be up to 10 cm long and the inflorescence 1–2.5 cm long.

References

Sharma, H.M., Dwivedi, C., Dalter, B.C., Abou-Issa, H. (1991) Antineoplastic properties of Maharishi Amrit Kalash, an Ayurvedic food supplement against 7,12 dimethylbenz (a) anthracene-induced memory tumours in rats. *Journal of Research and Education in Indian Medicine*, 10, 1–8.

Shekhani, M.S., Pir Muzzam Shah, Afshan Yasmin, Rabia Siddiqui, Shahnaz Perveen, Khalid Mohammed Khan, Shana Urooj Kazmi, Atta-ur Rehman (1990) An immunostimulant sesquiterpene glycoside from Sphaeranthus indicus. *Phytochemistry*, 29, 2573–2576.

Vaidya, A.R. *The Ancient Indian System of Rejuvenation and Longevity.* Indian Book Center Delhi India 1998.

38 Musli

In Ayurveda two types of *musli*, black and white are recognized.

MUSLI BLACK

Curculigo orchioides Gaertn.
Family: Amaryllidaceae

THE PLANT AND ITS DISTRIBUTION

The plant grows as an under-shrub in the forests of south and east India. The herb has 3–4 leaves, 15–50 cm long and 3–5 cm broad, emerging from the soil (Fig. 30A). Flowers are bluish-yellow in colour, in two rows. The fruits are slightly bigger than 1 cm and oval in shape. The rootstock (Fig. 30B) is straight, about 1 cm thick, black from outside but white internally, with prominent nodes. The root has a mucilaginous bitter taste, it is rich in mucilage and contains oleogum resin.

USES IN FOLKLORE AND AYURVEDA

It is mainly used for diseases of the urinogenital system in both males and females (Yadav *et al.* 1974). It may be used as follows:

As a diuretic

It helps in polyurea, dysuria, gonorrhoea, menorrhagia, leucorrhoea and piles.

For erectile dysfunction (impotence)

It is considered a nutritive and aphrodisiac, for which 3–6 g of root powder is given twice daily.

As a geriatric tonic

It is used for gastroenteritis, hepatitis and as an anti-inflammatory agent. For most of the diseases, 25–50 g of dry root in powdered form is boiled in milk, with sugar

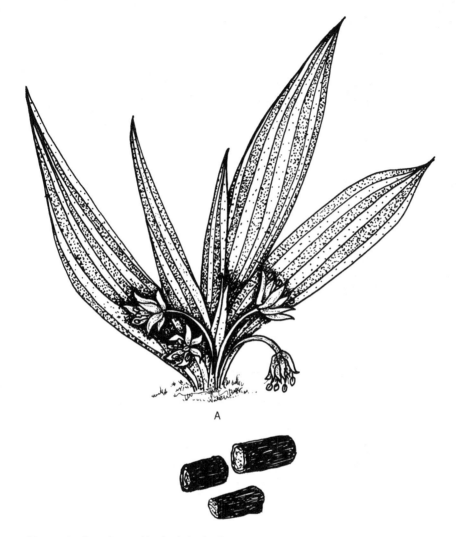

Figure 30 Curculigo orchioides **A** herb, **B** root.

according to taste. In this way it exudes mucilage and has a demulcent activity, which helps convalescent geriatric patients.

It is also used by pulverizing equal parts of *Asparagus racemosus, Curculigo orchioides, Sphaeranthus indicus, Abrus precatorius* and *Butea frondosa.*

Dose 2–5 g of powder with honey or *ghee.*

Ayurvedic preparation

Musalyadi churn

Method Pulverize equal quantities of *Curculigo, Tribulus, Bombax, Mucuna* and *Tinospora* (starch).

Dose 10–20 g with milk.

Uses In gynaecological problems due to general debility.

THERAPEUTIC INDICATIONS AND PHARMACOLOGICAL STUDIES

Fan *et al.* (1996) observed the inhibitory effect of the root on hepatitis virus B replication. Rao and Mishra (1996) noted anti-inflammatory and hepatoprotective activity in it.

MUSLI WHITE

It may be obtained from one or more of the following plants:

Asparagus adscendens Roxb. (Family: Liliaceae)
A. filicinus Ham.
Chlorophytum arundinaceum Baker (Family: Liliaceae)
C. tuberosum Baker
Roscoea purpurea Royle (Family: Scitaminae)

In commerce the drug consists of white tubular translucent pieces, up to 5 mm thick and 15 cm long. Before marketing, these are boiled in water and the outer root coat removed. This process gelatinizes starch and on cooling the root gives a waxy translucent appearance. When immersed in water the root regains its original shape by absorbing water. These roots are leathery on chewing, slightly mucilaginous, with a pleasant taste and smell.

White *musli* is considered a nutritive tonic and is used in place of *Orchis*. Tubers (12 g) boiled in milk are used for sexual inadequacies in both males and females.

Dua *et al.* (1992) observed adaptogenic activity in *Asparagus adscendens*, which protects the animals against blood pressure problems following ischaemia.

References

Dua, P.R., Tandon, M., Shukla, Y.N., Thakur, R.S. Adaptogenic activity of *Asparagus adscendens* *Proceedings of 25th Indian Pharmacologocal Society*, Muzafarpur, Bihar, India, 5–8 December 1992.

Fan Tao, Fu Xi Xian, Zhang Guo Qing (1996) The inhibitory effect of some Chinese herbs on hepatitis B virus replication in vitro and its mechanism (in Chinese). *Chinese Journal of Experimental and Clinical Virology*, 10, 27–30.

Rao, K.S., Mishra, S.H. (1996) Studies on *Curculigo orchioides* Gaertn. for antiinflammatory and hepatoprotective activity. *Indian Drugs*, 33, 20–25.

Yadav, B.B.L., Tiwari, K.C., Tiwari, V.P. (1974) A scientific study on *Cucrculigo orchioides* Gaertn. *Journal for Research in Indian Medicine*, 9, 109–123.

39 Neem

Azadirachta indica A. Juss
Family: Meliaceae

THE PLANT AND ITS DISTRIBUTION

It is an evergreen tree, growing mainly in south Asian countries, but has recently been introduced in the other drier parts of the world. Younger trees in dry localities may become leafless for a month or so in February to March. The leaves are exstipulate, alternate on a long slender petiole (Fig. 31A). The tree mainly flowers in May or June. Flowers are whitish pink (Fig. 31D) and fruit 1–2 cm long, ovoid and drupe (Fig. 31C), enclosing a shrivelled kernel (Fig. 31B).

USES IN FOLKLORE AND AYURVEDA

A monographic account of this tree has been given by Puri (1999), so only salient features about *neem* are given here.

According to Indian mythology, the tree is of divine origin. It originated from drops of nectar from heaven. The word *neem* is derived from Sanskrit *nimba* which means *to bestow health*. Other synonyms of this name are: *neta* – leader of medicinal plants, *pichumarda* – antileprotic, *ravisamba* – has healing effect like that of sunrays, *arishta* – resistant to insects, *krimighan* – antimicrobial, *sheetal* – has a cooling effect on the human system. Since ancient times, it came into prominence due to the part it played in rural daily life in India and for its healing power in chronic and obstinate diseases. It has been called *Village Pharmacy*, *Heal all*, and even *Nature's Drugstore*.

In earlier times the patients suffering from incurable and chronic diseases were advised to live under *neem* and eat all parts of the tree. Since it is considered *cool* in its effect, patients were advised to avoid all things hot in nature like animal products, alcohol, sex, spices, etc. Milk as a part of the diet was allowed. It was so popular in ancient India that some scholars think that, at that time, more than 50 per cent of the Ayurvedic preparations contained *neem* as an ingredient. In the nineteenth century a *neem* bark decoction was used for all types of fever, mainly malaria.

Even today in the Indian sub-continent *neem* is a household name for treating skin diseases. It is a common practice to take a bath in the decoction of its leaves or to chew tender leaves as a blood purifier. The fatty oil obtained from the seed is applied

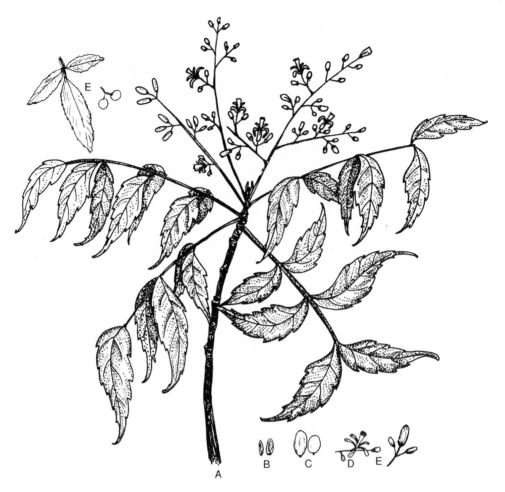

Figure 31 Azadirachta indica: **A** twig, **B** dry kernel, **C** fresh fruit, **D** flowers, *Melia azedarach*:
E leaf and fruit.

externally on skin diseases or is mixed with other ingredients. The stem sap, which is sometimes exuded by the old *neem* tree, is very much esteemed for general physiological health.

THERAPEUTIC INDICATIONS AND PHARMACOLOGICAL STUDIES

Anthelmintic activity

It is effective against a large number of nematodes and in ankylostomiasis. It gave good results as an ingredient of an anti-filarial compound.

Anti-microbial activity

It has been used as a disinfectant. Some recent studies have indicated that *neem* extract significantly inhibited many pathogenic organisms. Bark and leaf extracts suppressed fungal spore formation and in some cases were fungicidal. This activity may be due to sulphurous compounds or the limonoid gedunin in the tree.

Neem preparations have schizonticidal activity against various *Plasmodium* spp. and *Trypanosoma* spp., which cause malaria and other protozoal infections. A purified fraction of *neem* oil in a cream base has been found effective in leucorrhoea caused by *Chlamydia trachomatis*. It was highly effective in clearing infection from the cervico-vaginal region. A cream of *neem* was effective against *Candida albicans*, *Gardnerella vaginalis* and human papilloma 16 virus infecting the female genital tract. It was pro-phylactic against septicaemia caused by *Salmonella typhi*. The water extract of tender leaves has shown anti-viral activity in some cases, so *neem* preparations are being tried against HIV infection.

Anti-diabetic activity

The *neem* oil and the bitter principle nimbidin have significant anti-diabetic activity, which is comparable to that of sulphonyl urea. *Neem* oil lowered the blood glucose levels of normoglycaemic and hypoglycaemic rats.

Some commercial herbal preparations containing *neem* are available in India for treating diabetes.

Anti-inflammatory activity

It is common practice to use *neem* oil, or a decoction and poultice made from leaves and bark, for external application in gout, rheumatism, arthritis, pains, etc. Two bitter compounds, nimbin and nimbinin, obtained from the oil were comparable to cortisone in their action. The bark showed anti-inflammatory effect due to polysaccharides and gallic acid.

Anti-tumour activity

An intraperitoneal administration of polysaccharides from bark showed *in vitro* activity against Sarcoma 180 ascites tumour. In cases of mouth cancer its cytocidal effect on malignant cells has been documented. Cytotoxic effects of limonoids have also been reported.

Anti-ulcerogenic activity

A mixture of *neem* bitters had anti-gastric activity. It protected patients with Shay ulceration and duodenal lesions.

Hepatoprotective effect

An Ayurvedic preparation *Neemtwagadi kashyam*, with *neem* bark and other herbs, is specific for jaundice. In some experiments, *neem* was found effective for hepatotoxicity.

Immunomodulator property

Earlier anti-stress properties was recorded for *neem* oil, but recent studies confirmed that bark has an immunomodulator property. The compounds responsible for the inhibition of chemiluminescence production by activated human polymorphonuclear leucocytes have been isolated and identified. The anti-malarial effect of *neem* also appears to be due to the body mobilizing the immune system to suppress infection.

Chemical studies

Recently limonoids have been studied extensively. Azadirachtin is an important compound out of these.

Toxicological studies

Neem preparations have been considered safe because the leaves are used as fodder by ruminants. Recent studies indicated that extracts of leaf, bark and isolated limonoids have very low toxicity, but seed oil is not very safe in the prescribed doses.

Substitutes

The *neem* tree is sometimes confused with China berry, *Melia azedarach*, but can be easily differentiated from this tree by leaf morphology and shape of the seed (Figs. 31D, E).

Reference

Puri, H.S. *Neem The Divine tree, Azadirachta indica*. Harwood Academic Publishers, Amsterdam, Holland 1999.

40 Peepali

Piper longum L
P. peepuloides Roxb.
P. retrofractum Vahl.
Family: Piperaceae

THE PLANTS AND THEIR DISTRIBUTION

P. longum is an underground creeper or under-shrub which roots from the nodes and grows in the sub-tropical climate of the Indian subcontinent. The leaves are alternate, ovate, 5–12 cm long, acuminate and have a cordate base (Fig. 32A). Flowers are unisexual, green or yellow with berries (Fig. 32B) crowded in a black spike, 1–2 cm long and 2–3 mm in diameter. When chewed it is greenish, slimy with a spicy odour and mild pungent smell, slightly different from that of black pepper. *P. peepuloides* (Fig. 32C) has a mulberry-like fruiting spike, while in *P. longum* it is compact.

The fruiting spike used as *peepali* is mainly obtained from various cultivars of *P. longum* and allied species. Fruiting spikes are aborted in one of the cultivars, which is known as *Navsari peepal* in the trade. Another cultivar, growing in east India has globular fruiting spikes. The fruiting spike of *P. retrofractum* (Fig. 32D), called *bari peepal* (*bari* is big, in this case fruiting spikes are more than double the size of common *peepali*), is probably imported from Malaysia and Indonesia. Some people probably prefer this because of its bigger size and pungency. The root of *Piper* species, under the name *peeplamul*, is widely used in Ayurvedic medicines. Another Ayurvedic herb called *gaj pipal* (*gaj* means elephant), is also known which has a big fruiting spike. It is obtained from *Scindapsus officinalis*. The tree *Ficus religiosa* is also known as *peepal*, so sometimes there is confusion between *peepal* and *peepali* as both the plants have cordate, acuminate leaves.

USES IN FOLKLORE AND AYURVEDA

In Ayurveda it is considered a digestant, a *Rasayana*, sweet, slightly hot, bitter, anti-*kaph* and is a laxative. It is said to be useful in bronchial troubles, stomach diseases, fevers, leprosy, diabetes, piles, arthritis and inflammation. The detailed uses of *peepali* are:

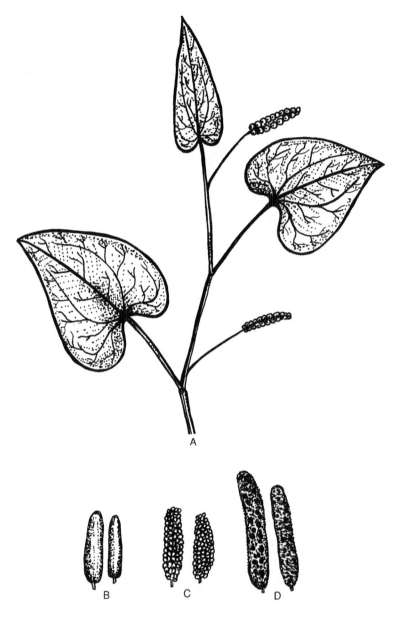

Figure 32 Piper longum: **A** twig, **B** fruiting spike, **C** *P. peepuloides*: fruiting spike,
D *P. retrofractum*: fruiting spike.

For respiratory problems

Equal parts of honey with *peepali*, or double quantity of raw sugar with *peepali*, helps
fevers and respiratory problems. For coughs with phlegm, fry *peepali* in *ghee* and
powder it. Take half a tablespoon of this powder with 1 g of salt and two table-
spoons of honey thrice daily. *Peepali*, when boiled in milk, is a smooth muscle relaxant,

anti-allergic and used for prophylaxis of asthma. Boil one fruiting spike in milk on the first day and eat it with the milk. On the second day take two fruiting spikes, three on third day and so on, increasing the number every day until intolerable. This treatment relieves chronic respiratory diseases but may cause heartburn.

For flatulence

Take 1 g of *peepali* powder and 2 g salt, mix in yogurt and drink. It causes the gas to escape from the stomach and thus provides relief for motions. It also helps appetite less.

For piles and haemorrhoids

In piles with or without blood, take 1/2 g of the *peepali* powder, 1 g of roasted cumin, add salt as per taste, mix in yogurt milk and drink.

For sciatica

Take half a tablespoon of finely powdered *peepali* along with two teaspoons of castor oil, twice daily.

For obesity

Take 1/2 spoon *peepali* powder with honey twice daily, for 2–3 months.

For conjunctivitis

Make a fine powder of 5 g *peepali* and 10 g *haritaki*. Moisten these powders with water and after kneading turn it into a candle-like structure and dry. Before use grind this candle on a wet rough stone and apply the paste onto the eyelids.

For gastroenteritis

Take an equal quantity of *peepali* and dried young *haritaki* fruit. Make a fine powder of these. Take one tablespoon of this mixture.

As an anthelmintic

For worm infestations, one part take *peepali* powder, two parts raw sugar, mix and take a dose of half a tablespoon with water.

Ayurvedic preparations

Peepali quath

Boil 20 g of coarse *peepali* powder with one glassful of water until reduced to half. Divide the resultant decoction into three equal doses and add honey. Drink thrice daily for chronic fevers and spleen enlargement until cured.

Pachak peepali

Soak *peepali* in lime juice, add salt and keep for seven days. Chew two of these *peepali* in the morning and evening for indigestion, lack of appetite, etc.

Peepali churn

Method   Make a fine powder of 50 g each of *peepali, Cyperus scariosus, Aconitum heterophyllum* and *Pistacia lentiscus* gall.

Dose   1 g with honey.

Use   For fevers, loose motions, gastroenteritis, vomiting, coughs, colds, etc. in infants and children.

Peepali pak

Method   Boil 100 g of finely powdered *P. longum* in two litres of milk until the whole mass turns semi-solid. Roast it in *ghee* and add half a kilogram of sugar syrup, heat until solid. Make candy balls of 10–20 g each.

Dose   Take one candy ball with milk after food.

Use   It increases digestive power.

Peepali assav

Method   Take 125 g *Woodfordia* flowers, 750 g dry black grapes, 3.85 kg sugar and 5 g each of coarsely powdered long and black pepper, *Piper cubeba*, turmeric, *Plumbago zeylanicum* root, *Cyperus scariosus, Embelia ribes, Piper betle*, areca nut, *Symplocos racemosus, Cissampelos pareira, Emblica officinalis*, aloe juice dry, *Vetiveria, Santalum album, Saussurea*, clove, valerian, *Nardostachys grandiflora*, cinnamon, cardamom, *Cinnamomum* spp. leaves, *Mesua ferrea* and *Callicarpa macrophylla*. Crush grapes and add the above herbs and sugar in a pot with 5.25 litres of water and let it ferment for 45 days. When ready, filter and pour it into bottles.

Dose   25 ml.

Use   It is a general tonic, particularly useful in digestive and respiratory problems.

Contraindication

Preparations containing *peepali* should not be used in the case of blisters, dryness and persistent bitter taste in the mouth, red eyes, hot and watery face, inflammation of the body and sleeplessness.

THERAPEUTIC INDICATIONS AND PHARMACOLOGICAL STUDIES

Tripathi *et al.* (1996) reviewed *Piper* spp. for the phytochemistry and biological activity. The important aspects of this study are given below.

Trikatu

In Ayurveda, a composition consisting of long pepper, black pepper and ginger is very often incorporated into various formulations under the name *Trikatu*. In some research (Atal *et al.* 1981) it was found that *Trikatu* enhanced the bioavailability of other therapeutic agents. Zutshi and Kaul (1982) observed that individual members, as well as *Trikatu* collectively, increased the bioavailability of vaccines by 300 per cent when orally ingested. The same effect was seen in long and black pepper, and it was found that this activity is due to the alkaloid piperine. Lee *et al.* (1984) carried out a pharmacological study on piperine. Bano *et al.* (1987) noted that piperine altered the pharmacokinetic parameters of phenytoin. Majumdar *et al.* (1990) also observed that piperine makes pentabarbitone more potent and thus increases sleeping time by inhibiting liver enzymes. Annamalai and Manavalan (1990) also confirmed that *Trikatu* enhanced the therapeutic activity by reducing acid secretion and preventing the degradation of active medicaments by gastric acids. Majeed *et al.* (1996) patented the use of piperine for gastro-intestinal absorption and its systemic utilization in nutritional supplements. Shoba *et al.* (1998) confirmed that *Trikatu* enhanced the bioavailability of drugs.

Anti-allergic action

Dahanukar *et al.* (1984) observed this activity of *peepali* in childhood asthma when fed to children both under and above the age of five. This treatment reduced the severity of attacks. It reduced passive cutaneous anaphylaxis and protected against antigen-induced bronchiospasm (Dahanukar and Karandikar, 1984).

Vasodilator effect

Shoji *et al.* (1986) isolated a compound dehydropperonaline from it, which possessed coronary vasodilating activity.

Analgesic activity

Eun (1986) fed piperine from *P. longum* to experimental rats to study the mechanism of its analgesic action. This alkaloid showed profound analgesia, it increased the level of β-endorphin in the midbrain and decreased opiate binding.

Anti-cancerous property

Reen and Singh (1991) noted that piperine caused the inhibition of pulmonary cytochrome P 450 both *in vitro* and *in vivo*. It protected against AFBI-induced cytotoxicity and micronuclei formation in H4IIEC3 rat hepatoma cells. It markedly reduced the toxicity of mycotoxins. It was capable of counteracting AFBI toxicity by suppressing cytochrome P-450 mediated bioactivation of mycotoxins (Singh *et al.* 1994).

Anti-ulcer activity

Gursahani and Vasudevan (1994) observed anti-nuclear activity in piperine. Oral administration of this alkaloid significantly inhibited ulceration. It had a protective action on gastric mucosa.

Hepatoprotective effect

Koul and Kapil (1993) noted that piperine inhibited the metabolism of drugs by the liver. It also had a liver protective effect.

A marketed Ayurvedic preparation containing *Thespesia populnea*, cardamum, ginger, liquorice, long pepper and honey showed marked anti-hepatotoxicity activity in the laboratory as well as in clinical studies (Shirwalke *et al.* 1990).

Anti-microbial activity

Kapil (1993) tried piperine against *Leishmania donovani*, which causes kala-azar or black fever and found it a potent inhibitor of this pathogen. Ghoshal *et al.* (1996) found anti-amoebic activity in *P. longum* fruit, against *Entamoeba histolytica* caecal amoebiasis. The ethanol extract cured 90 per cent of rats.

Anabolic effect

Singh and Guru (1972) noted an anabolic effect in the preparation *Pippali Rasayna*. Singh *et al.* (1973) found analeptic activity in the alkaloids. Tripathi *et al.* (1989) noted a thyrogenic response in long pepper. It increased the basal metabolic rates with significant enhancement in the tissue's oxygen uptake and thyroid peroxidase activity.

In bronchial asthma

Anshuman (1984) tried an Ayurvedic preparation *Vardhman Peepali* (peepali boiled in milk) and found it effective for respiratory disorders and in bronchial asthma.

In dysentery

Aggarwal *et al.* (1994) tried *Pippali Rasayana* prepared from *Peepali* and *Butea* seed for chronic dysentery and worm infestation. The preparation was tested for anti-giardial and immunostimulating activity. There was up to 80 per cent recovery from infection. It did not kill parasites directly but by host resistance, by inducing significant activity on macrophages, as was indicated by increased macrophage migration index and phagocytic activity. Agrawal *et al.* (1997) carried out further studies of *Pippali Rasayana* on giardiasis. After 15 days of treatment there was complete disappearance of *Giardia lamblia* (*G. duodenalis*) and a reduction of mucus and pus cells. The recovery rate was 92 per cent with no abdominal discomfort.

In muscular weakness

Dasture (1994) tried two Ayurvedic herbomineral preparations containing *Trikatu* for muscular weakness. Both of these potentiated electrically induced contractions. D'Hooge *et al.* (1996) observed anti-convulsant properties in piperine. It significantly blocked convulsions induced by receptor agonists.

Chemical studies

It contains 0.7 per cent essential oil, the alkaloids piperine and piplartine, as well as the other compounds sesamin and pillasterol. In the root, piperine, piplartine and piperlonguimine alkaloids are present (Thakur *et al.* 1989).

Substitutes

The roots of *Piper longum* are well known under the name *piplamul*. It is said to be mild but inferior in effect, compared with *peepali*. It is available in small cylindrical pieces of nodal and internodal pieces, about 2 mm thick. The nodal pieces are considered superior to internodal ones.

References

Agarwal, A.K., Singh, M., Gupta, N., Saxena, R., Puri, A., Verma, A.K. (1994) Management of giardiasis by an immunomodulatory herbal drug Pippali rasayana. *Journal of Ethnopharmacology*, 44, 143–146.

Agarwal, A.K., Tripathi, D.M., Sahai, R., Gupta, N., Saxena, R.P., Puri, A., Singh, M., Misra, R.N., Dubey, C.B., Saxena, K.C. (1997) Management of giardiasis by a herbal drug *Pipali Rasayana*: a clinical study. *Journal of Ethnopharmacology*, 56, 223–236.

Annamalai, A.R., Manavalan, R. (1990) Effect of *Trikatu* and its individual components and piperine on gastrointestinal tracts: Trikatu-a bioavailable enhancer. *Indian Drugs*, 27, 595–604.

Anshuman, P.S., Singh, K.P., Aasra, K.G. (1984) Effect of Vardhman Pippali (*Piper longum*) on patients with respiratory disorders. *Sachitra Ayurveda*, 37, 47–49.

Atal, C.K., Zutshi, U., Rao, P.G. (1981) Scientific evidence on the role of Ayurvedic herbals on bioavailability of drugs. *Journal of Ethnopharmacology*, 4, 229–232.

Bano, G., Amla, V., Raina, R.K., Zutshi, U., Chopra, C.L. (1987) The effect of piperine on pharmacokinetics of phenytoin in healthy volunteers. *Planta Medica*, 53, 568–569.

Dahanukar, S.A., Karandikar, S.M. (1984) Evaluation of antiallergic activity of *Piper longum*. *Indian Drugs*, 21, 377–383.

Dahanukar, S.A., Karandikar, S.M., Desai, M. (1984) Efficacy of *Piper longum* in childhood asthma. *Indian Drugs*, 21, 384–388.

Dasture, A.V. (1994) Screening of two Ayurvedic preparations for usefulness in treatment of muscular weakness. *Deerghayu International*, 1, 3–8.

D'Hooge, R., Pei, Yinquan, Raes A., Lebrun, P., Bogaert, P.P. van, Deyn, P.P. de (1996) Anticonvulsant activity of piperine on seizures induced by excitatory amino acid receptor agonists. *Arzneimittel Forschung*, 46, 557–560.

Eun, J.S. (1986) A study on the mechanism of analgesic action of piperine. *Yakhak Hoeji*, 30, 169–173.

Ghoshal, S., Prasad, B.N.K., Laksmi, V. (1996) Antiamoebic activity of *Piper longum* fruits against *Entamoeba histolytica* in vitro and in vivo. *Journal of Ethnopharmacology*, 50, 167–170.

Gursahani, H.I., Vasudevan, T.N. Antiulcer activity of piperine. *Proceedings 46th Indian Pharmaceutical Congress*, Chandigarh, India, 28–30 December 1994.

Kapil, A. (1993) Piperine: a potent inhibitor of Leishmania donovani in vitro. *Planta Medica*, 59, 474.

Koul, I.B., Kapil, A. (1993) Evaluation of the liver protetctive potential of piperine, an active principle of black and long peppers. *Planta Medica*, 59, 413–417.

Lee, E.B., Shin, K.H., Woo, W.S. (1984) Pharmacological study on piperine. *Archives Pharm. Research*, 7, 127–132.

Majumdar, A.M., Dhuley, J.N., Deshmukh, V.K., Raman, P.H., Thorat, S.L., Naik, S.R. (1990) Effect of piperine on pentobarbitone-induced hypnosis in rats. *Indian Journal of Experimental Biology*, 28, 485–487.

Majed, M., Badmaev, V., Rajendran, R. Use of piperine to increase the bioavailability of nutritional compounds. *Patent to Sabinasa Corporation*, Piscataway, N.J., U.S. Patent 5,536,506, dated 19 July, 1996.

Ray, K.P.S. (1979) Pepper. *Indian Drugs*, 16, 199–203.

Reen, R.K., Singh, J. (1991) In vitro and in vivo inhibition of pulmonary cytochrome, P 450 activity by piperine, a major ingredient of Piper species. *Indian Journal of Experimental Biology*, 29, 556–573.

Shirwalker, A., Kumar, A.V., Sreenivasan, K.K., Gundu Rao, P. Evaluation of a marketed antihepatotoxic Ayurvedic preparation. *Proceedings of 42nd Annual Indian Pharmaceutical Congress*, Manipal, 28–30 December 1990.

Shoba, G., Joy, D., Joseph, T., Majeed, M., Rajendra, R., Srinivasan, P.S.S.R. (1998) Influence of piperine on the pharmcokinetics of curcumin in animals and human volunteers. *Planta Medica*, 64, 353–356.

Shoji, N., Umajawo, A., Saito, N., Talemoto, T., Rajiwara, A., Ohizumu, Y. (1986) Dehydropperonaline: an amide possessing coronary vasodilating activity isolated from *Piper longum* L. *Journal of Pharmaceutical Science*, 75, 1188–1189.

Singh, I.P., Guru, L.V. (1972) A preliminary study on the effect of alcoholic extractive of Pippali Rasayna on serum proteins of experimental animals. *Journal of Research in Indian Medicine*, 7, 81–84.

Singh, J., Reen, R.K., Wiebel, F.J. (1994) Piperine, a major ingredient of black and long peppers, protects against AfB1-incuded cytotoxicity and micronuclei formation in H4IIEC3 rat hepatoma cells. *Cancer Letters*, 86, 195–200.

Singh, N., Kulshrestha, Srivatava, R.K., Kohli, R.P. (1973) Studies on the analeptic activity of some *Piper longum* alkaloids. *Journal of Research in Indian Medicine*, 8, 1–9.

Tripathi, A.K., Jain, D.C., Sushil Kumar (1996) Secondary metabolites and their biological and medicinal activities of *Piper* species plants. *Journal of Medicinal and Aromatic Plant Sciences*, 18, 302–321.

Tripathi, P., Tripathi, G.S., Tripathi, Y.B. (1989) Thyrogenic response of *Piper nigrum*. *Fitoterapia*, 60, 539–542.

Zutshi, U., Kaul, J.L. (1982) The impact of ayurvedic herbals on drug bio-availability. *Indian Drugs*, 19, 476–479.

41 Punernava

Boerhaavia diffusa L.
Family: Nyctagenaceae

THE PLANT AND ITS DISTRIBUTION

It is a common prostate or ascending creeping weed, purple in colour (Fig. 33A), which grows throughout the warmer parts of India on sandy and rocky soil. The stem is thickened at the nodes. The leaves are ovate or suborbicular, rounded at the apex, 2–4 cm long, margin entire, pink, with a base that is rounded to subcordate. Flowers are very small (4–6mm), in umbels arranged in panicles.

In Ayurvedic literature two types of *punernava*, red and white, are mentioned. *B. diffusa* and the allied species *B. repanda* and *B. erecta* with reddish leaves and commonly with violet pink flowers are considered the source of the red variety but there is controversy about the correct identification of white *punernava*. At one stage *Trianthema monogyna* L., which is a prostate, succulent herb that grows in the rainy season in damp places and has both pink and white flowers was thought to be white *punernava* (Singh and Udupa, 1972a). However *B. verticillata* R. Br. has now been identified as the source of this drug. It is a robust form but very rare in nature.

Punernava (Fig. 33B) is a woody rootstock, fibrous, twisted like rope, usually less than 1 cm thick and brownish in colour. When pressure is applied to it, it liberates white powder which causes a light itching. It has no characteristic taste or smell. To confirm the source of commercial samples, Surange *et al.* (1973) carried out a comparative pharmacological study on the genuine root and commercial samples and found that both have the same activities.

USES IN FOLKLORE AND AYURVEDA

In Ayurveda *punernava* is used as antidote to toxins, a rejuvenator and a *Rasayana* as follows:

For cardiac problems

In oedema, it is given with equal quantities of *Picrorhiza*, *Swertia* and ginger. It is said to have a *Digitalis*-like effect.

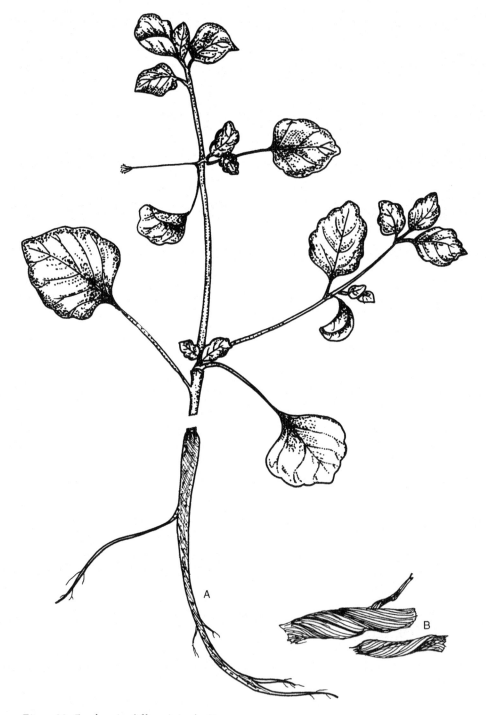

Figure 33 Boerhaavia diffusa **A** herb, **B** root.

For bronchial troubles

For coughs with sputum and inflammation, it is given with equal quantities of calamus and ginger. This medicament causes nausea but clears the bronchial tubes of all extraneous matter.

For liver problems

The distillate from the herb is considered effective in controlling cirrhosis of the liver.

As a diuretic

It is used for oedema, inflammation, nephrotic conditions, jaundice, ascites and for scanty urine.

Ayurvedic preparation

Punernava mundur

Method   Pulverize 200 g of following mixture of herbs in equal quantities: *Boerhaavia*, *Operculina turpethum*, ginger, black pepper, long pepper, *Embelia ribes*, *Cedrus deodara*, *Saussurea lappa*, turmeric, *Plumbago zeylanica*, *Terminalia bellirica*, *T. chebula*, *Emblica officinalis*, *Baliospermum montanum*, *Piper cubeba*, *Holarrhena antidysentrica* seed, *Picrorhiza kurroa*, *Piper longum* root, *Cyperus scariosus*, *Pistacia lentiscus*, *Carum carvi*, *Ptychotis* and *Myrica nagi*. Take 400 g of processed iron rust in 1,600 ml of cow's urine in an iron pot. (Iron rust is processed by first heating it strongly on coal and immersing in cow's urine when red hot. This treatment is repeated seven times. The rust is powdered and mixed with an infusion of *Triphala*. The whole mixture is dried and heated thirty times. In the end a brick-red coloured iron compound is obtained.) Boil the rust in the urine until it is reduced to one-fourth. Add the powder of herbs prepared above to this rust and heat the whole mixture until it is thick enough for making pills of pea size.

Dose   2–4 pills twice daily with raw sugar, followed by water.

Uses   It is prescribed for hepatic diseases, such as inflammation, swelling accompanied by flatulence, mild fever, indigestion, anaemia, spleen enlargement and weakness. It helps excretion of both urine and faeces, and increases respiratory rate. It stimulates blood circulation, which results in reduced swellings of the liver and spleen, as well as reducing oedema.

THERAPEUTIC INDICATIONS AND PHARMACOLOGICAL STUDIES

As a diuretic

The ash of the plant is rich in potassium nitrate and for a long time it was considered that the diuretic action of the herb was attributed to this (Thakur *et al.* 1989). Earlier studies indicate that *punernava* increased urinary output but decreased urinary albumin and specific gravity. Singh and Udupa (1972 a, b, c) observed that the best results with this herb were seen in oedema due to renal diseases. It had a urinary antiseptic effect and improved the pattern of renal recovery. It showed cardiotonic, hypertensive and smooth muscles relaxant effects. These authors postulated that it increased urine output due to its cardiotonic effect. The increase in the cardiac output raised the blood pressure, leading to an increase in the renal blood flow and improved glomerular filtration rate. It was useful in nephrotic syndrome. The root extract studied by Mudgal (1974, 1975) had a better diuretic, anti-inflammatory property and it improved renal recovery faster. When given to patients of nephrotic syndrome by Singh (1991), the root, in powder form, was as effective as cortisone and modern diuretics. *Punernava* increased serum protein and immunoglobulin levels but reduced urinary protein excretion (Singh *et al.* 1992).

As an anabolic agent

Appa Rao *et al.* (1967, 1969) studied the *Rasayana* effect of the powdered root on human volunteers. A moderate decrease in the mean levels of blood urea and serum acid phosphates was observed. Rajgopalan *et al.* (1977) observed that it caused nitrogen retention through its action on the liver, which helped growth and longevity.

Anti-hepatotoxic activity

Chakraborti and Handa (1989) found anti-hepatotoxic activity in petroleum ether, chloroform and methanol extracts of *B. repand* root. Rawat *et al.* (1997) tried powders and aqueous extracts of various sized roots. The aqueous extract (2 ml/kg) of a root of diameter 1–3 cm, collected in May, was more effective compared with the other root powders.

In ulcers due to stress

Sharma *et al.* (1991a) observed that the herb protected animals from stress and haemorrhagic ulcers. It had differential effects on the GABA levels of various regions of the brain (Sharma *et al.* 1991b). Mungantiwar *et al.* (1997) found that the alkaloid fraction of the root possessed restorative activity against stress-induced changes in plasma and cortical levels in rats. It significantly augmented the antibody production in stressed rats.

Effect on enzymatic systems

Goswami and Sarma (1992) administered crystalline alkaloids of this herb to experimental animals to study catalase and adenosine triphosphatase (ATPase) activity. In the initial stages there was no alteration in catalase activity, but it decreased significantly after two hours. ATPase activity, after the administration of the alkaloids, increased after 45 minutes and reached its peak after 135 minutes.

Cardiotonic effect

Punarnavoside, a new anti-fibrinolytic agent, has been isolated from the root by Jain and Khanna (1989). A lignan isolated from the roots exhibited a significant calcium channel antagonistic effect in a frog's heart single cell (Lami *et al.* 1991).

In sexual inadequacy

The root powder in a dose of 500 mg, twice daily for 15 days, was effective against leucorrhoea and spermatorrhoea (Singh, 1991).

Toxicological studies

The ethanol extract was administered twice daily in pregnant female albino rats during the entire period of gestation. It did not have any teratogenic effect or foetal abnormality (Singh *et al.* 1991).

References

Appa Rao, M.V.R., Rajagopalan, S.S., Srinivasan, V.R., Sarangan, R. (1969) Study of Mandookparni and Punernava for their Rasayana effect on normal healthy adults. *Nagarjun*, 12, 33.

Appa Rao, M.V.R., Usha, S.P., Rajagopalan, S.S., Sarangan, R. (1967) Six months' result of double blind clinical trial to study effect of Mandookparni and Puneranava on normal adults. *Journal of Research in Indian Medicine*, 2, 79.

Chakraborti, K.K., Handa, S.S. (1989) Antihepatotoxic investigations on *Boerhaavia repand* Willd. *Indian Drugs*, 27, 161–166.

Goswami, P., Sarma, T.C. (1992) Effect of *Boerhaavia diffusa* Linn. extracts on the activities of enzyme systems. *Journal of Research in Ayurveda and Siddha*, 13, 135–140.

Jain, G.K., Khanna, N.M. (1989) Punarnavoside, a new antifibrinolytic agent from *Boerhaavia diffusa* Linn. *Indian Journal of Chemistry*, 28B, 163–166.

Lami, N., Kadota, S., Kikuchi, T., Momose, Y. (1991) Constituents of the roots of *Boerhaavia diffusa* L. III Identification of Ca 2+ channel antagonistic compound from the methanol extract. *Chemical and Pharmaceutical Bulletin*, 39, 1551–1555.

Mudgal, V. (1974) Comparative studies on the anti-inflammatory and diuretic action with different parts of the plant *Boerhaavia diffusa* Linn. (Punernava). *Journal of Research in Indian Medicine*, 9, 57–58.

Mudgal, V. (1975) Studies on medicinal properties of *Convolvulus pluricaulis* and Boerhaavia diffusa. *Planta Medica*, 28, 62–68.

Mungantiwar, A.A., Nair, A.M., Shinde, U.A., Saraf, M.N. (1997) Effect of stress on plasma and adrenal cortisol levels and immune responsiveness in rats: modulation by alkaloidal fraction of Boerhaavia diffusa. *Fitoterapia*, 68, 498–500.

Rajagopalan, S.S., Appa Rao. M.V.R., Rao, T.K., Sitaraman, R., Lakshmipathi, A. (1977) Effects of *Punernava* on longevity, growth and tissue composition of albino rats. *Nagarjun*, 20, 23–27.

Rawat, A.K.S., Mehrotra, S., Tripathi, S.C., Shome, U. (1997) Hepatoprotective activity of *Boerhaavia diffusa* L. roots – a popular Indian ethnomedicine. *Journal of Ethnopharmacolgy*, 56, 61–66.

Sharma, K., Pasha, V.K., Dandiya, P.C. (1991a) Effect of *Boerhaavia diffusa* on behavioural, biochemical and pathological manifestations of stress. *Proceedings 24th Indian Pharmacological Society Conference*, Ahmedabad, 29–31 December 1991.

Sharma, K., Pasha, V.K., Dandiya, P.C. (1991b) Effect of *Boerhaavia diffusa* Linn on GABA levels of the brain during stress (abstract). *Conference of Pharmacology and Symposium on Herbal drugs*, New Delhi, 15 March 1991.

Singh, A., Singh, R.G., Singh, R.H., Mishra, N., Singh, N. (1991) An experimental evaluation of possible teratogenic potential in *Boerhaavia diffusa* in albino rats. *Planta Medica*, 57, 315–316.

Singh, R.H., Udupa, K.N. (1972a) Studies on the indigenous drug Punernava (*Boerhaavia diffusa* Linn.). Part I Identification and pharmacognostical studies. *Journal of Research in Indian Medicine*, 7, 1–12.

Singh, R.H., Udupa, K.N. (1972b) Studies on the indigenous drug Punernava (*Boerhaavia diffusa* Linn.). Part III. Experimental and Pharamacological studies. *Journal of Research in Indian Medicine*, 7, 17–27.

Singh, R.H., Udupa, K.N. (1972c) Studies on the indigenous drug Punernava (*Boerhaavia diffusa* Linn.). Part IV. Preliminary controlled trials in nephrotic syndrome. *Journal of Research in Indian Medicine*, 7, 28–33.

Singh, R.P., Shukla, K.P., Pandey, B.L., Singh, R.G., Usha Singh, R.H. (1992) Recent approach in clinical and experimental evaluation of diuretic action of Punarnava (*Boerhaavia diffusa*) with special reference to nephrotic syndrome. *Journal of Research and Education in Indian Medicine*, 11, 29–36.

Singh, S.P. (1991) Therapeutic activity of Punarnava (*Boerhaavia repanda* Willd) root powder. *Journal of Research and Education in Indian Medicine*, 10, 23–25.

Surange, S.R., Pataskar, R.D., Pendse, G.S. (1973) Comparative pharmacological studies on roots of genuine and commercial samples of Boerhaavia diffusa Linn. (Punernava). *Journal of Research in Indian Medicine*, 8, 4.

Thakur, R.S., Puri, H.S., Akhtar Hussain *Major Medicinal Plants of India*. Central Institute of Medicinal and Aromatic Plants, Lucknow, India 1989.

42 Pushkarmul

Inula racemosa Hook f.
Family: Asteraceae (Compositae)

THE PLANT AND ITS DISTRIBUTION

The herb (Fig. 34A) may grow up to 2 m tall. The leaves are big, 20–40 cm long and 12–20 cm broad. The outer surface of its leaves are rough, lower hirsuate and margin dentate. Inflorescence is 4–5 cm in diameter. Its root (Fig. 34B) is thick tuberous, horny, with a slight orris-camphoraceous smell. It grows in the alpine region of the western Himalayas, along with *Saussurea lappa* and very often one is substituted for the other.

The Ayurvedic name of the plant, *pushkarmul* (*Pushkar* is sun, and *mul* root in Sanskrit), is often used in a corrupted form, *pohkarmul*, in Indian trade. Genuine root is hard to obtain and very often *S. lappa* root is supplied instead. Some people consider orris root obtained from *Iris germanica* or even *I. florentina* a source of *pushakarmul*, while others think that *I. racemosa* is the source of another Ayurvedic herb, *rasna* (Chunekar and Pandey, 1969).

USES IN FOLKLORE AND AYURVEDA

It is considered a diuretic, stimulant, digestant, anti-inflammatory, anthelmintic and bronchodilator. It causes contraction of the uterus and the respiratory system, relieves swellings, backache and rheumatic pain. It is an antidote to poison (*ama*) developed within the body. For skin diseases such as ringworm and itching, decoction of the root is used for washing, and the root macerated in cow's urine is applied externally as a cataplasm.

THERAPEUTIC INDICATIONS AND PHARMACOLOGICAL STUDIES

In heart diseases

Tripathi *et al.* (1984a, 1988) assessed the adrenergic beta blocking activity of root powder in ischaemic heart diseases. Petroleum ether extract of the root lowered

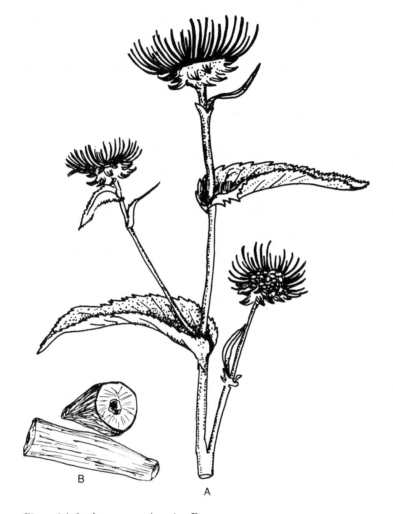

Figure 34 Inula racemosa **A** twig, **B** root.

plasma insulin and glucose levels within 75 minutes of oral administration. It counteracted adrenaline and induced hyperglycaemia in rats. Sati and Sharma (1990) tried it for congestive cardiac failure. Arora *et al.* (1995) evaluated the cardioprotective activity of the drug in coronary artery diseases, hypertension and diabetes mellitus.

Pushkar Guggal (2 g), a mixture of *Commiphora* and *Inula*, was administered three times daily for 4 months in angina pectoris and in the management of ischaemic heart diseases. By this treatment periodical pain, discomfort and dysphonia were controlled. It decreased mean serum cholesterol (Sharma and Gupta, 1983, Tripathi *et al.* 1984b, Sharma *et al.* 1986a,b, Singh *et al.* 1991, 1993).

Dwivedi *et al.* (1987) tried a polyherbal preparation containing *pushkarmul, Saussurea lappa* and *Terminalia arjuna* for heart diseases. It enhanced the aortic prostaglandin E2.

In diabetes

Singh *et al.* (1985) used this root with *Cinnamomum tamala* leaves and found it to be very effective for diabetes. Tripathi and Chaturvedi (1995) observed that alcohol extract lowered blood glucose and enhanced liver glycogen without an increase in plasma insulin. It may be due to enhanced insulin synthesis. It had no effect on the adrenal gland. Chaturvedi *et al.* (1995) studied its effect on glucose levels in albino rats. Ethanol extract, 400 mg/kg, lowered plasma glucose level four hours after administration. It increased the concentration of liver glycogen and reduced the concentration of plasma insulin, which returned to normal after four hours.

Hepatoprotective effect

Rao and Mishra (1997) found that the root was effective in liver diseases.

Anti-asthmatic effect

Singh *et al.* (1980) observed its anti-asthmatic, anti-spasmodic activity. The alcohol extract of the root protected against bronchiospasms induced by histamines, pollen, etc.

As a hypolipidaemic agent

It reduced fatty acids, triglycerides, total serum lipids and cholesterol (Ojha *et al.* 1977). Singh *et al.* (1993) tried *Pushkar guggal* on 200 hypolipidaemia patients and observed good results.

Anti-microbial property

The essential oil from *I. helenium* was effective against bacteria and fungi (Bourrel *et al.* 1993). Note: This root also contains inulin, and some of the above pharmacological activities, as detailed under *Saussurea lappa*, may be due to this compound.

Chemical studies

The root contains inulin and essential oil. The other active constituent is alantolactone.

Toxicological studies

In large doses it causes nausea and vomiting.

References

Arora, R.C., Agarwal, N., Arora, S., Kanchan, S.N. (1995) Evaluation of CT (cardioprotective drug) in subjects of coronary artery diseases, hypertension, and diabetes mellitus. *Flora and Fauna*, 1, 203–205.

Bourrrel, C., Vilarem, G., Perinean, F. (1993) Chemical analysis, bacteriostatic and fungistatic properties of the essential oil of Elecampane (*Inula helenium* L). *Journal of Essential Oil Research*, 5, 411–417.

Chaturvedi, P., Shukla, S., Tripathi, P., Chaurasia, S., Singh, S.K., Tripathi, Y.B. (1995) Comparative study of Inula racemosa and Saussurea lappa on the glucose levels in albino rats. *Ancient Science of Life*, 15, 62–70.

Chunekar, K.C. Pandey, G.S. *Bhavprakash Nighantu* (in Hindi). Chowkhamba Vidyabhawan, Varanasi India, 1969.

Dwivedi, S., Chansouria, J.P.N., Mani, P.N., Udupa, K.N. (1987) Influence of certain indigenous drugs on the prostaglandin E2 like activity in the ischaemic aorta. *Indian Drugs*, 24, 378–382.

Ojha, J.K., Sharma, P.V., Bajpai, H.S. (1977) Inula racemosa (pushkarmul) – a hypolipid agent, an experimental and clinical study. *Indian Journal of Pharmacy*, 39, 176.

Rao, K.S., Mishra, S.H. (1997) Hepatoprotective activity of *Inula racmosa* root. *Fitoterapia* 68, 510–514.

Sati, R.B., Sharma, R.K. (1990) Management of congestive cardiac failure with cardiac drugs. *Aryavaidyan*, 4, 123–126.

Sharma, S.D., Gupta, V.K. (1983) A clinical assessment of *Commiphora mukul* (Guggulu) and *Inula racemosa* (Pushkarmula) for the treatment of coronary heart disease (Hridroga). *Journal National Integrated Medicine Association*, 25, 384–393.

Sharma, S.D., Upadhyay, B.N., Tripathi, S.N. (1986a) A new Ayurvedic compound for the management of ischaemic heart disease (Hrdyroga). *Ancient Science of Life*, 5, 161–167.

Sharma, S.D., Upadhyay, B.N., Tripathi, S.N. (1986b) Ayurvedic therapy for coronary heart disease (hridyaroga). *Journal National Integrated Medical Association*, 26, 249–253.

Singh, N., Nath, R., Gupta, M.L., Kohli, R.P. (1980) An experimental evaluation of anti-asthmatic potentialities of *Inula racemosa*. (Puskar Mul). *Quarterly Journal of Crude Drug Research*, 18, 89–96.

Singh, R., Singh, R.P., Batliwala, P.G., Upadhyaya, B.N., Tripathi, S.N. (1991) Pushkar Guggal an antianginal and hypolipidemic agent in coronary heart disease (CHD). *Journal of Research in Ayurveda and Siddha*, 12, 1–18.

Singh, R.P., Singh, R., Ram, P., Batliwala, P.G. (1993) Use of Pushkar Guggal, an indigenous, antischemic combination in the management of ischaemic heart disease. *International Journal of Pharmacology*, 31, 147–160.

Singh, T.N., Upadhyay, B.N., Tewari, C.M., Tripathi, S.N. (1985) Management diabetes mellitus (Premeha) with *Inula racemosa* and *Cinnamoum tamala*. *Ancient Science of Life*, 5, 9–16.

Tripathi, S.N., Upadhyaya, B.N., Gupta, V.K. (1984) Beneficial effect of *Inula racemosa* (Pushkarmoola) in Angina pectoris: A preliminary report. *Indian Journal of Physiology and Pharmacology*, 28, 73–75.

Tripathi, S.N., Upadhyay, B.N., Sharma, S.D., Gupta, V.K., Tripathi, Y.B. (1984a) Role of Pushkara Guggal in the management of ischaemic heart disease. *Ancient Science of Life*, 4, 9–19.

Tripathi, T.B., Tripathi, P., Upadhyay, B.N. (1988) Assessment of the andenergic beta-blocking activity of *Inula racemosa*. *Journal of Ethnopharmacology*, 23, 3–9.

Tripathi, Y.B., Chaturvedi, P. (1995) Assessment of endocrine response of *Inula racemosa* in relation to glucose homeostasis in rats. *Indian Journal of Experimental Biology*, 33, 686–689.

43 Salai Guggal

Boswellia serrata Roxb. ex Colebr.
Family: Burseraceae

THE TREE AND ITS DISTRIBUTION

The tree grows wild in forests of hilly areas of central India. It has smooth, yellow or ash coloured bark with alternate, imparipinnate leaves (Fig. 35) which are crowded at the end of branches. Leaflets are sessile and opposite, in 8–15 pairs. Flowers are in axillary racemes. The fruit is three-angled, splitting into three valves.

Two varieties of the tree have been recognized:

var. *serrata* with pubescent leaves.

var. *glabra* with entirely glabrous leaves. (It is sometimes wrongly identified as *B. glabra*.)

The gum is obtained by removing small patches of the bark from the tree trunk. The resin from the stem, on drying, gets deposited along the sides of the bark after a few days, and is collected from there. The gum is pooled at collection centres and is sorted by hand into various qualities. The gum pieces are globular, club shaped, stalactitic drops of pale yellow to brown, which may coagulate to form bigger lumps. The gum has a typical odour. In trade the oleo-gum resin is known as *Kundru, Dhup, Loban*, Indian olibanum or frankincense. Some times the gum of *B. carterii* Birdw. imported from north Africa or Arabia is also supplied as *Kundru*.

USES IN FOLKLORE AND AYURVEDA

In Ayurveda the gum is considered anti-dysentric, anti-pyretic, and is used mainly in rheumatism and convulsions, but also in various nervous diseases. It is an astringent and anti-inflammatory agent when applied externally. It is not a constituent of important Ayurvedic products. It is sometimes used as a substitute for *guggal* gum.

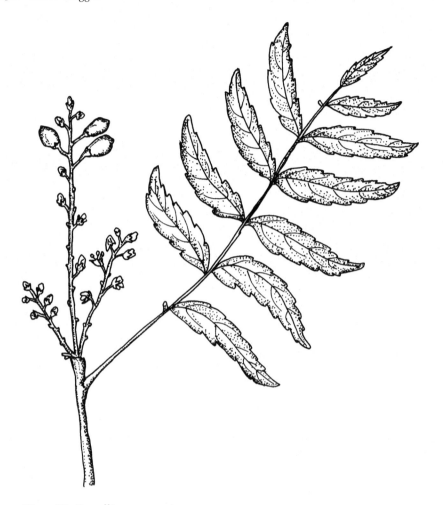

Figure 35 Boswellia serrata twig.

THERAPEUTIC INDICATIONS AND PHARMACOLOGICAL STUDIES

Tranquillizing property

The non-phenolic fraction of the gum was tried on rats by Menon and Kar (1971).

The animals showed a reduction in spontaneous motor activity and the closing of eyelids. The rats became alert at the slightest disturbance but returned to a state of sedation after a few minutes, showing a tranquillizing effect. The non-phenolic fraction acted like morphine. It produced marked and long-lasting hypotensive activity in anaesthetized dogs (Kar, 1977).

As an anti-inflammatory agent

Pachnanda *et al.* (1980) administered gum to patients with musculoskeletal rheumatism, including rheumatoid arthritis and ankylosing spondylitis, and achieved good results. Gupta *et al.* (1987) found that defatted alcohol extract was effective against rheumatoid arthritis and related ailments such as osteoarthritis, juvenile rheumatoid arthritis, soft tissue fibrositis and spondylitis. The mechanism of action was similar to the non-steroidal group of anti-arthritic drugs and it was free from gastric irritation and ulcerogenic activity. It improved the blood supply to the joints and restored the integrity of vessels internally damaged or obliterated by spasms. Singh and Atal (1986) also confirmed that the alcoholic extract of gum exhibited a marked anti-inflammatory activity in oedema in rats without any ulcerogenic effect. Singh *et al.* (1992) showed that the active constituent, boswellic acid, had a novel mode of action and formed a new category of anti-inflammatory drug. Duwiejua *et al.* (1993) observed the anti-inflammatory effects. Singh *et al.* (1996) noted on further studies that boswellic acid elicited inhibitory action on vascular permeability. It did not have an analgesic or ulcerogenic effect but had good anti-pyretic activity. Ammon *et al.* (1992, 1993) found boswellic acid a potent inhibitor of prostaglandin. It inhibited the formation of 5-lipxygenase products in polymorphonuclear neutrophils in a dose related manner.

Immunomodulator activity

Sharma *et al.* (1988, 1996) studied the effect of boswellic acid on cell-mediated and humoral components of the immune system and its immunotoxicological potential. It enhanced the phagocytic function of the adherent macrophages. Prolonged oral administration increased body weight, total leucocyte count and humoral antibody titres in rats. It was not cytotoxic and did not have immunosuppression effects. Knaus and Wagner (1996) found that β-boswellic acid, the major constituent of resin, possessed anti-complementry activity in the classical and alternative pathways through their effects on complement-dependent immunohaemolysis of erythrocytes. A special extract of gum resin was tried on joint swelling, pain, erythrocyte sedimentation rate and stiffness. It was found effective in rheumatoid arthritis. Etzel (1996) concluded that it is not only a good analgesic but a disease modifying agent which could replace other such products.

A clinical trial of a herbomineral compound containing *Withania, Boswellia*, turmeric and zinc was carried out on osteoarthritis patients by Kulkarni *et al.* (1991). It produced a significant drop in the severity of pain and disability score. Another form of the above preparation without zinc, when tried for 3 months, relieved pain, decreased morning sickness, and brought about a drop in erythrocyte sedimentation. Radiological assessment did not show any significant changes (Kulkarni *et al.* 1992).

In leukaemia

Shao *et al.* (1998) observed the inhibitory activity of boswellic acids against human leukaemia HL-60 cells in culture. It inhibited the synthesis of DNA, RNA and proteins in human leukaemia in a dose-dependent manner.

In hyperlipidaemia

It decreased serum cholesterol and triglycerides (Zutshi *et al.* 1986).

Review

Gupta *et al.* (1987) gave an account of gum chemistry and pharmacology.

Chemical studies

Mainly terpenoids, boswellic acid and other related pentacyclic triterpenic acids have been reported.

Toxicological studies

The gum extract is safe, well tolerated and can be used in long-term therapy (Etzel, 1996).

References

Ammon, H.P.T., Safayhi, H., Mack, T., Sabieraj, J. Potent inhibitors of prostaglandin and/or leucotriene synthesis from turmeric and Salai Guggal. *International Seminar-Traditional Medicine*, Calcutta, 7–9 November 1992.

Ammon, H.P.T., Safayhi, H., Mack, T., Sabieraj, J. (1993) Mechanism of antiinflammatory actions of curcumin and boswellic acids. *Journal of Ethnopharmacology*, 38, 113–119.

Duwiejua, M., Zeitlin, I.J., Waterman, P.G., Chapman, J., Mahnago, G.J., Provan, G.J. (1993) Antiinflammatory activity of resin from some species of plant family Burseraceae. *Planta Medica*, 59, 12–16.

Etzel, R. (1996) Special extract of *Boswellia serrata* (H-15) in the treatment of rheumatoid arthritis. *Phytomedicine*, 3, 91–94.

Gupta, V.N., Yadav, D.S., Atal, C.K. (1987) Chemistry and Pharmacology of gum resin of *Boswellia serrata* (Salai Guggal). *Indian Drugs*, 24, 221–223.

Kar, A. (1977) Effect of the gum resin of *Boswellia serrata* Roxb. on the cardiovascular system and isolated tissues. *Indian Drugs and Pharmaceutical Industry*, 12, 17–20.

Knaus, U., Wagner, H. (1996) Effects of boswellic acid of *Boswellia serrata* and the other triterpenic acids on the complement system. *Phytomedicine*, 3, 77–81.

Kulkarni, R.R., Patki, P.S., Jog, V.P., Gandage, S.G., Patwardhan, B. (1991) Treatment of osteoarthritis with a herbomineral formulation: a double blind, placebo-controlled, cross-over study. *Journal of Ethnopharmacology*, 33, 91–95.

Kulkarni, R.R., Patki, P.S., Jog, V.P., Gandage, S.G., Patwardhan, B. (1992) Efficacy of an Ayurvedic formulation in rheumatoid arthritis: A double blind placebo controlled cross over study. *Indian Journal of Pharmacology*, 24, 98–101.

Menon, M.K., Kar, A. (1971) Analgesic and psychopharmacological effects of gum resin of *B. serrata*. *Planta Medica*, 19, 333–341.

Pachnanda, V.K., Shashi Kant, Deedar Singh, Singh, G.B., Gupta, O.P., Atal, C.K. (1980) Clinical evaluation of Salai guggal in patients of arthritis. *XIII Annual Conference of Indian Pharmacological Society*, Chandigarh, 26 December 1994.

Shao Yu, Ho, VhiTang, Chin CheeKok, Badmaev, V., Ma Wei, Huang MouTuan (1998) Inhibitory activity of boswellic acids from *Boswellia serrata* against human leukemia HL-60 cells in culture. *Planta Medica*, 64, 328–331.

Sharma, M.L., Kharjuria, A., Kaul, A., Singh, S., Singh, G.B., Atal, C.K. (1988) Effect of Salai guggal ex *Boswellia serrata* on cellular and humoral immune responses and leucocyte migration. *Agents and Actions*, 24, 161–164.

Sharma, M.L., Kaul, A. Khajuria, A., Singh, S., Singh, G.B. (1996) Immunomodulatory activity of boswellic acids (pentacyclic triterpene acids) from *Boswellia serrata*. *Phytotherapy Research*, 10, 107–112.

Singh, G.B., Atal, C.K. (1986) Pharmacology of an extract of Salai Guggal ex-*Boswellia serrata*, a new non-steroidal anti-inflammatory agent. *Agents Actions*, 18, 407–412.

Singh, G.B., Surjeet Singh, Sarang Bani (1996) Anti-inflammatory actions of boswellic acids. *Phytomedicine*, 3, 81–85.

Singh, G.B., Surjeet Singh, Sarang Bani., Kaul, A. (1992) Boswellic acid: a new class of anti-inflammatory drugs with a novel mode of action. *International Seminar-Traditional Medicine-Calcutta, India*, 7–9 November 1992, 81–82.

Zutshi, U., Rao, P.G., Ravi, S., Singh, G.B., Surjeet Singh, Atal, C.K. (1986) Mechansim of cholesterol lowering effects of Salai guggal ex *Boswellia serrata* Roxb. *Indian Journal of Pharmacology*, 18, 182–183.

44 Salep

Orchis latifolia L.
Syn: *Dactylorhiza hatagirea*
Family: Orchidaceae

THE PLANTS AND THEIR DISTRIBUTION

The source of salep is tubers of many species of orchids, such as *Orchis latifolia* L., *O. laxiflora* Lam., *O. maculata, O. militaris* L., *O. mario* L., *O. mascula* L., *O. pyramidalis* L., *O. sambucina* and *O. simia* L. In Russia, salep is obtained from *Orchis* spp., *Gymnadenia* spp. *(Habenaria), Anacamptis* spp. and *Platanthera* spp.

In Turkey and Iran, these tubers have been collected for many centuries and exported under the Arabic name *Sahlep*, which changed to salep in Europe and to *Salem* in India. Salep has been mentioned in Greek and Roman mythology as a talisman under the name *Satyrion.* In western Asian and adjoining European countries, it is very much valued as a tonic, restorative and aphrodisiac. Gypsies call the root *Karengro* and use it as an aphrodisiac and as love amulet. It is highly nutritious. It has a sweetish taste and unpleasant smell. Salep is said to be hot, humid as per the concept of traditional healers and so is well esteemed for impotency and nervous disorders in the *Unani-Tibb* (Greco-Arabic system of medicine) where the following varieties of tuber have been recognized: *Salam punja* if palm-like, *Salam lahsunia* if garlic-like, *Salam mishri* if translucent and globular like sugar candy and *Salam Badshah* (*Badshah* is emperor) if big or round.

The Sanskrit name of salep is probably *munjatak* (Trivedi *et al.* 1974) but this name is not used now. In India, salep is broadly classified into *salem panja* – when it is like the palm of a hand and s*alem mishri* – when globular or oval. It is obtained from many orchids but the common sources are: *O. latifolia., O. mascula, Eulophia hormusjii* Duthie *E. campestris* Wall., *E nuda* Lindll, *Habenaria commelinifolia* Wall. Ex Lindl., *Cymbidium aloifolium,* and *Satyrium nepalensis* (Puri, 1970). *E. hormusjii* is of interest because it is a tuberous orchid which grows in the plains of Punjab and at one time was identified as *Salam Lahori* (after Lahore which is in Pakistan now, earlier it was the capital of united Punjab). In *O. latifolia*, the tuber may be palmate or two dichotomously branched tubers joined together. In *E. camapestris*, the tuber is irregularly branched and often lobed, while in *E. nuda* it is spherical and smooth, like potato. *O. latifolia* grows in the Himalayas, while the other *Orchis* spp and *Salam Badshah* (*Allium macleanii*) are imported to India from Iran and Afghanistan.

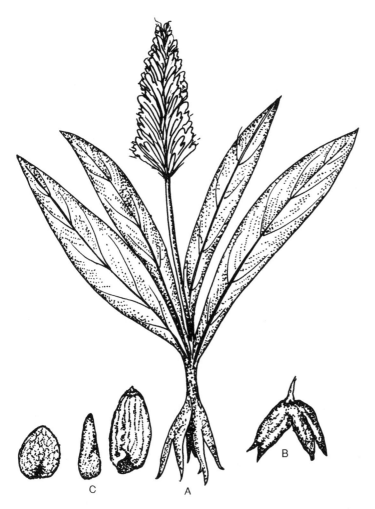

Figure 36 Orchis latifolia **A** herb, **B** dry root, **C** Salep, commercial samples.

O. latifolia (Fig. 36A) grows at a height of 3,000–3,500 m in the western Himalayas. It is a small herb, 5–15 cm long, with lanceolate or linear oblong leaves and a spike about 5 cm long with purple flowers. The bracts are longer than the flowers. In Kashmir, the herb is known as *Narmada*, (male female) and in the central Himalayas *Hathjori* (like hand). The root (Fig. 36B) is like aconites. The daughter tuber originates from the side of the mother tuber and both the tubers become slightly bifurcated at the tapering ends so they look like legs. When fresh these tubers may form a human configuration, very much like that of ginseng tubers.

When the plants mature and the flowers dry, the roots are removed from the soil. In commercial centres, the tubers are blanched in saline boiling water. When soft they are peeled by macerating by hand and dried again. This treatment gelatinizes the starch and gives a waxy, horny texture to the tubers (Puri, 1971a). In commerce

(Fig. 34C) s*alam mishri* tubers are round to oval, dirty white to pale yellow, slightly wrinkled or smooth, waxy, hard, whereas tubers of *salam panja* are like a human hand, 1–3 cm long, about 0.5 cm thick and joined at the top. Sometimes potato starch mixed with acacia gum is made into the shape of salep and boiled in water to gelatinize the starch. When dry these fake tubers, acquire the texture and shape of the genuine drug and are used as an adulterant. Keeping this adulteration in mind, Puri (1971a) provided the pharmacognostic characters of *O. latifolia* and *Eulophia hormuji* (Puri, 1971b) to differentiate genuine tubers from the adulterants.

USES IN FOLKLORE AND AYURVEDA

As a nutrient

The fine powder of the root contains up to 48 per cent mucilage, which becomes thick and mucilaginous when boiled in milk, so that one teaspoon of salep in a cup of milk forms a nutritious drink. It is useful for nervous debility, mental and physical exhaustion, hemiplegia and for paralytic affections. It helps weak digestion which is due to the sluggishness of the digestive system, loose motions and hyperacidity.

In mediaeval times, the sailors used to have 2 teaspoons of salep daily during sea voyages, boiled in a glass of water and sweetened. It kept their bodies strong and active. It was also added to sherbet.

For sexual inadequacy

It is an ingredient of many aphrodisiac preparations used for increasing the quantity, quality and retention time of semen in the body. A recipe is made by pulverizing 100 g *Orchis*, and 200 g almond kernel. It is used by both sexes, taking 10 g everyday on an empty stomach in the morning and before sleep in the evening.

For diabetes

Pulverize 100 g each of *Orchis, Chlorophytum, Curculigo* and use half a teaspoon twice daily in the morning on an empty stomach and before retiring in the evening. These herbs may not act directly on sugar metabolism but will provide energy to the body due to the loss of sugar absorption.

For leucorrhoea

Make a fine powder of 50 g each of *Orchis, Asparagus, Chlorophytum, Curculigo* and *Withania*. When one teaspoon is used before retiring to bed, there is symptomatic relief of backache due to leucorrhoea. It can be used after childbirth.

For general lethargy (fibromyalgia)

Salep can be used for any type of body weakness, apathy towards work and sleep, incapability of doing physical work and exercise, body ache, muscular pains, etc. Make a fine powder of equal quantities of *Orchis* and long pepper, take 5 g of it with goat's milk, twice daily.

To allay irritation in gastro-intestinal canal

A mucilage is prepared and used by shaking one part of powdered salep with 10 parts of cold water until dispersed. Add 90 parts of boiling water to it and shake the whole mass. Drink it like sherbet.

Ayurvedic preparations

Vidyriadi churn

Method Mix 50 g each of finely powdered *Pueraria, Orchis, Withania, Pedalium, Chlorophytum,* and *Anacyclus.*

Dose One teaspoon twice daily with milk.

Indications It makes the body strong. It helps semen retention, premature ejaculation, nocturnal emission and spermatorrhoea.

A slight variation of this preparation is *Rativallabh churn*, used for the same purpose. (Note: *Rativallabh Churn* significantly differs from *Rativallabh Pak*.)

Salam pak

Method Take 400 g *Orchis*, 200 g pistachio, 200 g almond, 100 g *Buchanania latifolia* kernel, 100 g walnut, 100 g *Chlorophytum*, 50 g *Pedalium* and 20 g each of *Withania, Hygrophila, Asparagus, Pistacia lentiscus* oleo-gum resin, *Mucuna* seed without its seed coat, 10 g each of saffron, nutmeg, clove, mace, *Piper cubeba*, bamboo manna, cinnamon, *Cydonia vulgaris* seed, 1250 g sugar and 400 g *ghee*. Grind the salep separately into a fine powder and roast it with a low heat with a small amount of *ghee* until the salep turns light brown in colour. Make a paste of the remaining dry fruits and fry them in the remaining *ghee*. Make a sugar syrup and add it to the above cooked salep, dry fruits, herbs and spices. Make candy balls of 20 g each.

Dose 10–20 g as per the digestive power, twice daily, chew thoroughly and drink milk afterwards.

Use It is used as a winter tonic for all types of sexual inadequacy, mental and physical weaknesses, laziness and low digestion.

Salam pak forte

For an additional tonic effect and for increasing disease resistance, immunity and mental power, particularly for middle-aged patients, add to *Salam Pak*, 10 g *Ras sindur* (red sulphide of mercury), 20 g mica compound and 20 g tin compound before making the candy balls. The dose of *Salam Pak Forte* should be 10 g or less, compared with the original preparation is 20 g and it should be used for 60 days, in winter only.

THERAPEUTIC INDICATIONS AND PHARMACOLOGICAL STUDIES

As a sex tonic

Ageel *et al.* (1994) studied the effect of ethanol extract of *O. maculata* tuber on the sexual behaviour of male rats using a number of tests including penile erection, homosexual mounting, stretching, yawning, aggressiveness, copulatory behaviour and orientational activities. The extract at a dose of 500 mg/kg enhanced sexual arousal in male rats. It produced a significant increase in all the parameters.

Khan and Rehman (1994) tried a polyherbal preparation, with *Orchis* as the main ingredient, to study the sexual behaviour of adult male albino rats, at a dose of 500 mg/100 g weight, for five days. When the treated male rats were exposed to female rats there was an improvement in their sexual functions.

Chemical studies

It contains 48 per cent mucilage, 2.7 per cent starch, nitrogenous substances (5 per cent) and a bitter glucosidic substance (Nadkarni, 1954).

References

Ageel, A.M., Islam, M.W., Ginawi, O.T., Al Yahya, M.A. (1994) Evaluation of the aphrodisiac activity of the *Litsea chinensis* (Lauraceae) and *Orchis maculata* (Orchidaceae) extracts in rats. *Phytotherapy Research*, 8, 103–105.

Khan, N.A., Rahman, S.Z. The effect of Majoon Salab on male sexual function. *Proceedings National Seminar on Unani Medicine*, Hyderabad (India), 22–24 July 1994.

Nadkarni, K.M. *Indian Materia Medica*, Vol I. Popular Prakashan, Bombay 1954.

Puri, H.S. (1970) Salep: The drug from orchids. *American Orchid Society Bulletin.* 39, 723.

Puri, H.S. (1971a) Pharmacognostic investigations on the root of *Orchis latifolia. Indian Drugs*, 8, 15–18.

Puri, H.S. (1971b) Macro- and micromorphology of the tuber of *Eulophia hormusjii* Duthie. *American Orchid Society Bulletin*, 40, 704–706.

Trivedi, V.P., Dixit, R.S., Lal, V.K., Joshi, P. (1974) Clues for identification of a controversial drug (Mumjataka) from ancient literature. *Journal of Research in Indian Medicine*, 9, 56–63.

45 Semal Musli

Bombax ceiba L.
Syn: *B. malabaricum* DC.
Salmalia malabarica (DC) Schott. & Endl.
Family: Bombacaceae

THE TREE AND ITS DISTRIBUTION

It is a tall deciduous tree, common up to 1,500 m throughout warmer parts of India. It has a buttressed trunk, with grey bark and sharp conical prickles on the young stem. The branches are in whorls. Leaves (Fig. 37A) are large with 5–7 lanceolate leaflets, each 10–20 cm long. Flowers (Fig. 37C) are crimson red, 10–15 cm in diameter, appearing before the new leaves. Capsules are dirty brown and when open the seeds float on the air with the help of pappus.

In Ayurveda it is mainly the gum, known as *mochrus*, and the young root called *semal musli* (Fig. 37B) which are used in medicine. *Mochrus* consists of lustrous brown-red particles. *Semal musli* is obtained from young roots and the adjoining stem pieces of 1–2 year old trees. It is 5 cm or so thick, dull brick-red in colour with circular striation and a papery covering. There is no characteristic smell but it has a mucilaginous taste.

USES IN FOLKLORE AND AYURVEDA

The gum is astringent, constipating, a nutrient, anabolic, a blood purifier and strengthens the vital fluid and other vital systems. It is very effective for gastroenteritis and loose motions. It coagulates the blood and so helps stem bleeding, particularly excessive bleeding during menstruation and pulmonary tuberculosis. It prevents threatened miscarriage. It is prescribed with ginger, dry fruits, etc. in the form of candies, to ladies after childbirth.

Semal musli is a geriatric tonic, nutrient, *Rasayana*, with a stimulating action on the generative organs. As an aphrodisiac 12 g of root powder with 12 g sugar and 12 ml of water is taken twice daily.

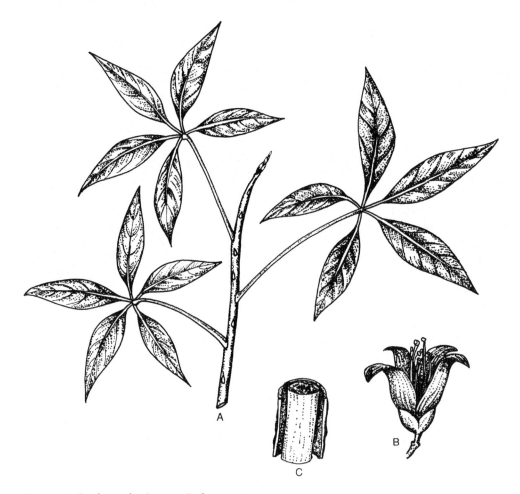

Figure 37 Bombax ceiba **A** twig, **B** flower, **C** root piece.

Ayurvedic preparation

A nutritive tonic

Method   Mix fine powders of 200 g *mochrus*, 300 g poppy seed, 400 g *Abroma augusta* dry leaves, 300 g *Mucuna*, without its seed coat, 500 g *Chlorophytum*, 400 g *Asparagus* and 300 g *Pistacia lentiscus* gum.

Dose   650–1,000 mg, twice daily with water.

Use   In female sexual debility.

Chemical studies

The gum mainly consists of catechutannic acid. The root bark has various naphthalene derivatives related to gossypol (Thakur *et al.* 1989).

Reference

Thakur, R.S., Puri, H.S., Akhtar Hussain *Major Medicinal Plants of India.* Central Institute of Medicinal and Aromatic Plants, Lucknow India 1989.

46 Shankhpushpi

Convolvulus pluricaulis Choice
Family: Convolvulaceae

THE PLANTS AND THEIR DISTRIBUTION

According to Ayurveda, it is a small annual herb, with conch shell-like flowers (*shankh* is conch and *pushp* flower). Three varieties of *shankhpushpi*, with white, red or blue-coloured flowers, are recognized but the variety with white flowers (*C. pluricaulis*) is considered genuine. It is a spreading climber, with a woody stem, 10–60 cm long branches with trichomes, leaves up to 4 cm long and white or pink flowers. It grows during the rainy season in the hotter parts of India. The other herbs (Upadhye and Kumbhojkar, 1993) which are used as *shankhpushpi* are:

Convolvulus arvensis L. (Fig. 38A)
C. microphyllus Sieb. ex Spreng.
Evolvulus alsinoides L. (Fig. 38B)
Clitoria ternatea L.
Conscorea decussata Schult.

USES IN FOLKLORE AND AYURVEDA

According to the ancient Indian author Vagbhatta, it is the best of the three herbs in the *Medha Rasayana* group used as a brain tonic. It has a cooling effect on the brain. The herb increases the vital fluid; it is hot in effect, so is a digestive, appetizer and carminative. It cures skin diseases and is an antidote to poisons. The other uses of this herb are:

As a mental tonic

The herb is considered good for the brain, it is said to sharpen memory, intellect, brain power, cure mental diseases and impart deep sleep. It is used as follows:

1. In epilepsy and cerebral ischaemia, use one teaspoon of juice twice a day.

2. The fine powder of the whole herb, one teaspoon twice daily with milk, is a mental tonic for students and intellectuals.

3. In high fevers, when mental balance is lost, one teaspoon of the powder with water is given 3–4 times in a day.

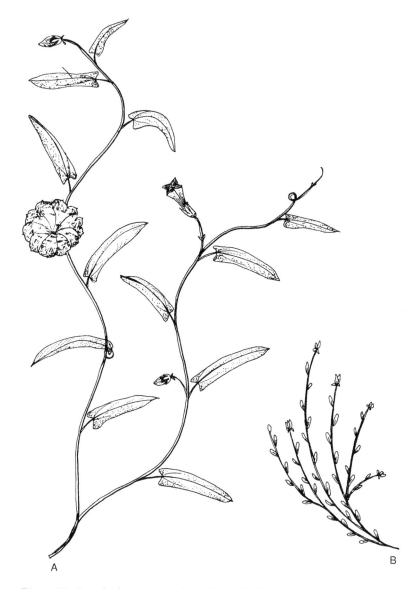

Figure 38 Convolvuls arvensis **A** herb, **B** *Evolvulus alsinoides.*

4. In enuresis (bed wetting) half a teaspoon of powder of the herb with honey, followed by milk or water is given for 1–2 months.

5. For nervous debility and memory loss, an infusion of one part of the herb in 40 parts water, in a dose of 50–100 ml is used with cumin and milk.

For diabetes

One teaspoon of *shankhpushpi* mixed with half teaspoon of black pepper is administered twice daily.

For high blood pressure

Make a decoction by boiling two teaspoons of the herb in 400 ml of water until reduced to 100 ml. Filter it. Drink this decoction for 2–3 days along with one teaspoon of dry powder of the herb. Continue this treatment for 1–2 weeks until the blood pressure is normal.

Ayurvedic preparations

Shankhpushpi syrup

Method　Soak 125 g *Convolvulus* and 25 g *Centella* or *Bacopa* in 3 litres of water until reduced to 2.5 litres, macerate the herbs in water and filter to remove water insoluble matter. In the filtrate dissolve sugar (5 kg) and citric acid (1 g).

Dose　1–2 teaspoonful

Use　As a mental tonic, it stimulates the nervous system and enhances memory. It relieves headaches due to mental exertion. It helps other nervous diseases like epilepsy, convulsions and hysteria.

Shankhpushpi pills

Method　Take 1,000 ml of *Convolvulus* and *Withania juice*, and 100 g of fine powdered *Centella, Glycyrrhiza, Tinospora, Asparagus, Eclipta, and Acorus calamus*. Boil the juices until reduced to half, filter and concentrate to obtain 250 ml of fluid. Add to this fine powders of the rest of herbs, mix thoroughly and make pills of 125 mg each.

Dose　Adults 2 pills, children 1 pill with milk, for 4–5 months.

Uses　For increasing mental powers and treating various nervous diseases like insomnia, depression and high blood pressure.

THERAPEUTIC INDICATIONS AND PHARMACOLOGICAL STUDIES

In anxiety neurosis

Prasad *et al.* (1974) tried it for experimental stress. The herb had effect on various glands through neurohumours, particularly acetylcholine. Mudgal *et al.* (1977) studied neurohumoral changes in the body under the influence of this herb. Mudgal and Udupa (1977b) noted that the herb had a distinct psychotropic effect, which was anti-anxiety in its nature, and resulted in improved mental function (Singh and Mehta, 1977). In other experiments, the herb was found to induce a feeling of well-being, good sleep, relief from anxiety, nervousness, palpitation and increases in memory spasm. It caused a reduction in neuroticism and mental fatigue. The herb showed a significant barbiturate hypnosis potentiation effect, a rise in the levels of

5-hydroxytryptamine, histamine, and a reduction in the levels of acetylcholine and catecholamine in all brain tissue (Singh *et al.* 1977a, b). Because of these activities, the herb was used before anaesthesia (Deshpande and Lalta Prasad, 1978). Shukla (1981) recommended it as an anti-anxiety agent. Sinha *et al.* (1989) put forth the view that the memory potentiation and learning effect of the herb may be due to protein synthesis. The herbs collected during spring showed the maximum hypnosis potentiating activity (Mishra *et al.* 1995).

Hypotensive effect

Mudgal *et al.* (1972), Mudgal and Udupa (1977a) observed maximum activity in the leaves.

In Fabry's disease

Goldman *et al.* (1996) postulated that the nortropane alkaloid isolated from this herb was a glycosidase inhibitor and may be of help in Fabry's disease, which is caused by lack of α-galactosidase activity.

Anti-ulcerogenic effect

Purohit *et al.* (1996) observed that the alcoholic extract of the whole plant of *E. alsinoides* significantly reduced the incidence of ulcers.

In schizophrenia

An indigenous psychotropic preparation made from the extracts of *E. alsinoides*, *Centella*, *Withania*, *Glycyrrhiza*, *Saussurea*, calamus, *Rauvolfia* and *Myristica*, in a dose of 100 mg was tried on untreated schizophrenia patients. It showed improvement in 50 per cent cases without side effects (Parikh *et al.* 1984). In patients of depressive illness, a dose of 25 ml *Shankhpushpi* syrup showed a positive anti-depressant effect (Kushwaha and Sharma, 1992). It also helped in catatonia (Purohit *et al.* 1996).

Intercation with phenytoin

A polyherbal Ayurvedic preparation containing *Convolvulus pluricaulis*, *Centella asiatica*, *Nepeta hindostana*, *N. elliptica*, *Nardostachys jatamansi* and *Onosma bracteatum* reduced the anti-epileptic activity of phenytoin (Dandekar *et al.* 1992).

Chemical studies

Tropane alkaloids like pseudotropine, polyhydroxy tropanes, tropinone and pyrrolidine have been isolated (Todd *et al.* 1995).

Toxicological studies

Horses exhibited weight loss, colic and vascular sclerosis of the small intestine when grazed on *C. arvensis* (Todd *et al.* 1995).

References

Dandekar, U.P., Chandra, R.S., Dalvi, S.S., Joshi, M.V., Gokhale, P.C., Sharma, A.V., Shah, P.U., Kshirsagar, N.A. (1992) Analysis of a clinically important interaction between phenytoin and Shankhpushpi, an Ayurvedic preparation. *Journal of Ethnopharmacology*, 35, 285–288.

Deshpande, P.S., Lalta Prasad (1978) Role of indigenous drugs before anaesthesia. *Journal of Research in Indian Medicine, Yoga and Homoeopathy*, 13, 9–12.

Goldman, A., Message, B., Tepfer, D., Molyneux, R.J., Duclos, O., Boyer, F.D., Pan, Y.T., Elbein, A.D. (1996) Biological activities of the nortropane alkaloid, calystegine B2, and analogs: structure–function relationships. *Journal of Natural Products*, 59, 1137–1142.

Kushwaha, H.K., Sharma, K.P. (1992) Clinical evaluation of Shankhpushpi syrup in the mangement of depressive illness. *Sachitra Ayurveda*, 45, 45–50.

Mishra, A.S., Verma, J., Kumari, N. (1995) Studies on medicinal properties of *Convolvulus pluricaulis* and *Boerhaavia diffusa*. *Biojournal*, 61, 31–36.

Mudgal, V., Rai, V., Singh, R.H., Udupa, K.N. (1977) Neurohumoral changes under the influence of Shankhpushpi. *Journal of Research in Indian Medicine, Yoga and Homoeopathy*, 12, 58–61.

Mudgal, V., Srivastava, D.N., Singh, R.H., Udupa, K.N. (1972) Hypotensive action of *Convolvulus pluricaulis*. *Journal of Research in Indian Medicine, Yoga and Homoeopathy*, 7, 74–77.

Mudgal, V., Udupa, K.N. (1977a) Hypotensive activity with different doses of extracts of various parts of *Convolvulus microphyllus* (Shankhpushpai). *Journal of Research in Indian Medicine, Yoga and Homoeopathy*, 12, 124–126.

Mudgal, V., Udupa, K.N. (1977b) Anti-convulsive action of Shankhpushpi. *Journal of Research in Indian Medicine, Yoga and Homoeopathy*, 12, 127–129.

Parikh, M.D., Pradhan, P.V., Shah, L.P., Bagadia, V.N. (1984) Evaluation of indigenous psychotropic drugs – a preliminary study. *Journal of Research in Ayurveda and Siddha*, 5, 12–17.

Prasad, G.C., Gupta, R.C., Srivastava, D.N., Tandon, A.K., Wahi. R.S., Udupa, K.N. (1974) Effect of Shankhpushpi on experimental stress. *Journal of Research in Indian Medicine*, 9: 19–27.

Purohit, M.G., Shanthaveerappa, B.K., Shrishailappa, B., Swamy, H.K.S. (1996) Antiulcer and anticatatonic activity of alcoholic extract of *Evolvulus alsinoides* (Convolvulaceae). *Indian Journal of Pharmaceutical Sciences*, 58, 110–112.

Shukla, S.P. (1981) Anti-anxiety agents of plant origin. *Probe*, 20, 201–208.

Singh, R.H., Agrawal, V.K., Mehta, A.K. (1977a) Studies on the effect of Medhya Rasayana drug, Shankhpushpi (*Convolvulus pluricaulis*). Part III. Pharmacological studies. *Journal of Research in Indian Medicine, Yoga and Homoeopathy*, 12, 48–52.

Singh, R.H., Mehta, A.K. (1977) Studies on psychotropic effect of the Medhya Rasayana drug, Shankhpushpi (*Convolvulus pluricaulis*). Part I. Clinical Studies. *Journal of Research in Indian Medicine, Yoga and Homoeopathy*, 12, 18–25.

Singh, R.H., Mehta, A.K., Sarkar, F.H., Udupa, K.N. (1977b) Studies on psychotropic effects of the Medhya Rasayana drug, Shankhpushpi (*Convolvulus pluricaulis* Chois.). Part II. Experimental Studies. *Journal for Research in Indian Medicine, Yoga and Homoeopathy*, 12, 42–47.

Sinha, S.N., Dixit, V.P., Madnawat, A.V.S., Sharma, O.P. (1989) The possible potentiation of cognitive processing on administration of *Convolvulus microphyllus* in rats. *Indian Medicine*, 1, 1–6.

Todd, F.G., Stermitz, F.R., Schultheis, P., Knight, A.P., Traub-Dargatz, J. (1995) Tropane alkaloids and toxicity of *Convolvulus arvensis*. *Phytochemistry*, 39, 301–303.

Upadhye, A.S., Kumbhojkar, M.S. (1993) Studies on the Ayurvedic drug Shankhpushpi from western Maharashtra: Medico-botanical aspect. *Bulletin of Medico-Ethnobotanical Research*, 14, 64–69.

47 Shatawari

Asparagus racemosus Willd.
(Family: Liliaceae)

The herb in some of the earlier Indian floras has been wrongly identified as *A. officinalis*.

THE PLANT AND ITS DISTRIBUTION

It is a small shrub or a woody climber and grows in all parts of India at a low altitude in the shade and in tropical climates. The rootstock has fascicled tuberous roots. Branches are angular, leaves (Fig. 39A) reduced to spinescent scales and 0.4–0.6 mm long. Flowers are white, solitary, clustered in a raceme. The fruit is a subglobose berry with 1–6 smooth black seeds.

The roots of *A. adscendens* Roxb. (Fig. 39D) and *A. gonoclados* Baker (Fig. 39E) are also known as *shatawari*. *A. sarmentosus* Willd. has a bigger root so is called *mahashatwari* or big *shatawari*. *A. filicinus* Ham. which grows in the temperate Himalayas and has a bunch of tuberous roots is sometimes used as *shatawari* but is a source of another Ayurvedic root, *safed musli*.

The root is dried after harvesting and may be boiled, peeled and cut into pieces. The root is very rich in mucilage and on pulverizing, the powder forms hard lumps by absorbing moisture.

In trade there are two varieties, one is pale brown, slightly resinous and said to come from Nepal (Fig. 39B) whilst the other is dirty white, horny, spongy and probably from south India (Fig. 39C). The Ayurvedic physicians prefer the root from Nepal as it is said to be more effective.

USES IN FOLKLORE AND AYURVEDA

According to Ayurveda, *shatawari* is heavy, cold, bitter, nutritive; it relieves *vata* and *pitta* and is a *Rasayana*. In *pitta* 5 g of this root with honey and *ghee* is given twice daily. It helps fatigue, insomnia, weakness, laziness and in urinogenital disorders. In *vata* take an equal quantity of *Asparagus* and long pepper and use 5 g with honey twice daily.

In *kapha* use *Shatawari pak* – a compound preparation.

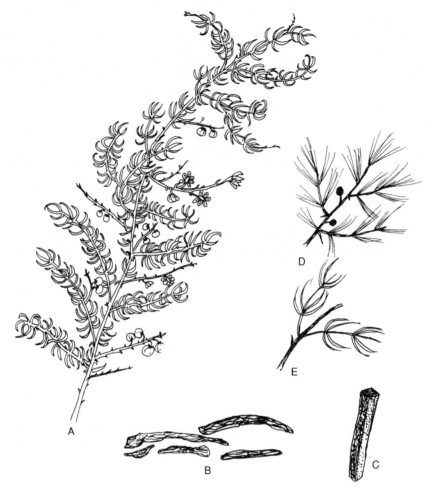

Figure 39 *Asparagus racemosus* **A** twig, **B** root from Nepal, **C** root from south India, *A. adscendens*: **D** twig, **E** *A. gonoclados*: twig.

Shatawari is said to help intelligence and weak eyesight. It is a blood purifier and an antiinflammatory agent. It is an important ingredient of many Ayurvedic formulations, mainly used for proper development of the body to make it more energetic. The major uses of *shatawari* are:

During pregnancy

It is used for breast development, proper embryonic growth and to rid genital organs of diseases. In the first eight months of pregnancy, it is prescribed in a powder form orally, but during the ninth month a swab of cotton dipped in oil made from *Asparagus* is inserted into the vagina daily before sleep. It acts as a lubricant, makes vaginal muscles strong and elastic, which helps a painless delivery.

For leucorrhoea

Mix 5–10 g powdered *Asparagus* with equal amount of *ghee*, swallow it and drink sweet, warm milk afterwards. Continue this treatment twice daily for 40 days.

As a galactagogue

Five to ten gram of *Asparagus* powder followed by warm milk is recommended to pregnant ladies and to lactating mothers during the lactation period.

For dry coughs

For both infants and mothers, take equal quantities of powdered *Asparagus*, *Adhatoda* leaves and sugar. Before use, boil 10 g of this mixture in 200 ml of water and when the water is reduced to half, filter to remove insoluble matter. Boil the decoction further until reduced to one-fourth (50 ml). For mothers the dose is 2–3 teaspoon of the decoction, and for infant 3–4 drops, three to four times a day.

For throat problems

Pulverize equal quantities of the roots of *Asapargus*, *Acorus calamus* and *Sida cordifolia*. Use 5 g of this powder, 2–3 times a day.

Ayurvedic preparations

A galactagogue

Each capsule contains extracts of 200 mg *Asparagus*, 100 mg *Withania*, 50 mg *Glycyrrhiza*, 50 mg *Trigonella* and 20 mg garlic.

Dose   One capsule three times a day.

Use   It develops breasts (Sholapurkar, 1986). After childbirth it stimulates lactation and increases the milk yield.

Shatawari Pak

Ingredients   100 g each of *Sida cordifolia*, *Asparagus* and *Cassia tora*; clove, cardamom, nutmeg, mace, raisins, 200 g almond, 1 kg sugar made into thick syrup, 900 g milk solid matter (condensed milk) and 450 g *ghee*.

Method   Make a fine powder of the first three ingredients. Separately roast the condensed milk in *ghee* until brown in colour, add the sugar syrup and heat some more to further dry the mixture. When still hot add the powdered herbs, spices and chopped dry fruits. Stir the whole mass for some time. When still warm, make candy balls of 20–25 g each.

Dose   As per digestive power, 20–25 g in the morning with milk.

Use It makes both male and female bodies strong. This preparation increases the bioavailability of *shatwari* to the patients.

Shatawari ghrit

Ingredients 400 ml *Shatawari* juice, 400 ml milk, 200 g *ghee*, A*stvarga* (eight herbs used together, see *Chavanprasha* under *amalaki* for their names), black grapes, *Uraria picta*, *Desmodium gangeticum*, *Glycyrrhiza*, *Pueraria tuberosa* and *Pterocarpus santalinus*, all in equal quantities. (Note: If *Asparagus* juice is not available then steep 400 g of dry *Asparagus* powder in 800 ml of water and keep for 24 hours. Macerate the root in water and pass through muslin – this filtrate is equivalent to juice of *Asparagus*.)

Method Grind the herbs, make a thick paste of these with juice, add 25 g each of sugar and honey. Cook all the herbs in milk and *ghee* until all water evaporates and only fatty matter is left. On cooling, mix the remaining sugar and honey.

Dose 1–2 teaspoon with milk in the evening.

Uses It is an aphrodisiac and is beneficial to the sexual systems of both males and females. For males, it is spermatogenic, imparts strength, increases the retention time of ejaculation and dissipates excess body heat. In females, it helps pain and inflammation due to vaginal diseases. It regularises menstruation, helps dysmenorrhoea and conception. According to an Ayurvedic concept, normal conception does not take place in some women because of excessive body heat. This preparation helps conception by keeping the sperm alive for longer due to its cooling effect.

Contraindications

Any activity which generates body heat, for example non-vegetarian or heavy food, meals which are hot in nature, tobacco, sleeping during the day, excessive work, sexual intercourse and exercise.

THERAPEUTIC INDICATIONS AND PHARMACOLOGICAL STUDIES

In ulcers

Kishore *et al.* (1980) tried the root in the treatment of duodenal ulcers. There was a definite cure in many cases. It also helped hyperacidity. When Dahanukar *et al.* (1983) tried *Asparagus* with *Terminalia chebula*, they found that the preparation had a cytoprotective effect on gastric mucosa in acute gastric ulceration. Duodenal ulcers were prevented and the ulcer index was diminished. Dahanukar *et al.* (1986) found it to have a protective effect against abdominal sepsis. When Singh and Singh (1986) tried 12 g of root, in three divided doses, for six weeks on duodenal ulcer patients, it relieved symptoms in most of the cases. Pande and Rajgopalan (1994) found the herb effective in acid dyspepsia with or without ulcers. Bharti Mahashweri and Tewari

(1996) prescribed 20 g of the root, in three divided doses, with milk for one month, to duodenal ulcer patients. Some were suffering from hyperchlorohydria and hyperacidity, whilst other had normal levels of gastric acidity. This treatment reduced both total acid and free hydrochloric acid in all the patients.

Immunomodulating activity

Thatte *et al.* (1987) observed that pre-treating patients with *Asparagus* produced leucocytosis, indicating the herb has an immunomodulating property. It brought immunotherapeutic modifications of *E. coli*-induced abdominal sepsis. In another preparation Seena *et al.* (1993) also noted that *shatawari* might be playing the role of an immunomodulator.

Galactagogue activity

Tennekoon *et al.* (1987) observed this activity in *Asparagus falcatus*. Vihan and Panwar (1988) fed *shatawari* to lactating goats to study the galactagogue activity. There was substantial increase in milk yield by a dose of 100g /kg/day of *shatawar* powder. Khurana *et al.* (1996) gave a preparation containing *Leptadenia*, *Nigella*, fennel, *Pueraria*, *Glycyrrhiza*, cumin and *Asparagus* to healthy buffaloes. It resulted in significant increase in milk yield. The effect was evident after 7 days, peaked on the 21st day and was sustained for 35 days.

In male infertility

Samanta (1992) studied the modulation of male infertility by *Asparagus*, *Astercantha* and *Curculigo*, by prescribing 8–10 g per day of a mixture of these herbs, divided into three doses with milk and sugar, for three months to patients with oligospermia, necrospermia and with less motile, unhealthy sperm. After one month of treatment some changes in sperm morphology were observed. There was a considerable improvement in the number and motility of the sperm, and immaturity was reduced. After three months the sperm became normal in 80 per cent of patients.

In nausea and vomiting

Siddiqui and Hakim (1994) prescribed a 6 g mixture of *Asparagus*, *Amomum subulatum*, *Carum carvi* and *Glycyrrhiza* extract in two equally divided doses for 6 weeks. Relief from pain and burning in epigastrum, nausea and vomiting, and distension of abdomen was observed.

Anti-tumour activity

Sekin *et al.* (1994) mentioned that a polycyclic alkaloid from this root showed anti-tumour activity on various tumour models *in vitro*. The same alkaloid also showed anti-oxytocin activity *in vitro* (Sekin *et al.* 1995). Shao *et al.* (1996) observed that the crude saponins from the root inhibited the growth of human leukaemia cells in culture, in a dose- and time-dependent manner. Saponins were cytostatic at low concentration but at higher levels the effect was cytocidal. Dhuley (1997) studied the effect of *A. racemosus* on the function of macrophages obtained from mice treated with the carcinogen ochratoxin A. The chemotactic activity of murine macrophages was significantly decreased. The production of interlukin-1 and tumour necrosis factor was also markedly reduced.

As a general tonic

Dhatriyadi yoga, a polyherbal preparation containing *Emblica officinalis*, *Asparagus* and *Nardostachys grandiflora*, when given to pregnant women, maintained optimal levels of haemoglobin and serum protein. The preparation was quite safe and as effective as an allopathic tonic (Dwivedi and Tewari, 1991).

Chemical studies

Asparagus contains steroidal sapogenins and steroidal glycosides.

References

Bharati Maheshwari, C.M., Tewari, S.K. (1996) A clinical study of Parinamasula and its treatment with Satavari (*Asparagus racemosus* Willd). *Ancient Science of Life*, 15, 162–165.

Dahanukar, S.A., Date, S.G., Karandikar, S.M. (1983) Cytoprotective effect of *Terminalia chebula* and *Asparagus racemosus* on gastric mucosa. *Indian Drugs*, 20, 442–445.

Dahanukar, S.A., Thatte, U., Pai, N., More, P.B., Karandikar, S.M. (1986) Protective effect of *Asparagus racemosus* against-induced abdominal sepsis. *Indian Drugs*, 24, 124–128.

Dhuley, J.N. (1997) Effect of some Indian herbs on macrophage functions in ochratoxin A treated mice. *Journal of Ethnopharmacology*, 58, 15–20.

Dwivedi, M., Tewari, P.V. (1991) Dhatriyadi Yoga in obstetrics-efficacy and cost. *Sachitra Ayurved*, 44, 360–362.

Khurana, K.L., Balvinder Kumar, Khanna Sudhir, Maniya Anju. (1996) Effect of herbal galactagogue Payapro on milk yield in lactating buffaloes. *International Journal of Animal Sciences*, 11, 239–240.

Kishore, P., Pandey, P.N., Pandey, N.S., Dash, S. (1980) Treatment of duodenal ulcer with *Asparagus racemosus* Linn. *Journal of Research in Ayurveda and Siddha*, 1, 409–416.

Pande, T.N., Rajgopalan, S.S. (1994) Comparative study of three regimen containing Satavari on Amlapitta (acid dyspepsia with or without ulcer). *Journal of Research in Ayurveda and Siddha*, 15, 23–24.

Samanta, S.K. Modulation of male infertility by Ayurvedic drugs. *International Seminar on Traditional Medicine*, Calcutta, 7–9 November 1992.

Seena, K., Kuttan, G., Kuttan, R. (1993) Anticancer activity of selected plant extracts. *Amala Research Bulletin*, 13, 41–45.

Sekine, T., Ikegami, F., Fukaswa, N., Kashimagi, Y., Aizawa, T., Fuji, Y., Ruangrungsi, N., Murakoshi, I. (1995) Structure and related steriochemistry of a new polycyclic alkaloid asparagamine A showing anti-oxytocin activity, isolated from *Asparagus racemosus*. *Perkin Transection 1*, No 4, 391–393.

Sekine, T., Kukasawa, N., Kashiwagi, Y., Ruangrungsi, N., Murakoshi, I. (1994) Structure of asparagamine A, a novel polycyclic alkaloid from *Asparagus racemosus*. *Chemical and Pharmaceutical Bulletin*, 42, 1360–1362.

Shao, Yu, Chin Cheekok, Ho Chi Tang, Ma Wei, Garrison, S.A., Hunag, Mou Tuan (1996) Anti tumour activity of the crude saponin obtained from Asparagus. *Cancer Letter*, 104, 31–36.

Sholapurkar, M.L. (1986) Lactare: for improving lactation. *Indian Practitioner*, 39, 1023–1926.

Siddiqui, M.Y., Hakim, M.H. (1994) Effect of Safoof-e-Satawar in acid peptic disorder (Hurqat-e-Meda). *Hamdard Medicus*, 37, 131–136.

Singh, K.P., Singh, R.N. (1986) Clinical trial on Satavari (*Asparagus racemosus* Willd.) in duodenal ulcer disease. *Journal of Research in Ayurveda and Siddha*, 7, 91–100.

Tennekoon, K.H., Karunanayake, S.H., Mahindaratna, M.P.D. (1987) Evaluation of the galactagogue activity of *Asparagus falcatus. Ceylone Journal of Medical Science*, 30, 63–67.

Thatte, U., Chhabria, S., Karandikar, S.M., Dahanukar, S. (1987) Immunotherapeutic modification of *E. coli*-induced abdominal sepsis and mortality in mice by Indian medicinal plants. *Indian Drugs*, 25, 95–97.

Vihan, V.S., Panwar, H.S. (1988) A note on galactogogue activity of *Asparagus racemosus* in lactating goats. *Indian Journal of Animal Health*, 27, 177–178.

48 Som Ras

In *Rig-Veda*, one of the oldest repositories of human knowledge, a long-cherished substance of the *vedic* people, *somras*, the *soma* juice, is mentioned. Out of over 1,000 hymns in *Rig-Veda*, 120 are devoted exclusively to *soma*. It was a god-narcotic of ancient Indians, which attained an exhalted place in the magico-religious ceremonies of the Aryans (Schultes and Hofmann, 1992). For a long time, it was considered by some to be a herb, the juice of which could lead to the attainment of superhuman power. It was a divine bliss, which gave pleasure to human beings. It was a juice of immortality, comparable to present day tonics, ambrosia, nectar, elixir, panacea or the most recently introduced adaptogens, smart drugs or mood elevators. According to Schultes and Hofmann (1992) when the culture changed from hunting to pastoralism and agriculture, the use of *soma* died out and was forgotten long ago, so its source became a mystery.

The source of *soma*, on the basis of vague descriptions given in ancient texts, was identified as a dark coloured, leafless milky sap-containing creeper. These characteristics resembled *Periploca aphylla* (Fig. 40A) and *Sarcostemma brevistigma* (Fig. 40C) of the Asclepiadaceae family but these herbs lacked the physiological effects on the human body ascribed to *soma*, so some authors thought that it might be from hallucinogenic plants such as *Cannabis* or *Peganum harmala*, or a stimulant like *Ephedra vulgaris* (Fig. 40B) (Puri, 1977).

Wasson (1972), after an extensive ethnobotanical study of hallucinogenic fungi of South America, considered *soma* to be the fly agaric mushroom, *Amanita muscaria* (Fig. 40D), family Amanitaceae. This fungus is found in the western Himalayas at an altitude of approximately 2,000 m in the rainy season on rotting organic matter. When mature, the fructification is crimson red in colour and looks like a beautiful flower. Insects are attracted to it by its colour and get killed on contact, due to the fungus's poisonous nature. The crimson umbrella has white scales and contains the remains of dead insect bodies. When fully mature the fructification is 7–20 cm in diameter, the central stalk is 20–25 cm long with a broad bulbous base and has numerous hair-like fibres spread all over the soil. The stalk is on off-white colour, fleshy when young but becoming horny on maturity. The base of the stem has white valves adhered to it. On the ventral side of the umbrella are numerous gills, which enclose spores and disperse them on maturity.

Wasson (1972) provided coloured photographs of all the developmental stages of fly agaric and compared them with the descriptions given in the *vedas*. The author also concluded that the use of *soma* was comparable to the hallucinogenic fungi used by some tribes of Mexico for religious rites. A *soma*-like drink is still consumed in some areas of Central Asia and Siberia, the areas from which Aryans probably migrated to India.

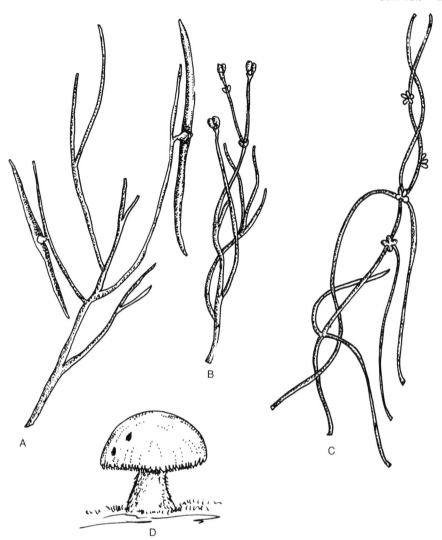

Figure 40 **A** *Periploca aphylla*, **B** *Ephedra vulgaris*, **C** *Surcostemma bravitigma*,
      D *Amanita muscaria* (diagrammatic).

Chemical studies

It contains hallucinogenic compounds like muscimol, muscarin, ibotenic acid and
tropane alkaloids. During the drying of fly agaric, ibotenic acid changes to muscimol
(Schultes and Hofmann, 1992).

Toxicological studies

In small doses *Amanita* extract relaxes the body and imparts peace of mind but after
some time the hallucinogenic effect begins. The body becomes semi-conscious with

the stimulation of the nervous system, vivid dreams, recollection of old memories and supernatural feelings. Long-term use of this herb is harmful.

References

Puri, H.S. *Medicinal Plants of India* (in Punjabi). Punjab State University Text Book Board, Chandigarh India 1977.
Schultes, R.E., Hofmann, A. *Plants of the Gods. Their Sacred, Healing and Hallucinogenic Powers.* Healing Arts Press, Rochester, Vermont 1992.
Wasson, R.G. *Soma: Divine Mushroom of Immortality.* Harcourt Blace Jovanovich Inc. USA 1972.

49 Sonth

Zingiber officinale Roscoe
Family: Zingiberace

THE PLANT AND ITS DISTRIBUTION

It grows in hot, humid, sub-tropical climates in many parts of the world. The herb has broad leaves, arising from the ground (Fig. 41A). It rarely flowers. The fresh root is called *adrak* and the dried root *sonth* in most parts of India (Fig. 41B). Before drying, the rhizome is boiled in water and the outer corky layers are scrapped. It is cut longitudinally and dried. Sometimes calcium is added to the water before boiling.

USES IN FOLKLORE AND AYURVEDA

As per Ayurveda, it is pleasant anti-*ama*, anti-*vata*, digestant, pungent, light, oily, hot in effect, laxative and anti-inflammatory. It makes food tasty and increases vital fluids. It helps bronchial troubles, nausea, vomiting and heart diseases.

Throughout the whole of Asia, from China to Turkey, ginger has a reputation of being a powerful aphrodisiac. A masticate of a mixture of ginger, cinnamon, *Piper cubeba* and *Anacyclus pyrethrum* is often recommended for this purpose. Ginger juice is an aphrodisiac if taken with honey and half boiled egg at night for a month. It is said to strengthen the sex organs and cure impotence.

In traditional Chinese medicine dry ginger rhizome is used to expel interior cold, while fresh ginger disperses exterior cold (Bone, 1997).

Ayurvedic Formulation

Subhagya Shunthi Pak

Method Take 750 g ginger, 750 g *ghee* and 25 g each of *Asparagus*, *Pueraria*, *Chlorophytum*, *Tribulus*, *Sida* root, *Tinospora* starch, cinnamon, cardamom, *Cinnamomum* spp. leaves, Indian thyme, *Abies* leaves, celery, fennel, *Pluchea lanceolata*, *Inula racemosa*,

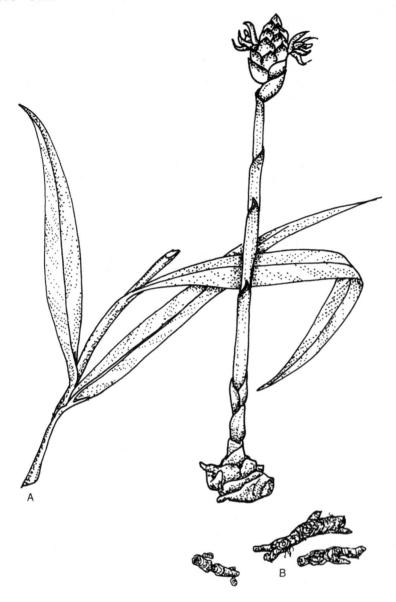

Figure 41 Zingiber officinale **A** herb, **B** dry rhizome.

bamboo manna, *Cedrus deodara* wood, dill, *Hedychium spicatum*, *Nardostachys grandiflora*, calamus, *Butea* gum, *Mesua ferrea*, mace, fenugreek, *Glycyrrhiza*, *Santalum album*, *Pterocarpus santalinus*, *Embelia ribes*, *Vetiveria*, *Adhatoda*, coriander, *Randia dumetorum*, *Cyperus scariosus* and 3.25 kg sugar. Make fine powders of all the herbs and ginger separately. Fry ginger in *ghee*, and when warm add the powdered herbs, sugar and make balls of about 20 g each.

Dose   Half to one ball with one teaspoon of *ghee*, twice daily with milk, for 90 days.

Use   It makes women's bodies strong and healthy, giving them a good shape. It increases breast size and cures diseases of the generative system. It clears pimples, acne, blemishes, etc. from the face and makes the skin smooth and lustrous. If used by lactating mothers, the breastfed infant receives all the beneficial effects of ginger.

THERAPEUTIC INDICATIONS AND PHARMACOLOGICAL STUDIES

It is used in tonic preparations for women, mainly after confinement. It is an anti-oxidant, anti-microbial and acts as a preservative. Puri (1988) and Bone (1997) have given a review of the medicinal uses of ginger. The important points given in these articles and additional information are as follows:

As an anti-inflammatory agent

Ginger extract reduced swelling and was as active as aspirin. Patients suffering from rheumatoid arthritis received relief using it. The pungent active constituent, gingerol, inhibited prostaglandin and leukotriene synthesis (Kiuchi *et al.* 1992). It was a more potent inhibitor of prostaglandin biosynthesis than indomethacin. The essential oil of ginger inhibited chronic adjuvant arthritis in rats (Bone, 1997).

As a digestive agent

Ginger has a proteolytic enzyme action similar to papain. It has a stimulating action on bile, saliva production, gastric secretion and helps digestion by increasing metabolism (Sambiah and Srinivasan, 1989, 1991).

Anti-ulcer activity

It inhibited experimentally-induced gastric ulcers. Through its anti-microbial activity it prevented ulceration and inhibited the manufacture of prostaglandin (Bone, 1997).

As an anti-microbial agent

It was effective against both gram-positive and gram-negative bacteria in various culture experiments. At the dose of 3 g, thrice daily, it had a significant effect on *Entamoeba histolytica* and *Giardia* spp. Anti-viral, anti-fungal, anthelmintic, anti-filarial and molluscicidal activities have also been observed (Bone, 1997, Billing and Sherman, 1998).

As a cardiotonic

Ginger has a tonic effect on the heart's action (Shogi, 1982). It can increase blood pressure by restricting blood flow in the peripheral area of the body. It has anti-platelet activity and a positive inotropic effect (Bone, 1997).

For lowering cholesterol

It lowered cholesterol both in the blood and in the liver by impairing its absorption. It suppressed appetite, which further decreased cholesterol intake (Giri *et al.* 1984, Bhasakar *et al.* 1984). The effect was not immediate. Tanabe *et al.* (1993) isolated a compound from ginger, which had an inhibitory effect on cholesterol biosynthesis.

In hepatotoxicity

It countered liver toxicity by increasing bile secretion (Sambiah and Srinivasan, 1991).

Anti-tumour effect

Ethanol extract showed a biphasic effect on the secretion of cytokines by human peripheral blood mononuclear cells *in vitro* (Cheng *et al.* 1995).

Anti-emetic effect

Many studies have shown that it increased bile secretion, prevented nausea and motion sickness. It had central nervous system depressant, cough suppressant, anti-vomiting, anti-convulsant and prostaglandin synthesis inhibition properties (Bone, 1997).

As an immunomodulator

Ginger had a stimulating effect on the immune system (Bone, 1997).

In migraine headaches

It helped neurological disorders, particularly migraines (Mustafa and Srivastava, 1990).

As an anabolic agent

In malabsorption syndromes, it improved body weight, appetite and increased haemoglobin percentage (Nanda *et al.* 1985, 1993).

Hypo-uricaemic effects

Maheshwari *et al.* (1995) administered water and alcohol extract of ginger for 30 days and observed a significant fall in the level of serum uric acid. Alcohol extract was more effective.

Chemical studies

It contains 1.0–2.5 per cent essential oils, pungent principles gingerols and shogaols (Bone, 1997).

Toxicological studies

It should be used with care during pregnancy.

References

Bhaskar, P.A., Rao, K.S., Rao, M.V.R., Venkatachalam, M.S. (1984) Effect of spices in food on blood cholesterol. *Current Medical Practitioner*, 29, 96–97.

Billing, J., Sherman, P.W. (1998) Antimicrobial functions of spices, why some like it hot. *Quarterly Review of Biology*, 73, 3–49.

Bone, K. (1997) Ginger. *British Journal of Phytotherapy*, 4, 110–120.

Cheng, C.P., Chang, J.Y., Wang, F.Y., Chang, J.G. (1995) The effect of Chinese medicinal herb *Zingiber rhizome* extract on cytokine secretion by human peripheral blood mononuclear cells. *Journal of Ethnopharmacology*, 48, 13–19.

Giri, J., Sakthi Devi, T.K., Meerarani, S. (1984) Effect of ginger on serum cholesterol levels. *Indian Journal of Nutrition and Dietetician*, 21, 433–436.

Kiuchi, F., Iwakami, S., Shibuya, M., Hanaoka, F., Sankawa, U. (1992) Inhibition of prostaglandin and leukotriene biosynthesis by gingerols and diarylheptanoids. *Chemical and Pharmaceutical Bulletin*, 40, 387–392.

Maheshwari, A.K., Tiwari, M.P., Pant, M.C. (1995) Hypouricemic effect of *Zingiber officinlae* (ginger) extract. *Indian Journal of Hospital Pharmacy*, 32, 18–20.

Mustafa, T., Srivastava, K.C. (1990) Ginger (*Zingiber officinale*) in migraine headache. *Journal of Ethnopharmacology*, 29, 267–273.

Nanda, G.C., Tewari, N.S., Prem Kishore (1985) Clinical studies on the role of Sunthi in the treatment of Grahni Roga. *Journal of Research in Ayurveda and Siddha*, 6, 78–87.

Nanda, G.C., Tewari, N.S., Prem Kishore (1993) Clinical evaluation of Sunthi (*Zingiber officinale*) in the treatment of Grahni Roga. *Journal of Research in Ayurveda and Siddha*, 14, 34–44.

Puri, H.S. (1988) Ginger: nature's remedy for heart patients. *Quarterly Newsletter of American Herb Association*, 6, 8–9.

Sambiah, K., Srinivasan, K. (1989) Influence of spices and spice principles on hepatic mixed function oxygenase system in rats. *Indian Journal of Biochemistry and Biophysics*, 26, 254–258.

Sambiah, K., Srinivasan, K. (1991) Secretion and composition of bile in rats, fed diet containing spices. *Journal of Food Science and Technology*, 28, 35–38.

Shogi, N. (1982) Cardiotonic principles of ginger (*Zingiber officinale*). *Journal of Pharmaceutical Sciences*, 71, 1174–75.

Tanabe, M., Chen, U.D., Saito, K.I., Kano, Y. (1993) Cholesterol biosynthesis inhibitory component from *Zingiber officinale*. *Chemical and Pharmaceutical Bulletin*, 41, 710–713.

50 Talamkhana

Hygrophila spinosa T. And.
Syn: *Astercantha longifolia* Nees.
Hygrophila auriculata (Schum.) Hiene
Family: Acanthaceae

THE PLANT AND ITS DISTRIBUTION

It is a spinescent herb (Fig. 42) which grows in marshy land, along rivers and in ponds in warm areas. It may grow up to 1 m tall, with yellow, sharp spines up to 2 cm long. The leaves are coarse, lanceolate, in a spiral of six, of which the outer two leaves are longer, maybe up to 20 cm long, while the inner four leaves are 4 cm long. Flowers are bluish to violet, about 3 cm long and in pairs of four. The fruit is flat, 8 mm long, rectangular, sharp, consisting of 4–8 seed. The seeds are red and hirsuate. When chewed the seeds are tasteless but there is a secretion of tenacious mucilage.

USES IN FOLKLORE AND AYURVEDA

The seed is considered diuretic, a tonic, augmentative, an aphrodisiac and spermatogenic. It is used for inflammation and allied diseases of the liver, urino-genital problems and sexual inadequacies. It affords strength, virility and increases seminal retention ability. The seed is hard to digest, causes constipation and so is used with milk and sugar.

In general debility and impotency, 10 g of *talamkhana* seed with an equal quantity of processed *Mucuna* seed or a powder of 10 g each of *talamkhana*, *gokshru* and *shatawari* is prescribed with milk.

THERAPEUTIC INDICATIONS AND PHARMACOLOGICAL STUDIES

As a hepatoprotective agent
Singh and Handa (1995) tried methanolic extract for this purpose.

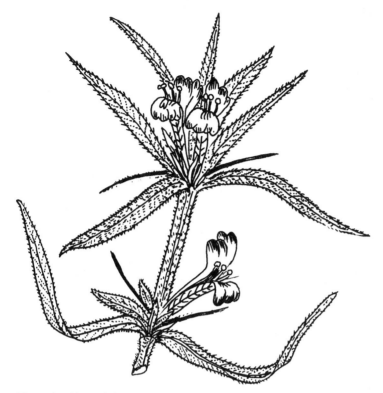

Figure 42 Hygrophila spinosa twig.

Anti-tumour activity

Mazumdar *et al.* (1997) observed that the petroleum ether extract from the root inhibited anti-tumour activity in mice with Ehrlich ascites carcinoma and sarcoma 180.

Chemical studies

The seed has 23 per cent fatty oil. It also contains the enzymes diastase, lipase and protease.

References

Mazumdar, U.K., Malaya Gupta, Maiti, S., Mukherjee, D. (1997) Antitumour activity of *Hygrophila spinosa* on Ehrlich ascites carcinoma and sarcoma 180 induced in mice. *Indian Journal of Experimental Biology*, 35, 473–477.

Singh, A., Handa, S.S. (1995) Hepatoprotective activity of *Apium graveolens* and *Hygrophila auriculata* against paracetamol and thioacetamide intoxication in rat. *Journal of Ethnopharmacology*, 49, 119–126.

51 Tulsi

Ocimum tenuiflorum L.
Syn. *O. sanctum* L.
Family: Lamiaceae (Labiate)

In scientific literature, the name *Ocimum sanctum* is commonly used for this herb. The same has been followed in this book. It is also known as Holy basil or Sacred basil.

THE PLANT AND ITS DISTRIBUTION

It is grown in most Hindu houses and is worshipped. *Tulsi* is allocated sixth place amongst eight objects of worship in Hindu rituals. It is *satvik*, having spiritual uplifting qualities. Five types of *tulsi* have been recognized in ancient texts. Of these *Ram* (green) and *Krishna* (black) are varieties of *O. tenuiflorum*. The identification of other types is doubtful.

The herb (Fig. 43) is very branched, slightly woody and often pale purple in colour. The leaves are ovate, elliptic, oblong, 3 to 4.5 cm long and 1.5 to 2 cm broad, hairy, with minute dots and margin entire. Flowers are purple-pink and whorled in racemes.

The herb survives only in a warm climate in summer.

USES IN FOLKLORE AND AYURVEDA

Tulsi is widely prescribed for diseases due to *vata*. The other uses are:

Antidote to poisons

Tulsi destroys the poisons (*ama*) generated in the body due to irregularities in dietary habits, indisciplined lifestyle, lack of self control or weakness. It is also an antidote for environmental pollutants.

For skin diseases

External application of the leaf paste helps minor skin infections, such as acne, etc.

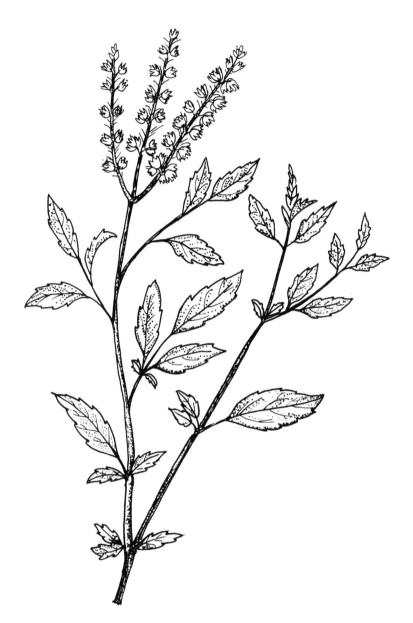

Figure 43 Ocimum tenuiflorum twig.

For incurable diseases

It is helpful in diseases such as cancer and high blood pressure. If a rigid regulated lifestyle is followed, it may be effective in leukaemia.

As a general tonic

The juice is sharp and bitter. It stimulates the digestive system, prevents vitiation of blood, rejuvenates the body, increases vital fluid (semen) and cures nervous weakness. Five grams of the leaf juice, twice daily has a *Rasayana*-like effect.

As an anti-stress agent

Tulsi, in the form of a tea, helps stress-related diseases due to physical, chemical or biological causes. It is particularly useful for peptic ulcers, heart diseases, hypertension, colitis, post-operative complications and even asthma.

As a brain tonic

Tulsi beads have long been used for mental peace. *Tulsi* leaves improve memory by stimulating brain activity. It helps forgetfulness and irregular delirium. Through its use mentally retarded children show noticable improvement. As a brain tonic, swallow five leaves in the morning with water or crush 10 *tulsi* leaves, 5 black peppers and 4 almonds and mix in honey.

As an aphrodisiac

Various recipes for this purpose are:

1   Drink a decoction of leaves with a pinch of cardamom powder and 10 g of *Orchis* powder.
2   Mix a fine powder of 5 parts *tulsi* seed, 5 parts *Tribulus*, 3 parts *Mucuna*, 4 parts *Chlorophytum* and 6 parts sugar. The dose is 20 g.
3   Chew small pieces of the root.
4   Mix *tulsi* seed and sugar in equal parts. Take 5 g of this mixture for two months.
5   Make pills of 3 g each from mixture of powdered *tulsi* and unrefined sugar. Take one pill twice daily for 45 days.

For coughs, colds and flu

The juice of leaves is diaphoretic, antiperiodic, stimulating, antiseptic and expectorant. It is used in catarrh and bronchitis.

1   Influenza, boil 10–15 leaves in 200 ml of water until reduced to half. Add a pinch of salt and administer while warm. Repeat this medication 2–3 times daily. It will induce perspiration.
2   For coughs, colds, all throat problems and body aches, etc., boil 11 *tulsi* leaves, one black pepper, a pinch of ginger and a pinch of salt in a cup of water until reduced to half. Prescribe thrice daily.
3   For asthma, take the leaf juice in honey, 3–4 times a day.

For indigestion

An infusion of leaves is used in hepatic affections and gastric disorders in children.

For increasing appetite, make a mixture by pulverizing equal quantities of *tulsi* leaves, seeds of cardamom, cumin, ginger, cinnamon, Indian thyme, mint, black salt. The dose is 10 g of powder with 20–50 ml of water, every hour until cured. Drink yogurt products only. Do not use milk, sugar or honey.

In gynaecological practices

For stimulating lactation

Take 20 ml of *tulsi* juice, 20 ml of maize leaf juice, 10 ml of *Withania* juice and 10 g honey, for seven days, following childbirth.

For leucorrhoea

Take 20 ml *tulsi* juice with rice gruel. Do not use milk. Eat only rice.

For amenorrhoea

Take 125 g each of *tulsi* seed, sesame seed, tender shoots of cotton and bamboo plants and 250 g of unrefined sugar. Mix all these in a wet grinder until they are kneaded. Make pea-sized pills. Take one pill twice daily with water until the regularity of periods is restored.

For urinary problems

Seeds are prescribed for involuntary urination in children, burning sensation during urination and mucus discharge in urine, etc.

Contraindication

Tulsi is considered hot for women. Use it with other herbs that have a cooling effect.

Ayurvedic preparations

Laghu raahmriga

Ingredients   Take equal quantities of *tulsi* juice, *ghee* and black pepper.

Dose   One tablespoon.

Use   It helps all acute, chronic, and incurable diseases.

Tulsi arishta

Ingredients   Take 700 g *Acacia nilotica* bark, 80 g of whole *tulsi* plants, 500 g raw sugar, 80 g *Emblica officinalis* flower and 10 g each of black pepper, long pepper, cardamom seed, nutmeg, cinnamon, *Piper cubeba* seed, *C. tamala* leaves, and *Mesua ferrea* flowers.

Method   Boil bark in 15 litres of water until reduced to one-fourth, strain the decoction, store in an earthen pot and add the coarse powder of all the other ingredients. Make the pot airtight by sealing the lid. Let the content ferment for one month. Filter and store in the bottles.

Dose   12–15 ml twice daily.

Use   It provides nutrition to the body, imparts strength and vigour to the bronchial and digestive systems of patients. It is said to increase quantity and improve quality of semen.

Tulsi tea

Ingredients   500 g of shade-dried *Tulsi* leaves, 50 g cinnamon, 100 g cinnamon leaves, 100 g *Centella*, 25 g *Viola bicolor*, 250 g fennel, 150 g cardamom seed, 250 g *Pterocarpus santalinus* and 25 g black pepper.

Method   Make a coarse powder of all items.

Dose   Take 1 g powder in a cup of water, boil and make a tea.

Use   It increases digestion and provides required energy to the body against all diseases.

THERAPEUTIC INDICATIONS AND PHARMACOLOGICAL STUDIES

Immunomodulator activity

Tulsi has an immunosuppressing effect and modifies host resistance to a number of conditions including allergic, infectious disorders and stress-induced changes (Godhwani *et al.* 1988, Mediratta *et al.* 1988).

Effect on the nervous system

Sakina *et al.* (1990) studied the effect of an ethanol extract fraction on the central nervous system (CNS). All the actions resembled those of low doses of barbiturates. It could reduce the severity and duration of electric shocks, and pentylene tetrazole-induced convulsions. It decreased the apomorphine-induced fighting response. Singh *et al.* (1991) studied the biochemical changes brought about by *tulsi* during stress. Ahumada *et al.* (1991) observed the depressing effect of the extract on the mouse nervous system. There was a significant increase in the narcosis time, which was dose dependent. It had a clear synergism with pentobarbitol in depressing the mouse's CNS response. It also had an anti-spasmodic effect. The crude aqueous extract potentiated hexabarbitone-induced hypnosis in rats. Singh and Agarwal (1991) tried it against induced pre-convulsive dyspnoea. Volatile oil from the leaves and fixed oil from the seed was effective. These also inhibited hind paw oedema in rats. Singh and Majumdar (1995) noted that the analgesic activity of the herb's fixed oils was related to the peripheral system and was not centrally mediated like morphine. The effect may be due to prostaglandin inhibition.

Anti-pyretic activity

Tandan *et al.* (1989) observed that the essential oils had significant anti-pyretic activity.

Hypotensive effects

Subbulakshmi and Sarvaiya (1991) noted this effect.

Adaptogenic properties

Bhargava and Singh (1981) and Dadekar *et al.* (1988) noted anti-stress activity in the herb, while Singh *et al.* (1989) studied it for anoxia tolerance. Ahumada *et al.* (1991) observed an adaptogenic effect in-induced narcosis in rats. It enhanced the physical endurance and survival time, and protected against modulated humoral immune responses. Bhattacharya *et al.* (1994–1995) studied the modulation of blood sugar levels in stress-induced rats by this herb. Trivedi *et al.* (1995) carried a clinical evaluation of the leaf powder for laryngo-pharyngitis, bronchial asthma and in stress-related hypertension. It was found to be a highly efficacious immunomodulator in humans. It increased cell-mediated immune response. Kozlovskaya (1996) studied the psychotropic effects of an essential oil and water extract on the behaviour of rats under acute emotional stress and on the status of the lymphoid organs (thymus, adrenal glands and spleen); both the water extract and essential oil had a similar effect in correcting behavioural as well as somatic reactions to stress. Sadekar *et al.* (1998) carried out research on the immunomodulating effect of dry leaf powder on humoral response in poultry, naturally infected with infectious bursal disease, IBD virus. The powder had a positive immunostimulatory effect and it overcame the immunosuppressive effect of the IBD infection.

Anti-ulcerogenic effect

Singh *et al.* (1991) observed the slowing effect of the herb on intestinal transit, which may be useful in emotional tension where intestinal motility is usually increased. This was attenuated to different degrees. Mandal *et al.* (1993) observed that the administration of the leaves reduced the ulcer index, and both free and total acidity in acute and chronic cases. Pre-treatment for seven days increased mucous secretion.

In skin diseases

Savargaonkar *et al.* (1990) tried a mixture of *tulsi* and *Nyctanthes arbor-tristis* on eczema by applying it externally. Bantwal and Mardikar (1990) clinically tried the black variety of the herb on leprosy patients.

Hypoglycaemic effect

The leaf extract was studied using normal and diabetic rats (Chattopadhaya, 1993).

Anaphrodisiac effect

Kantak and Gogate (1992) noted that higher doses of the leaves decreased the sexual behaviour of animals.

As an anti-cancerous agent

Prashar and Ashok Kumar (1995) investigated the chemopreventive activity of the ethanol extract of leaves against 2,12-dimethylbenz (a) anthracene (DMBA) induced papillomagenesis in the skin of mice. The extract had significant anti-neoplastic activity.

Radioprotective effect

Uma Devi and Ganasoundari (1995) studied the radioprotective effect of water or aqueous ethanol extract of the leaves before complete exposure of the body to gamma radiation in albino mice. Water extract was more effective than hydroalcohol menstrum. Intraperitoneal administration of these extracts gave the best protection. Furthermore Ganasoundari *et al.* (1997a,b) studied the modification of bone marrow radio sensitivity. An aqueous extract of the leaves was found to protect mice against lethal radiation levels. Ganasoundari *et al.* (1998) observed that the leaf extract enhanced bone marrow radioprotection and toxicity. Pre-treatment of tissues with *tulsi* resulted in a significant decrease in aberrant cells as well as different types of aberrations. It also acted as a detoxifier.

Anti-haemorrhagic effect

Jangde *et al.* (1996) noted that the aqueous and alcoholic extract of leaves significantly reduced the duration of bleeding in rabbits. The alcohol extract was more effective.

Antioxidant effect

Eugenol, one of the main ingredients of *tulsi* essential oil inhibited the accumulation of lipid peroxidation products in red blood cells, and maintained the activities of antioxidant enzymes. It protected free radical attack on the membrane and maintained the activities of antioxidant enzymes (Kumaravelu *et al.* 1996).

Chemical studies

The essential oil from the whole plant contained 71.3 per cent eugenol, 3.2 per cent carvacrol, 20.4 per cent methyl eugenol and 1.7 per cent caryophyllene.

References

Ahumada, F., Tricado, M.A., Arellano, J.A., Hancke, J., Wikman, G. (1991) Effect of certain adaptogenic plant extracts on drug-induced narcosis in female and male mice. *Phytotherapy Research*, 5, 29–31.

Bantwal, H.V., Mardikar, B.R. Clinical study of the effect of Krishna Tulsi to hospitalised leprosy patients (Abstract). *Proceedings of 42th Indian Pharmaceutical Congress*, Manipal, 28–30 December 1990.

Bhargava, K.P., Singh, N. (1981) Antistress activity of *Ocimum sanctum* Linn. *Indian Journal of Medical Research*, 73, 443–451.

Bhattacharya, P., Banerjee, R., Roy, U., Banerjee, B.P. (1994–1995) Modulation of blood sugar level of stress-induced albino rats with *Ocimum sanctum*. *International Conference on Progress in Medicinal and Aromatic Plant Research*, Calcutta, India. 30 December 1994.

Chattopadhyaya, R.R. (1993) Hypoglycaemic effect of *Ocimum sanctum* leaf extract in normal and strepozoticin diabetic rats. *Indian Journal of Experimental Biology*, 31, 891–893.

Dadkar, V.N., Joshi, A.G., Jagusta, V.S., Billimoria, F.R., Dhar, H.L. (1988) Antistress activity of *Ocimum sanctum* (Tulsi). *Indian Drugs*, 25, 172–175.

Ganasoundari, A., Uma Devi, P., Rao, B.S.S. (1998) Enhancement of bone marrow radioprotection and reduction of WR-2721 toxicity by *Ocimum sanctum*. *Mutation Research, Fundamental and Molecular Mechanisms of Mutagenesis* 397, 303–312.

Ganasoundari, A., Uma Devi, P., Rao, M.N.A. (1997a) Protection against radiation-induced chromosome damage in mouse bone marrow by *Ocimum sanctum*. *Mutation Research, Fundamental and Molecular Mechanisms of Mutagenesis*, 373, 271–276.

Ganasoundari, A., Zare, S.M., Uma Devi, (1997b) Modification of bone marrow radiosensitivity by medicinal plant extracts. *British Journal of Radiobiology*, 70, 599–602.

Godhwani, S., Godhwani, J.L., Vyas, D.S. (1988) *Ocimum sanctum*: a preliminary study evaluating its immunoregulatory profiles in albino rats. *Journal of Ethnopharmacology*, 24, 193–198.

Jangde, C.R., Ladukar, O.N., Maske, D.K., Patil, G.D. (1996) Effect of *Ocimum sanctum* Linn. on bleeding time in rabbits. *International Journal of Animal Sciences*, 11, 249–250.

Kantak, N.M., Gogate, M.G. (1992) Effect of short term administration of Tulsi (*Ocimum sanctum*) Linn. on reproduction behaviour of adult male rats. *Indian Journal of Physiology and Pharmacology*, 36, 109–111.

Kozlovskaya, M.M., Blednov, Y.A., Czabak-Garbacz, R., Kozlovksy, I.I., Arefolov, V.A. (1996) Stress correction effects of *Ocimum sanctum* L.: a psychopharmacological and neurochemical study. *Herba Polonica*, 42, 289–294.

Kumaravelu, P., Shanthi, S., Dakshinamoorhy, D.P., Devraj, N.S. (1996) The antioxidant effect of eugenol on CCl4-induced erythrocyte damage in rats. *Journal of Nutritional Biochemistry*, 7, 23–28.

Mandal, S., Das, D.N., Ray, K.D., Chaudhury, S.B., Sahana, C.C., Choudhuri, M.K. (1993) *Ocimum sanctum* Linn. A study of gastric secretion in rats. *Indian Journal of Physiology and Pharmacology*, 37, 91–92.

Mediratta, P.K., Dewan, V., Maiti, P.C., Sen, P. (1988) Effect of *Ocimum sanctum* Linn. on humoral immunoresponses. *Indian Journal of Medical Research*, 87, 384–386.

Prashar, Ritu., Ashok Kumar (1995) Chemopreventive action of *Ocimum sanctum* on 2,12 dimethylbenz (a) anthracene DMBA-induced papillomagenesis in the skin of mice. *International Journal of Pharmacognosy*, 33, 181–187.

Sadekar, R.D., Pimprikar, N.M., Bhandarkar, A.G., Barmase, B.S. (1988) Immunomodulating effect of *Ocimum sanctum* Linn. Dry leaf powder on humoral immune response in poultry naturally infected with IBD virus. *Indian Veterinary Journal*, 75, 73–74.

Sakina, M.R., Dandiya, P.C., Hamdard, M.E., Hameed, A. (1990) Preliminary psychopharmacological evaluation of *Ocimum sanctum* leaf extract. *Journal of Ethnopharmacology*, 28, 148–150.

Savargaonkar, V.V., Karanjkar, A.M., Kulkarni, P.H. (1990) Action of *Sushama* (Suksma medicine). *Deerghayu International*, 6, 5

Singh, N., Misra, N., Srivastava, A.K., Dixit, K.S., Gupta, G.P. (1991) Effect of antistress plants on biochemical changes during stress reaction. *Indian Journal of Pharmacology*, 23, 137–142.

Singh, N., Tomar, V.S., Chandra, T., Gupta, G.P. (1989) A comparative evaluation of the effects of some species of *Ocimum* on anoxia tolerance in albino rats. *Planta Medica*, 55, 95.

Singh, S., Agrawal, S.S. (1991) Anti-asthmatic and anti-inflammatory activity of *Ocimum sanctum*. *International Journal of Pharmacognosy*, 29, 306–310.

Singh, S., Majumdar, D.K. (1995) Analgesic activity of *Ocimum sanctum* and its possible mechanism of action. *International Journal of Pharmacognosy*, 33, 188–192.

Singh, V., Singh, A., Nath, R., Mishra, N., Dixit, K.S., Singh, N. (1991) Effect of some anti-stress plant drugs on the intestinal transit. *Journal of Biological and Chemical Research*, 10, 601–602.

Subbulakshmi, G., Sarvaiya, S.R. (1991) Hypotensive effect of *Ocimum sanctum*. *Bombay Hospital Journal*, 33, 39–43.

Tandan, S.K., Chandra, S., Jawahar Lal (1989) Pharmacological screening of the essential oil of *Ocimum sanctum* leaves. *Indian Journal of Pharmaceutical Sciences*, 51, 71–72.

Trivedi, V.P., Singh, S.K., Sharma, S.C., Singh, N. (1995) A clinical evaluation of Tulsi (*Ocimum sanctum* Linn) leaf powder in cases of laryngopharyngitis and coryza (common cold and cough). *Seminar on Research in Ayurveda and Siddha*, CCRAS, New Delhi, 20–22 March 1995.

Uma Devi, P., Ganasoundri, A. (1995) Radioprotective effect of leaf extract of Indian medicinal plant *Ocimum sanctum*. *Indian Journal of Experimental Biology*, 33, 205–208.

52 Vacha

Acorus calamus L.
Family: Araceae

THE PLANT AND ITS DISTRIBUTION

This herb originated in east Europe and adjoining areas. In India it grows in marshy and humid land in many places. It has sword-like leaves (Fig. 44A), arranged in a rosette, from the centre of which a bunch of blue or violet flowers may arise, hence the name *blue flag*. The root is about 1 cm thick, spreads prostrate within the soil and has distinct nodes and internodes. Numerous root fibres arise all over the internodes. During collection, the root (Fig. 44B) is removed from the soil, cut into 5 cm long pieces and dried. On drying it becomes rather flat with longitudinal striations. The central vascular portion is darker than the rest of the root. It has a distinct strong aromatic odour.

In Indian it is known as *vacha* or *ghorvacha* and it is distinguished from *balvacha* or *parsik vacha* (*khurasani vacha*) which does not have a central darker portion and is white throughout. It is obtained from *Iris germanica* L, which is cultivated in graveyards of Muslims in Kashmir. It is said that the root's smell keeps predators (rats) away, which would otherwise prey on the dead bodies. Tuberous roots of *Paris polyphylla* are also considered a source of this commodity.

USES IN FOLKLORE AND AYURVEDA

Since antiquity, calamus root has been used for medicinal baths, in incense and tea. In many areas magical effects are attributed to the plant. It is said that calamus root keeps people young, strengthens their health and boosts their sexual lives. A herbal bath with calamus is said to increase erotic desire. The original inhabitants of North America chewed the roots to ward off exhaustion or took it as snuff in a pulverized form (Ratsch, 1997). It is combined with *Centella* to stimulate sex and promote wisdom. It is commonly considered a hallucinogenic herb, but a number of people who tried the American strain (asarone-free) for this purpose did not have good experiences. In some cases the person required medical attention after ingestion. For pleasure, at least 30 cm of root has to be swallowed with a non-alcoholic beverage: carbonated drink, milk, etc. Alcohol counteracts its effect.

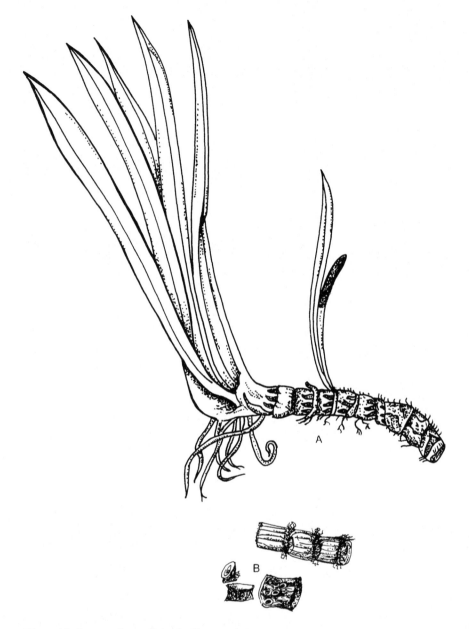

Figure 44 Acorus calamus **A** herb, **B** root pieces.

In Ayurveda the root is considered aromatic, bitter, hot, nauseating, anthelmintic, sudorific, mildly laxative and it is said to help inflammation, gaseous distension, and fevers. The details on these uses are as follows:

As a mental tonic

For intellectuals and students it is often prescribed with *Centella*, *Bacopa* and *Convolvulus* as a mental tonic. It increases memory and stimulates brain faculties. It helps unconsciousness, insanity, nervous breakdown, in physical debility and acts as a cerebral stimulant. It may be used by mixing half a teaspoon each of *vacha* and *ghee*, with milk for 2–3 months.

For pains and aches

Make a paste of the root by grinding it on a wet floor and apply it to the forehead. When applied externally it stimulates blood flow. It may be used on bruises and rheumatism in the same way.

For migraines

Make a very fine powder of *vacha* and long pepper and inhale a pinch of this mixture through nose.

For expelling worms

Heat 500 mg of asafoetida and add to it 3 g *vacha* powder. Swallow it with water. In acute cases use the mixture twice daily for 4–5 days.

An infusion of the root is sprinkled on the affected wound to drive away vermin.

For dry coughs

Briskly boil 25 g of coarse *vacha* powder in 250 ml of water. When warm, take 20 ml of this decoction, 3–4 times daily. It clears the throat and relieves dry throats and coughs. It stimulates the mucous membrane and salivary glands, which results in increased secretion.

For sinusitis

Sprinkle *vacha* powder on burning charcoal or a heater to produce smoke. Convert a piece of thick paper into a funnel-shaped structure, 15 cm in diameter at the broad end and about 1 cm at the tapered end (Fig. 45). Place the broader end slightly above the smoke source in such a way that the funnel does not catch fire but collects all the fumes. The tapering end should be placed near the nostrils so that the smoke is inhaled. Smoke is pungent but very effective. It clears the nose and through regular treatment surgical operations for sinusitis may even be avoided.

For stomach troubles

For digestive problems such as flatulence, dyspepsia and colic, boil 25 g of *vacha* in 500 ml of water and take 10–20 ml of decoction, depending on the severity of the case. For infants, grind *vacha* into mother's milk and give half a teaspoonful three times a day.

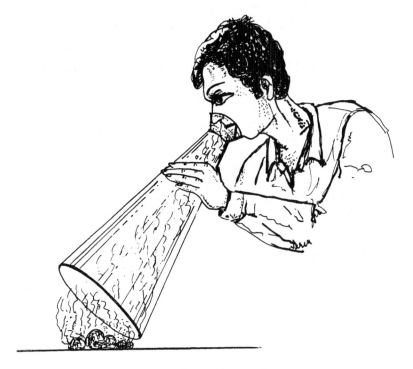

Figure 45 Method to inhale the fumes of the herb.

For spermatorrhoea

Pulverize 30 g *Triphala*, 10 g *Piper cubeba*, 10 g *vacha* and 5 g camphor. Take 2 g of this powder with cold water, lime water or with milk in the morning on an empty stomach, and two hours after meals in the evening. Continue until cured. This treatment makes the body physically strong, clears urine and helps digestion.

Contraindication

All items hot in nature, such as spicy, non-vegetarian food, alcohol, sex, etc. should be avoided during treatment with calamus.

Ayurvedic preparation

Sarswat churn

Ingredients   Pulverize equal quantities of *Centella*, *Convolvulus* and calamus. Moisten this mixture with *Centella* juice or decoction and let the powder dry. Repeat this process of moistening with juice three times. When fully dry use the powder.

Dose   3 g with milk for 3–4 months.

Use   As a general tonic, it increases mental and physical strength.

THERAPEUTIC INDICATIONS AND PHARMACOLOGICAL STUDIES

Relaxant activity

A papaverine-like relaxant, depressant and anti-spasmodic activity has been seen in the essential oil and in its isolated compounds asarone and β-asarone. It inhibited heart rhythms in frogs and dogs and relaxed the tone of isolated intestine. The neuropharmacological action of the oil revealed its sedative and tranquillizing effect. It caused a reduction in anxiety without dullness but with prolonged calming. It enhanced the activity of pentabarbitol and hexobarbital. Asarone antagonized the hyperactive and hallucinogenic effects of mescaline (personal communication). Both asarone and β-asarone are psychoactive, but hallucinogenic in higher doses. The essential oil-free alcohol extract had a sedative and analgesic property. The choloroform extract of the root had a cannabis-like activity, and the intraperitoneal administration of this extract brought about profound behavioural changes in monkeys (Dasgupta *et al.* 1977). Khare and Sharma (1982) observed anti-epileptic activity in it. Keller *et al.* (1985) noted that asarone had a spasmolytic activity against histamine. Aqueous alcohol extract reduced the severity of maximum shock-induced seizures but did not exhibit complete protection (Vohora *et al.* 1990). According to Martis *et al.* (1991) *Acorus* may be of use for epilepsy. Prasad and Chakraborty (1992) found it to be less tranquillizing but more hypotensive in nature. Zanoli *et al.* (1997) studied sedative and hypothermic effects induced by β-asarone and concluded that this compound cannot be considered a direct cannabinomimetic agent.

A polyherbal preparation containing ginseng, *Polygala*, *Calamus* and *Macrohyporia extensa* was given to thymectomized mice after the operation. It significantly ameliorated the learning and memory ability, which was impaired by thymecotomy. It acted on the cognitive process of the central nervous system (Zhou *et al.* 1992, Zhang *et al.* 1994).

For mental retardation

A polyherbal formulation consisting of *Centella asiatica*, *Calamus* and *Convolvulus* was given to mentally retarded children, in doses of 1,000 mg, 380 mg and 20 mg for one year. The treated group showed an appreciable increase in verbal mental age within seven and a half months, compared with the control. These herbs improved attention, activity levels and feed back, and controlled hyperactivity, aggressiveness, etc. (Rajagopalan, 1995).

Anti-inflammatory effect

The total extract had anti-inflammatory activity in acute and chronic models. It compared well with hydrocortisone and phenylbutazone (Sharma *et al.* 1989). Anti-pyretic, analgesic and anti-inflammatory activities were also observed in this root by Vohora *et al.* (1989) and by Siddiqui and Asif (1991).

In gastropathy

Rafatullah *et al*. (1994) observed anti-secretagogue, anti-ulcer and cytoprotective properties in the ethanol extract of the herb. It had the ability to inhibit gastric secretion, to protect gastroduodenal mucosa against injuries caused by pyloric ligation, indomethacin, reserpine, etc. It provided good protection against cytodestructive agents.

Anti-microbial properties

It exhibited anti-bacterial activities against *Mycobacterium tuberculosis* and other gram negative organisms (Alankar Rao and Rajendra Prasad, 1981).

The alcohol extract exhibited potent anti-viral activity in vitro against HSV-1 and HSV-2 virus types at well below a cytotoxic concentration. Host cells were not affected by the extract. The compound β-asarone, isolated from the extract, had a strong inhibitory activity against the replication of both virus types. This study justified the use of calamus as an anti-herpes agent (Badam, 1995).

In bronchial asthma

A preliminary report on the clinical trial has been given by Rajasekharan and Srivastava (1977).

In heart diseases

When *vacha* was used for three months in ischaemic heart disease, Mamagain and Singh (1994) observed an improvement in cases of chest pain, dyspnoea, reduced body weight index, serum cholesterol, and in electrocardiograms.

As an anthelmintic

A polyherbal treatment, including 250 g *Calamus* powder, three times a day was prescribed with *Embelia ribes* syrup (20 ml three times a day), *Semecarpus* oil (1 drop twice daily for two days), followed by purgation using 250 mg *Mallotus philippinensis* trichome powder twice daily, for two days, was highly effective against roundworm, threadworm and hookworm. When *vacha* was used alone, it was only effective against roundworm (Sharma *et al*. 1985).

Chemical studies

The root contains 1.5–3.5 per cent of yellow aromatic oil, mainly consisting of asarone and β-asarone, eugenol, asaraldehyde, galangin, etc. The composition of the oil from 2n, 3n and 4n varieties differs and β-asarone content increases with ploidy. The oil from the American 2n (diploid) race contains no asarone but in Indian varieties it is very high (Evans, 1988). β-Asarone is related to myristicin, the active constituent of nutmeg.

Toxicological studies

β-asarone is a hepatocarcinogen, mutagen and has a chromosome damaging property. Indian calamus oil fed to rats induced duodenal tumours (Bruneton, 1995).

References

Alankara Rao, G.S.J.G., Rajendra Prasad, Y. (1981) Antimicrobial property of *Acorus calamus* Linn. In vitro studies. *Indian Perfumers*, 15, 4–6.

Badam, I. (1995) In vitro studies on the effect of *Acorus calamus* extract and beta–asarone on Herpes viruses. *Deerghayu International*, 11, 16–18.

Bruneton, J. *Pharmacognosy, Phytochemistry, Medicinal Plants.* Lavoisier Publishing, Paris France 1995.

Dasgupta, S.R., Patra, B.B., Sikdar, S. (1977) Preliminary studies of the effect of chloroform extracted factor from *Acorus calamus* on the behaviour of conscious rhesus monkeys. *Science and Culture*, 43, 218–219.

Evans, W.C. *Trease and Evan's Pharmacognosy.* 18 Edition., Baillier and Tindall, London 1988.

Keller, K., Odenthal, K.P., Leng Peschlow, E. (1985) Spasmolytic activity of iso asorone from Calamus. *Planta Medica*, 51, 6–9.

Khare, A.K., Sharma, M.K. (1982) Experimental evaluation of antiepileptic activity of acorus oil. *Journal Scientific Research on Plants and Medicine*, 3, 100–103.

Mamgian, P., Singh, R. H. (1994) Controlled clinical trial of the Lekhaniya drug vaca (*Acorus calamus*) in cases of ischaemic heart diseases. *Journal for Research in Ayurveda and Siddha*, 15, 35–51.

Martis, G., Rao, A., Karanth, K.S. (1991) Neuropharmacological activity of *Acorus calamus*. *Fitoterpia*, 62, 331–337.

Prasad, H.C., Chakraborty, R. *Acorus calamus* Linn- A medicinal plant having hypotensive activity in experimental study. *International Seminar -Traditional Medicine*, Calcutta, 7–9 November 1992, p. 157.

Rafatullah, S., Tariq, M., Mossa, J.S., Al-Yahya, M.A., Al-Said, M.S., Ageel, A.M. (1994) Anti-secretagogue, anti-ulcer and cytoprotective properties of *Acorus calamus* in rats. *Fitoterapia*, 65, 19–23.

Rajagopalan, V. Effect of Ayushman-2 in Manasa Mandata (mental retardation). *Seminar on Research in Ayurveda and Siddha.* CCRAS, New Delhi, P 34, 20–22 March 1995.

Rajasekharan, S., Srivastava, P.N. (1977) Ethnobotanical study on vacha and its preliminary clinical trial in bronchial asthma. *Journal of Research in Indian Medicine. Yoga and Homoeopathy*, 12, 92–96.

Ratsch, Christian *Plants of Love. The History of Aphrodisiacs and a Guide to their Identification and Use.* Ten Speed Press, Berkeley CA, USA 1997.

Sharma, R.D., Chaturvedi, C., Tewari, P.V. (1985) Helminthiasis in children and its treatment with indigenous drugs. *Ancient Science of Life*, 4, 245–247.

Siddiqui, M.T.A., Asif, M. Anti-inflammatory activity of *Acorus calamus* Linn (Abstract). *Conference of Pharmacology and Symposium on Herbal drugs*, New Delhi (India), 15 March 1991.

Vohora, S.B., Shah, S.A., Dandiya, P.C. (1990) Central nervous system studies on ethanol extract of *Acorus calamus* rhizome. *Journal of Ethnopharmacology*, 28, 53–62.

Vohora, S.B., Shah, S.A., Sharma, K., Naqvi, S.A.H., Dandiya, P.C. (1989) Antibacterial, antipyretic, analgesic and antiinflammatory studies on *Acorus calamus* Linn. *Annals of the National Academy of Medical Sciences (India)*, 25, 13–20.

Zanoli, P., Avallone, R., Baraldi, M. (1997) Sedative and hypothermic effects induced by beta asarone, a main component of *Acorus calamus*. *Procedings of the Second International Symposium on Natural Drugs*, Maratea, Italy, 28 Sept.,–1 Oct., 1997. (edited by Capasso, F., Pasquale, R., Evans, F.J., Mascolo, N.J. (1998) *Phytotherapy Research*, 12 Supp. S114–116).

Zhang, Y.X., Saito, H., Nishiyama, N. (1994) Improving effects of DX- 9386, a traditional Chinese medicinal prescription on thymectomy-induced impairment of learning behaviour in mice. *Biological and Pharmaceutical Bulletin*, 17, 1199–1205.

Zhou Daxing, Li Changyu, Lin Qinnliang (1992) Facilitatory effects of *Acorus gramineus* on learning and memory in mice. *Traditional and Herbal Drugs*, 2, 417–419.

53 Vata Vriksh

Ficus benghalensis **L.** (It is sometimes wrongly spelt as *F. bengalensis*)
F. religiosa **L.**
Family: Moraceae

Both these trees along with other *Ficus* spp. are sometimes used for the same purposes.

Ficus benghalensis

THE PLANT AND ITS DISTRIBUTION

It is a native of the Himalayan and south Indian mountainous regions, but has been introduced as a sacred, shady tree in most parts of India, along village ponds or in community centres. It covers a vast tract of land by spreading its branches and by its prop roots, which hang from it and touch the soil to establish connections with it. As the tree ages, more and more branches and hanging roots arise. Leaves (Fig. 46B) are waxy, thick and leathery. Young buds are pink in colour. The fruit is red, enclosing numerous small seeds.

It appears that earlier, in Indian villages, businessmen (called *banya*) used to display their shop wares under the shade of this tree and at that time Englishmen named the tree after them, the *banyan* tree.

USES IN FOLKLORE AND AYURVEDA

In earlier Sanskrit literature, the tree has been considered on a par with *soma* (p. 262) in its effect. All parts of the tree, bark, root, latex and fruits were used. Fruits and young hanging roots were considered food for the elite to improve their memory power. For this purpose, *banyan* bark was dried in the shade, pulverized and mixed with double the quantity of sugar candy. Great importance was attached to the latex (called milk). It was considered rejuvenating, a stimulant and nourishing. It was collected from the tree by making a pit-like depression at the base of a large branch after sunset. The mouth of the pit was closed with a lump of raw sugar. Before sunrise, in the morning, the latex was collected in a vessel.

The other uses of the tree are as follows:

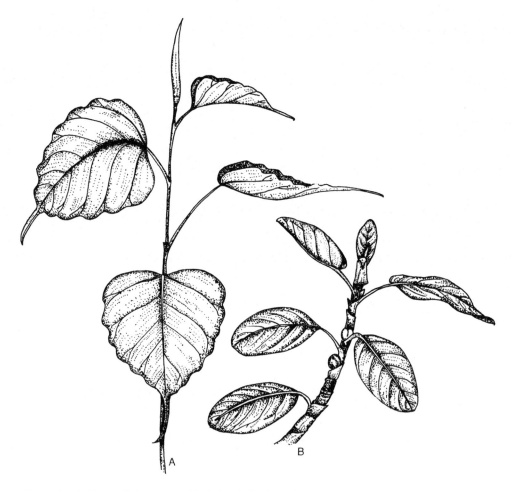

Figure 46 **A** *Ficus religiosa*, twig, **B** *F. benghalensis*, twig.

For sexual inadequacies

1   Pulverize dry tender shoots and hanging roots. Take a pinch of this powder at regular intervals for spermatorrhoea.
2   Macerate opium and nutmeg in the latex of the *banyan* tree. Four to five drops of this mixture on flat sugar candy helps premature ejaculation and nocturnal emission.
3   A decoction of *banyan* tree bark along with the other nourishing substances is said to have good effect on retention, quality and quantity of semen.
4   Six grams of the pulverized powder of twigs dried in shade, mixed with an equal quantity of sugar candy, when taken for seven days with 250–500 ml of milk first thing in the morning, thickens the semen and helps burning micturition.
5   The leaves also have a beneficial effect on human regenerative powers.
6   Unripe fruits dried in the shade, ground well and drunk are said to augment the urge for sex.

7 Fry 600 mg of asafoetida in *ghee* and mix one teaspoon of honey and one of *Ficus benghalensis* latex. Take this mixture twice daily for 40 days for impotence.

Contraindication

Do not use any sour or acidic things during treatment with this herb. Untoward thoughts should not arise in the patient's mind.

Ficus religiosa

THE PLANT AND ITS DISTRIBUTION

The tree grows wild in the forests of central India and Bengal but has been introduced in most parts of India as a sacred tree, where it is known as *peepal*. It is a spreading tree with cordate, acuminate, glabrous leaves (Fig. 46A). The fruits are small and enclose several seeds. The fruit is edible and is slightly sweet in taste.

USES IN FOLKLORE AND AYURVEDA

The decoction of the bark is considered cooling in effect (*shitavirya*, *shit* is cold and *virya* effect) and is prescribed in cases of sexual inadequacies and nervous debility which are supposed to have originated due to hotness in the body. The main uses are:

As a *Rasayana*

On the first day take 3 small *peepal* leaves and boil them in 125 ml milk and 125 ml water. On the next day increase the number of leaves to six and prescribe them as they were given on the first day. Increase the dose by three leaves every day until a dose of 30 leaves per day is attained. After this, follow the treatment in a descending order until a dose of three leaves a day is reached. This treatment is considered a *Rasayana* in its effect and is said to bring about changes in the vital fluid (*dhatu parivartana*) of the body, which is useful in cases of paralysis, chronic coughs and other chronic diseases.

For sexual inadequacies

a) Boil 500 g of tender twigs in 4 litres of water until the quantity of water is reduced to 500 ml. Cool and filter this decoction and add 2 kg sugar to make a linctus. Take 30 g of this linctus daily along with 250 ml milk, 60 g butter and sugar candy, according to taste.

b) Take one part of fresh green leaves and 8 parts of water. Crush the leaves and boil them in water, until the water is reduced to one-fourth. Filter, concentrate the decoction and add an equal quantity of sugar to it until a solid mass is obtained. Make pills of 60 mg each. The dose is 2–3 pills twice daily.

As a tonic for the nervous system

1   Dry fresh *peepal* bark in the shade, and pulverize it. Take this powder with milk and sugar. This increases memory and strengthens the nervous system. It is a brain tonic for weak memory and mental confusion.
2   In nervous debility, cook 120 g of young tender twigs, in half a litre of cow's milk three to four times. On cooling, strain the milk through cheesecloth. Add sugar candy to it as per taste and drink.
3   For insanity, boil 2–3 tender leaves in about 100 ml milk until the milk condenses. Add sugar according to taste.
4   For spasms and convulsion in children that arise due to involuntary muscle contraction, prepare a fine powder of the tree's hanging roots and mix it with an equal quantity of saffron. Give 60–120 mg of this mixture at half-hour intervals.

For syphilis

Take the young bud or bark after boiling it in milk.

As a healing agent

The decoction of bark is an astringent and is quite effective for healing wounds, ulcers, etc.

For psychoneurotic diseases

In cases of hysteria, emotional instability, intense craving, affections and wild emotions, etc., take 25 g of tender hanging roots, cut and pound them and add 12 g each of *Nardostachys jatamansi* (*N. grandiflora*), nutmeg, and 1.5 g musk. Macerate the whole mass in a blender and, when homogenous, make pills of 100 mg each. Prescribe one to four pills, thrice daily for four months. Avoid tension and hot food.

Ayurvedic preparation

Peepalavleh

Method   Take one part of *panchang* of *peepal* (five parts of tree, *i.e.* the root bark, leaves, fruit, tender shoots and fibrous hanging roots) and 16 parts of water. Macerate the herb in water and boil until reduced to one-fourth. Filter this decoction and dry the filtrate further until a thick paste is formed. Make pills of 250 mg each from this extract and wrap each pill in a piece of silver foil.

Dose   1–2 pills are to be taken with milk at night.

Use   These pills are said to be effective in all cases of nervous debility, mental confusion and mild insanity.

THERAPEUTIC INDICATIONS AND PHARMACOLOGICAL STUDIES OF F. *benghalensis* AND F. *religiosa*

Anti-diabetic effects

Neera Singh *et al*. (1992) observed that alcohol extract of *F. benghalensis* bark showed significant hypoglycaemic activity. It reduced levels of serum cholesterol and blood urea. Cherian and Augusti (1993) noted anti-diabetic activity in glycoside leucopelargonidin isolated from *F. benghalensis*. It demonstrated hypoglycaemic, hypolipidemic and serum insulin-raising levels in diabetic rats. It significantly enhanced the faecal secretion of sterols and bile acids. Vinod Kumar and Augusti (1993) showed that it had an insulin sparing action. Augusti *et al*. (1994) confirmed that the leucopelargonidin derivative showed significant hypoglycaemic and serum insulin-raising action in normal as well as in moderately diabetic dogs. Cherian and Augusti (1995) identified the effective compound as dimethyl ether of leucopelargonidin (3-o-alpha-L-rhamnoside). A low dose of insulin in combination with this compound maintained body weight, controlled urine blood sugar and ameliorated serum cholesterol and triglycerides.

Anti-diarrhoeal effect

The extract of *F. benghalensis* hanging roots and *F. racemosa* bark had an inhibitory effect against castor oil-induced diarrhoea. These extracts brought a reduction in gastrointestinal motility (Mukherjee *et al.* 1998).

Antioxidant effect

Daniel *et al.* (1998) isolated quercetin and polyphenolic flavonoids from the bark of *F. benghalensis* and evaluated their antioxidant action in hyperlipidaemic rats. These compounds showed a significant antioxidant effect and lowered serum lipids (cholesterol, phospholipids, triacylglycerols and free fatty acids).

Antigastroduodenal ulcer effects

A water decoction of *F. religiosa* bark protected the animals against induced gastric and duodenal ulcers (Bipul De, 1997).

Hypocholesterolaemic effect

Shukla *et al.* (1995) fed the water extract of *F. benghalensis* bark with cholesterol to rabbits. The bark extract not only prevented the elevation of serum cholesterol but brought its level down. There was an improvement in other parameters of lipid profiles. Daniel *et al.* (1998) confirmed this activity.

For leucorrhoea

Three grams of *F. benghalensis* bark, when administered five times a day for 30 days gave relief to patients with leucorrhoea (Sannd and Krishan Kumari, 1992).

Anti-tumour activity

The fruit extracts of *F. religiosa* and *F. benghalensis* exhibited anti-tumour and anti-bacterial activity (Mousa, 1994).

Toxicological studies

The leucopelargonidin derivatives did not show any toxic effects when administered for one month and and were not lethal, even at the high dose of 1.8 g/kg (Augusti *et al.* 1994).

References

Augusti, K.T., Daniel, R.S., Cherian, S., Sheela, C.G., Sudhakaran Nair, C.R. (1994) Effect of leucopelargonin derivative from *Ficus bengalensis* Linn on diabetic dogs. *Indian Journal of Medical Research*, 99, 82–86.

Bipul De, Maiti, R.N., Joshi, V.K., Agrawal, V.K., Goel, R.K. (1997) Effect of some Sitavirya drugs on gastric secretion and ulceration. *Indian Journal of Experimental Biology*, 35, 1084–1087.

Cherian, S., Augusti, K.T. (1993) Antidiabetic effects of a glycoside of leucopelargonidin isolated from *Ficus bengalensis* Linn. *Indian Journal of Experimental Biology*, 31, 26–29.

Cherian, S., Augusti, K.T. (1995) Insulin sparing action of leucopelargonidin derivatives isolated from *Ficus bengalensis* Linn. *Indian Journal of Experimental Biology*, 33, 608–611.

Daniel, R.S., Mathew, B.C., Devi, K.S., Augusti, K.T. (1998) Antioxidant effect of two flavonoids from the bark of *Ficus bengalensis* Linn in hyperlipidemic rats. *Indian Journal of Experimental Biology*, 36, 902–906.

Mandal, S.C., Maity, T.K., Das, J., Saha, B.P., Pal, M. (1998) *Ficus racemosa* affords antihepatotoxic activity against paracetamol-induced acute liver damage in rats. *Natural Product Sciences*, 43, 174–179.

Mousa, O., Vuorela, P., Kiviranta, J., Abdel Wahab, S., Hiltunen, R., Vuorela, H. (1994) Bioactivity of certain Egyptian *Ficus* species. *Journal of Ethnopharmacology*, 41, 71–76.

Mukherjee, P.K., Saha, K., Murugesan, T., Mandal, S.C., Pal, M., Saha, B.P. (1998) Screening of anti-diarrhoeal profile of some plant extracts of a specific region of West Bengal, India. *Journal of Ethnopharmacology*, 60, 85–89.

Neera Singh, Tyagi, S.D., Agarwal, S.C. (1992) Study of antidiabetic effects of alcoholic extract of *Ficus bengalensis* (Linn.) on alloxan diabetic albino rats. *Journal of Research in Ayurveda and Siddha*, 13, 56–62.

Sannd, B.N., Krishna Kumari (1992) A preliminary clinical trial of Vatavrakasha Curna on Svetapardara. *Journal of Research in Ayurveda and Siddha*, 13, 82–88.

Shukla, R., Anand, K., Parbhu, K.M., Murthy, S. (1995) Hypocholesterolemic effect of water extract of the bark of banyan tree, *Ficus bengalensis*. *Indian Journal of Clinical Biochemistry*, 10, 14–18.

Vinod Kumar, R., Augusti, K.T. Insulin sparing activity of a leucocyanidin derivative isolated from Ficus bengalensis Linn. *Amala Research Bulletin*, 13 August, 1993, pp. 32–36.

54 Vatsnabh

Aconitum spp.
Family: Ranunculaceae

THE PLANTS AND THEIR DISTRIBUTION

The plants, which yield aconite (*vatsnabh* of Ayurveda) grow in the alpine Himalayas. Earlier botanists identified these as *Aconitum napellus* L., but this identification was erroneous. The Indian aconites, which can be the source of *vatsnabh*, have been identified by Puri (1974a). The names of these, along with their natural distribution in India, are as follows: *Aconitum deinorrhizum* Stapf South Kashmir, *A. falconeri* Stapf Garhwal, *A. balfourii* Stapf Grahwal to Nepal, *A. ferox* Wall. ex Seringe, *A. spicatum* Stapf, and *A. laciniatum* Stapf, in Singalila Range, Darjeeling.

These plants are herbs, usually about 1 metre tall, but some plants of *A. spicatum* (Fig. 47A) may grow taller. The flowers are generally blue with a characteristic hood (Fig. 47B) and nectaries (Fig. 47C). The roots of these plants are characteristic (Fig. 47D) in that the mother tuber gives rise to the plant as well as to a daughter tuber (Fig. 47E). As the plant grows, the mother tuber shrivels due to nutrient depletion and the daughter tuber develops with an apical bud at the top. Puri (1975) provides a detailed botanical description of Indian aconites.

Aconite is one of the oldest herbs known to Indian physicians. It is a component of many Chinese preparations and in Tibet it is known as 'king of medicine' (Puri, 1974b). The poisonous nature of aconite is well known to Indians where the plant grows and they call it *vish* or *bikh*, which means poison. Earlier it was used as an arrow poison.

In the nineteenth century a root known as *Jadwar Khatai*, considered an antidote to poisons and sold at the price of gold, was much in demand. The British East India Company became interested in it as the source of a commercial commodity. On the basis of organoleptic characteristics it looked like some aconites, so Stapf was deputed by the East India Company to investigate the source of this precious herb, resulting in a monograph on Indian aconites (Stapf, 1905).

The dry roots of *vatsnabh* are brownish and horn-like (Fig. 47F), 6–12 cm long and 2–4 cm broad. The internal colour of the tuber may be off-white to brown to black. The fracture is horny and, on breaking the tuber, star-like cambium is visible. The root is starchy, has no smell but causes a tingling sensation when applied to the tip of the tongue. (Caution: it is very poisonous.) Since black aconite fetches a higher price, sometimes the off-white or brown aconite roots are boiled in ferrous sulphate dissolved

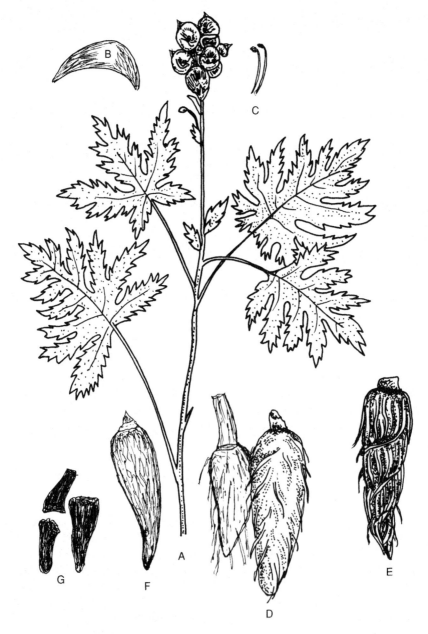

Figure 47 Aconitum spicatum **A** twig, **B** hood of flowers, **C** nectaries under hood,
D fresh root, daughter and mother tuber joined together, **E** fresh root,
F dry root, **G** treated root.

in cow's urine to give the root a black colour (Fig. 47G). Pharmacognostic details on
these aconites are described by Mehra and Puri (1970).

Aconite is one of the major nine poisons known in Ayurveda. For medicinal purposes
it is used after mitigation by breaking the root into pea-sized pieces. These pieces are
immersed in a pot containing cow's urine and the pot is kept in sunlight throughout

the day. Next day the old urine is discarded and replaced with fresh. This process is repeated three times and the root pieces are dried for future use. Sometimes the roots are boiled in cow's urine, instead of giving the above treatment.

USES IN FOLKLORE AND AYURVEDA

According to Ayurveda, *vatasnabh* after mitigation is hot and bitter but, if used in a proper way, it is a good *Rasayana* with anti-*tridosha* effects, mainly against *vata* and *kapha*. It increases internal fire (*agni*) within the body. It is an analgesic, anti-pyretic, cardiotonic and an anti-inflammatory agent. Earlier it was recommended in acute stages of venereal diseases, but now it is only used to a limited extent due to the lack of safety in therapeutic doses. As given by Puri (1974b) the various uses of mitigated aconites, at a dose of 7.5–15 mg, are as follows:

Anti-pyretic, anti-periodic and diaphoretic

It is used in various types of fevers.

For respiratory problems

Mainly used for asthma, where it provides good relief.

As a cardiotonic

For blood pressure problems, it is used as an hypotensive agent. It is a heart and nerve sedative and prevents heart palpitations. After mitigation in the Ayurvedic way, the roots lose their depressant action on the heart and develop a stimulating effect.

As a mental and physical tonic

It is prescribed as an aphrodisiac, particularly for involuntary urination and seminal ejaculation.

As an anodyne

It is used for neuralgia, trifacial neuralgia and rheumatism. It has a significant anti-inflammatory activity. In western pharmacopoeias, a preparation containing aconite, belladonna and chloroform was earlier very popular and applied externally to relieve pain.

THERAPEUTIC INDICATIONS AND PHARMACOLOGICAL STUDIES

General studies

Singh *et al.* (1985) studied the pharmacology of mitigated aconite for cardiotonic, analgesic, anti-pyretic and anti-inflammatory activity. The aconite showed all these activities and was not cardiotoxic. In another study Murayama *et al.* (1991) observed that processed aconite contained pyro-type alkaloids. These alkaloids had an analgesic and anti-inflammatory effect but were low in toxicity.

Cardiotonic effects

According to Dong and Chen (1995) the alkaloid showed therapeutic and prophylactic effects on different models of experimental arrhythmia without causing a marked effect on myocardial contractility.

Anti-cancerous property

The aconite extract increased the secretion of interlukin-1β tumour necrosis factor α and interleukin-6 in human mononuclear cells (Chang *et al.* 1994).

Chemical studies

The roots may contain 0.4–1.85 per cent of diterpenoid alkaloids, which resemble aconitine isolated from *A. napellus*. Some of the well known alkaloids from Indian aconites are bikhaconitine, pseudaconitine, aconitine, bishatisine and bishaconitine. Out of these pseudaconitine is the most toxic, bikhaconitine and indaconitine are more active than aconitine (Mehra and Puri, 1970).

Toxicological studies

POISONOUS and if used in excess of the prescribed dose it stops the heart.

References

Chang, J.G., Shih, P.P., Chang, C.P., Chang, J.Y., Wang, F.Y., Tseng, J. (1994) The stimulating effect of radix aconiti extract on cytokines secretion by human mononuclear cells. *Planta Medica*, 60, 576–578.

Dong, Y.L., Chen, W.Z. (1995) Effect of Guan-Fu base A on experimental cardiac arrhythmias and myocardial contractility. *Pharmeceutica Sinica* 30, 577–582.

Mehra, P.N., Puri, H.S. (1970) Pharmacognostic investigations on aconites of *Ferox* group. *Research Bulletin of the Panjab University* (N.S.) 21, 473–493.

Murayama, M., Mori, T., Bando, H., Amiya, T. (1991) Studies on the constituents of *Aconitum* species. IX. The pharmacological properties of pyro type aconitine alkaloids, component of processed aconite powder *Kako-bushimastu*, analgesic, antiinflammatory and acute toxic activities. *Journal of Ethnopharmacology*, 35, 159–164.

Puri, H.S. (1974a) Distribution of aconites in India. *Journal of Research in Indian Medicine*, 9, 41–43.

Puri, H.S. (1974b) Uses of aconites. *Journal d'Agriculture Tropicale et de Botanique Appliquée*, 21, 239–246.

Puri, H.S. (1975) Botanical studies on aconites. *Herba Hungarica*, 14, 123–133.

Stapf, O. (1905) The aconites of India. A monograph. *Annals Royal Botanical Gardens*, Calcutta (India), 10, 115–119.

Singh, L.B., Singh, R.S., Bose, R., Sen, S.P. (1985) Studies on the pharmacological action of aconite in the form used in Indian medicine. *Bulletin Medico Ethnobotanical Research*, 6, 115–123.

55 Vibhitaki

Terminalia bellirica (Gaertn.) Roxb.
Syn. *T. belerica* Roxb.
Family: Combretaceae

THE PLANT AND ITS DISTRIBUTION

It is a deciduous tree commonly known by the name *bahera*. It may grow up to 30 m in height. It grows throughout India except on very dry and marshy land. The leaves (Fig. 48A) are elliptic or broadly elliptic, obovate up to 7.5 cm long, crowded towards the end of the branches. Flowers are light greenish yellow, 1.25 cm across and have an offensive odour. The fruit (Fig. 48B) is a drupe, grey to light violet and 2–5 cm long.

USES IN FOLKLORE AND AYURVEDA

In Ayurveda, negative virtues are attributed to this tree, and the fruit is rarely used alone. In folklore, the unripe fruit is considered a laxative and the mature fruit an astringent. The fruit powder (2–10 g) is used for coughs, throat problems, fevers, and in gastroenteritis. The seed kernel is said to have analgesic, anti-inflammatory, aphrodisiac and narcotic effect. The seed oil is applied as a hair tonic. It is purgative, like castor oil. The fruit of this tree is one of the three ingredients of a very common Ayurvedic preparation *Triphala*.

THERAPEUTIC INDICATIONS AND PHARMACOLOGICAL STUDIES

An astringent, tonic, laxative and antipyretic effect have been seen in *vibhitaki* by Nandi *et al.* (1975), which may be of use for dropsy and leprosy. The other studies are as follows:

Anti-microbial properties

Four compounds isolated from the fruit exhibited anti HIV-1 activity, anti-malarial activity against *Plasmodium falciparum*, anti-fungal activity against *Penicillium expansum* and *Candida albicans in vitro* (Raghvan *et al.* 1997).

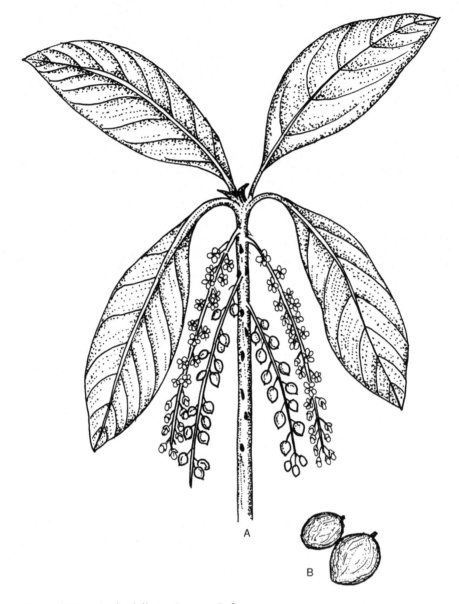

Figure 48 Terminalia bellirica **A** twig, **B** fruit.

Anti-diabetic activity

When Siddiqui (1961) injected ethanol extract, equivalent to one gram of dry fruit, intraperitonially into rabbits, it reduced blood sugar levels.

Hepatoprotective activity

Siddiqui (1963) found that it stimulated bile secretion. The fruit exhibited a significant hepatoprotective effect in a dose-dependent manner. A fraction of the fruit extract was tried on experimentally-induced hepatic injury in rats. The results were encouraging; it had both prophylactic and curative properties (Anand *et al.* 1994).

Anti-tussive and anti-asthmatic activity

The fruit exhibited bronchodilator, antispasmodic and anti-asthmatic effects. Trivedi *et al.* (1982) treated 93 cases of asthma using this fruit, 22 patients showed complete relief, in 22 cases there was a significant relief and in 35 cases there was moderate relief. It was effective in tropical pulmonary eosinophilia, with less relapse (Abhimanyu Kumar *et al.* 1994).

For myocardial necrosis

Tariq *et al.* (1977) used it along with *amalaki*.

Anti-mutagenic effect

The polyphenols isolated from the fruit showed this effect on *Salmonella tymphimurium* (Padam *et al.* 1966).

Anti-uraemic activity

Yokozawa *et al.* (1995) confirmed that tannins in the fruit have a uraemic decreasing effect.

Chemical studies

The fruit contains 21.4 per cent of both condensed and hydrolyzable tannins. Of these the important ones are gallic acid, ellagic acid and epigalates. In addition to these, saponins, nitrogenous crystalline principle phyllembin and a cardiac glycoside have also been isolated (Thakur *et al.* 1989).

Toxicological studies

It is very safe. No toxicity was seen, even up to a dose of 3.3 g/kg (Anand *et al.* 1994).

References

Abhimanyu Kumar (1994) Role of certain Ayurvedic herbal drugs in management of T.P.E. in children. *Indian Medicine*, 44, 5–10.

Anand, K.K., Singh, B., Saxena, A.K., Chandan, B.K., Gupta, V.N. (1994) Hepatoprotective studies of a fraction from the fruits of *Terminlia belerica* Roxb. on experimental liver injury in rodents. *Phytotherapy Research*, 8, 287–292.

Nandi, M., Sharma, R.C., Gupta, S.K., Arora, R.B. (1975) Chemical and Biological assay of *Terminalia belerica* Roxb. – A comparative study of three samples. *Journal of Research in Indian Medicine*, 10, 27–36.

Padam. S.K., Grover, I.S., Majar Singh (1996) Antimutagenic effects of polyphenols isolated from *Terminalia bellerica* myroblan in *Salmonella typhimurium*. *Indian Journal of Experimental Biology*, 34, 98–102.

Raghavan, V., Pushpagandan, P., Smitt, U.W., Andersewn, A., Christensen, S.B., Sittie, A., Nyman, U., Nileson, C., Olsen, C.E. (1997) New anti-HIV-1, antimalarial, and antifungal compounds from *Terminalia bellerica*. *Journal of Natural Products*, 60, 739–742.

Siddiqui, H.H. (1961) Studies on *Terminalia belerica* Roxb. *Indian Journal of Pharmacy*, 25, 297.

Siddiqui, H.H. (1963) Studies on *Terminalia belerica* Roxb. Effect on bile secretion and pharmacodynamic properties. *Indian Journal of Pharmacy*, 27, 297–302.

Tariq, M., Hussain, S.J., Asif, M., Jahan, M. (1977) Protective effects of fruit extracts of *Emblica officinalis* (Gaertn.) and *Terminalia belerica* Roxb., in experimental myocardial necrosis in rats. *Indian Journal of Experimental Biology*, 5, 485–486.

Thakur, R.S., Puri, H.S., Akhtar Hussain *Major Medicinal of Plants of India*. CIMAP, Lucknow India 1989.

Trivedi, V.P., Nesamany, S., Sharma, V.K. (1982) A clinical study of the antitussive and antiasthmatic effects of Vibhitakaphal Churna (*Terminalia belerica* Roxb.) in the cases of Kasa-Swasa. *Journal of Research in Ayurveda and Sidha*. 3, 1–8.

Yokozawa, T., Fujioka, K., Oura, H., Tanaka, T., Nonaka, G., Nishioka, I. (1995) Confirmation that tannin containing crude drugs have a uraemic decreasing action. *Phytotherapy Research*, 9, 1–5.

56 Vidari Kand

Pueraria tuberosa (Roxb. Ex Willd.) DC
Family: Fabaceae (Leguminose)

THE PLANT AND ITS DISTRIBUTION

It is a liana (Fig. 49A), found in sub-arid zones of India. The main tuber is like a big turnip and, in the soil, may be followed by smaller and smaller tubers in a chain. The tuber is brownish from the outside and dirty-white to pale yellow inside, which on drying may be thick on the outside, but with a flake-like structure inside or may be in the form of a barrel shape, in pieces 25–50 cm long and 25 cm thick. These dry papery wafers (Fig. 49B) have a liquorice-like taste. In south India, tubers of other plants, such as *Ipomoea digitata*, pith of *Cycas* and sometimes palms are considered *vidar kand*. In many instances in Ayurvedic literature, *vidari kand* has been identified as *I. digitata*.

USES IN FOLKLORE AND AYURVEDA

As per Ayurveda, it is a good nutrient, energizer, boosts vital energy and is an aphrodisiac. It is sweet in *ras*, a galactagogue, spermatogenic, cooling, greasy, diuretic and effective against all the three *kaphas*, calming burning sensations in the body. It is advisable to use it in cold areas or in cold weather. It is mainly used in the form of a fine powder for the following purposes;

As a galactagogue

For a lack of milk after childbirth, 5 g of powder is given to mothers in cow's milk.

As an anabolic agent

A weak child is given 2 g of powder with milk for digestion. For additional benefits, 2 g of *peepali* powder may be given along with it.

For digestive problems

Six grams of powder with *ghee* and sugar is given twice daily for enlargement of the liver and spleen.

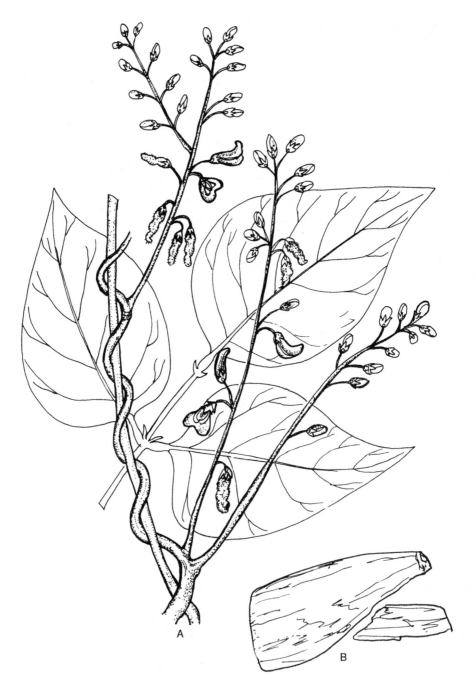

Figure 49 Pueraria tuberosa **A** twig, **B** pieces of tuber.

For excessive menstruation

Six grams of powder is used twice daily with honey.

For sexual debility

Fry crushed wheat or barley in *ghee* and add milk, honey, sugar and *vidari* powder to it.

For spermatorrhoea

1 Take pulverized *vidari* dried in its own juice and add almond, quince seed, clove, cardamom, nutmeg, *satavari*, *kawanch* and sugar. Take 6 g of this powder with milk.
2 Take juice of fresh root with cumin and sugar.

In Chinese traditional medicine

In the book written by Li Shih Chen in 1578, *Pueraria lobata* root (*kudzu* or *ko for*) has been mentioned for relieving thirst, for febrile conditions, as an anti-emetic, anti-toxic, for colds, snake bites and to counter the effect of excessive alcohol. It is said to help hypertension, stiffness of the neck, lack of perspiration, migraines, angina pectoris, hypoglycaemia and arterial diseases. For treating sudden deafness, alcohol extract of the tuber is prescribed, whilst for neck stiffness and hypertension a decoction is used.

Earlier *P. thomsonii* was used in China but *P. lobata* has been found to be richer in the active constituents, isoflavones. The tubers of these two species can be easily differentiated by their internal characters. Whereas the root of *P. thomsonii* is white due to the starch, *P. lobata* is yellow due to an excess of fibres. (It appears that tubers of *P. thomsonii* resemble that of *P. tuberosa*.)

Ayurvedic preparations

Maharasayana yoga

Method   Pulverized *vidari* tuber is saturated with the fresh juice of *vidari* and dried. This process is repeated 21 times and the powder is dried completely. If the fresh juice is not readily available, a decoction can be prepared by boiling coarse *vidari* powder in eight times as much water until water is reduced to one-fourth. After filtration, use this decoction in place of the juice.

Dose   5–10 g.

Use   An immunostimulant which increases the strength, power and sexual capacity in males.

THERAPEUTIC INDICATIONS AND PHARMACOLOGICAL STUDIES

As an anti-inflammatory agent

The peeled root, bruised into a cataplasm, reduced swelling. It was crushed and rubbed on the body for fevers and rheumatism. Nikam *et al.* (1977) isolated a steroidal neuromuscular blocking agent from the root. It was fully reversible, indicating that steroids act as an anti-depolarizing agent. Lee *et al.* (1994) studied the anti-inflammatory activity of flavonoids daidzein and puerarin. Both showed significant anti-inflammatory activity. Cho and Kim (1985) studied the product *Galgumn-tang* for anti-inflammatory and analgesic action. This product mainly consisted of *P. thunbergiana* and showed remarkable inhibition of inflammation.

For nervous diseases

Xiuxian and Xuiquin (1979) found that *Radix puerarie* was effective in 83 per cent of migraine cases. Shen *et al.* (1996) reported that the flavones from the root are antagonists or weak partial agonists of the benzodiazepine receptor.

For heart problems

Fan *et al.* (1985) carried out a pharmacological study on *radix puerariae* for acute regional myocardial ischaemia. It decreased the mean arterial pressure without decreasing the collateral coronary blood flow. Fang (1980) found that 100 mg of total isoflavones cured 90 per cent of hypertensive cases, 80 per cent of angina pectoris cases and 92 per cent of migraine cases. In the treatment of hypertension, total isoflavins injected into the carotid artery were capable of dilating the cerebral blood flow. It may be due to improved cerebral circulation that patients suffering hypertension, from migraines, and sudden deafness received relief. These compounds lowered catecholamine levels, decreased the oxygen supply and depressed lactic acid production by the oxygen-deficient heart muscles in angina pectoris. The compounds were not effective orally as they were destroyed in the body.

As an anti-spasmodic

Shibata *et al.* (1959) studied flavonoids and anthraquinones from *P. hirsuata* syn. *P. lobata*. They showed anti-spasmodic properties.

For gynaecological problems

It had emmenagogue, significant oestrogenic and progesteronogenic activities with no toxicity. The alcoholic extract was highly effective in dysmenorrhoea, dysfunctional uterine bleeding and in menopausal syndrome. Patients resistant to routine hormonal therapy responded remarkably to this treatment (Chandhoke *et al.* p.c.). Shukla *et al.* (1996) found that butanol extract had an oestrogenic mode of action. It increased glycogen content, protein concentration and total cholesterol in the reproductive organs of ovariectomized rats.

Khurana *et al.* (1996) studied the effect of a herbal galactagogue containing *Leptadenia*, fennel, *Glycyrrhiza*, *Pueraria*, *Asparagus* and cumin on the milk yield of lactating buffaloes. The preparation resulted in a significant increase in milk yield. The result was evident within seven days of treatment and was sustained for 35 days.

In alcoholism (antidipsotropic agent)

Keung and Vallee (1993) observed that the active constituents of the root, daidzin and daidzein, suppressed free-choice alcohol intake by Syrian golden hamsters. Overstreet *et al.* (1993) carried out further research. Keung *et al.* (1996) compared the effect of pure daidzin with that of crude daidzin contained in the methanol extract of the root, and concluded that this effect is not due to daidzin alone, but to the joint action of both isoflavone constituents daidzin and daidzein (Keung and Vallee, 1998).

Antioxidant effect

Sato *et al.* (1992) noted the antioxidant action of *Pueraria* isoflavonoids. These were able to scavenge free radicals involved in lipid peroxidation initiation. Speroni *et al.* (1996) confirmed this antioxidant effect.

Hepatoprotective effect

Sohn *et al.* (1985) noted that in the case of cadmium toxicity *P. thunbergiana* butanol extract had a diuretic and antidotal effect. Shukla *et al.* (1996) studied the protective action of butanol extract of the root on carbon tetrachloride-induced hepatotoxicity in rats. Treatment with *P. tuberosa*, seven days prior to administration of carbon tetrachloride protected rats against liver damage. Araro (1998) noted the preventive effects of nine saponins, isolated from the root, on the liver in *in vitro* immunological liver injury in primary cultured rat hepatocytes.

Chemical studies

Various isoflavones like puerarin, daidzein and daidzin have been reported.

Toxicological studies

Shukla (1995) studied in detail, the toxicity of the butanol extract of this tuber. Using this treatment the concentration of serum GPT (glutamic purvic transaminase) and GOT (glutamino oxaloacetic transaminase or aspartate transminase) were significantly higher. Significant changes were observed in the adrenal glands but there were no histopathological or functional effects.

References

Araro, T., Udayama, M., Kinjo, J., Nohara, T. (1998) Preventive effects of saponins from the *Pueraria lobata* root on in vitro immunological liver injury of rat primary hepatocyte cultures. *Planta Medica*, 64, 413–415.

Cho, E.H., Kim, I.H. (1985) Studies on the concurrent administration of medicine. I Anti-inflammatory and analgesic action of Galgun-tang and aspirin. *Korean Journal of Pharmacognosy*, 16, 7–11 (in Korean).

Fan, L., O'Keefe, D.D., Powel, W.J. Jr (1984) Effect of puerarin on regional myocardial blood flow and cardiac haemodynamics in dogs with acute myocardial ischaemia. *Acta Pharmaceutica. Sinica*, 19, 801–807.

Fan, L., O'Keefe, D.D., Powell, W.J. Jr. (1985) Pharmacologic studies on radix puerariae. Effect of puerarin on regional myocardial blood flow and cardiac hemodynamics in dogs with acute myocardial ischemia. *Chinese Medical Journal*, 98, 821–832.

Fang Qicheng (1980) Some current study and research approach relating to the use of plants in the traditional Chinese medicine. *Journal of Ethnopharmacology*, 2, 57–63.

Furusawa, J., Nohara, T. (1987) New ingredients of Puerariae radix. *Journal of Pharmaceutical Sciences*, 76, p S 197.

Keung, W.M., Lazo, O., Kunze, L., Vallee, B.L. (1996) Potentiation of the bioavailability of diadzin by an extract of Radix puerariae. *Proceedings of the National Academy of Sciences* USA, 93, 4284–4288.

Keung, W.M., Vallee, B.L. (1993) Daidzin and daidzein suppress free choice ethanol intake by Syrian golden hamsters. *Proceedings of National Academy of Sciences*, USA, 90, 10008–10012.

Keung, W.M., Vallee, B.L. (1998) Kudzu root: an ancient Chinese source of modern antidipsotropic agents. *Phytochemistry*, 47, 499–506.

Khurana, K.L., Balvinder Kumar, Khanna, S., Manuja, A. (1996) Effect of herbal galactagogue Payapro on milk yield in lactating buffaloes. *International Journal of Animal Sciences*, 11, 239–240.

Nikam, S.T., Sonurlikar, U.A., Bhide, M.B. (1977) Steroidal neuromuscular blocking agent from *Pueraria tuberosa*. *Indian Journal of Pharmacy*, 39, 161.

Overstreet, D.H., Lee, Y.W., Rezvani, A.H., Criswell, H.E. *Research Society on Alcoholism*. Symposium Skipper Bowles Centre for Alcohol Studies, University of North Carolina, Chapel Hill, USA 1993.

Sato, T., Kawamoto, A., Tarsumi, Y., Fujii, T. (1992) Mechanism of antioxidant action of *Pueraria* glycoside (PG)-1 (an isoflavonoid) and mangiferin (a xanthonoid). *Chemical and Pharmaceutical Bulletin*, 40, 721–724.

Shen, X.L., Witt, M.R., Nielsen, M., Sterner, O. (1996) Inhibition of (3H) flunitrazepam binding to rat brain membrane in vitro by puerarin and diadzein. *Acta Pharmaceutica Sinica*, 31, 59–62.

Shibata, S.T., Murakami, Y., Haroda, M. (1959) The constituents of *Pueraria* root. *Chemical and Pharmaceutical Bulletin*, 7, 134–136.

Shukla, Sangeeta (1995) Toxicological studies of *Pueraria tuberosa*, a potent antifertility plant. *International Journal of Pharmacognosy*, 33, 324–329.

Shukla, Sangeeta, Jonathan, S., Sharma, A. (1996) Protective action of butanolic extract of *Pueraria tuberosa* DC against carbon tetrachloride-induced hepatotoxicity in adult rats. *Phytotherapy Research*, 10, 608–609.

Sohn, D.H., Ann., H.S., Shin, S.D. (1985) Pharmacological effects of Puerarie radix butanol extract on cadmium toxicity in rats. *Yakhak Hoeji*, 29, 206–215.

Speroni, E., Guerra, M.C., Rossetti, A., Pozzeti, L., Sapone, A., Paolini, M., Cantelli-Forti, G., Pasini, P., Roda, A. (1996) Anti-oxidant activity of *Pueraria lobata* (Willd.) in the rats. *Proceedings of the VIII Congresso nazionale della Societa Italiana di Farmacognsia and 1st joint meeting of Belgian, Dutch, Spanish and Italian Research groups on Pharmacognosy*, Napels, Italy, 9–14th June 1996. Capasso, F., Evans, F.J., Mascolo, N. (eds.) *Phytotherapy Research* (Supplement 1), S 95–97.

Xiuxian, G., Xuiqin, L. (1979) Radix Puerariae in migraine. *Chinese Medical Journal*, 92, 260–262.

57 Vidhara

Argyreia speciosa Sweet
Syn: *A. nervosa* (Bulm f.) Bojes
Family: Convolvulaceae

In western countries, it is known as Baby Rosewood or Hawaiian Baby Rosewood.

THE PLANT AND ITS DISTRIBUTION

It mainly grows in deciduous forests but can be cultivated in warm climates. It is a liana with big cordate leaves (Fig. 50A) and a twining stem, with greenish violet-white flowers. The fruit is globular, enclosing three seeds. Each seed (Fig. 50B) is pyramidal in shape with a broad hilum.

In India, the genuine seeds are known as *bidhara beej asli* and are hard to obtain. These are very often substituted for similar types of seed of other members of Convolvulaceae. The plant is also known as *samunderphul*.

USES IN FOLKLORE AND AYURVEDA

In Ayurvedic formulations, the genuine seed is rarely used and are often substituted by the stem pieces of this plant, called *vidhara* root. It is considered an alterative, nervine tonic, aphrodisiac and is an important constituent of many commercial aphrodisiac preparations sold in India.

One of these preparations, *Ashwagandhadi Churn* (p. 49), is made by pulverizing equal quantities of *vidhara* stem with *ashwagandha*. Sometimes an equal quantity of *Hygrophila spinosa* seed powder is also added to it. Another product is prepared by soaking the pulverized root of *Argyreia* in *Asparagus* juice. After drying, when given in a dose of 3–6 g with *ghee*, for a month, it is said to improve intellect, strengthens the body and keeps old age away.

A psychedelic product, *Utopian Bliss Balls* is prepared by taking 5 *Argyreia* seed, 1 pinch of ginseng, 1 pinch of *gotu kola* and 1 teaspoon bee pollen. The mixture is stuffed into date palm pulp (Ratsch, 1997).

The seed is mainly used for the extraction of lysergic acid compounds, *d* lysergic acid amide and *d* isolysergic acid amide, both of which are closely related to LSD (*d*-lysergic acid diethylamide) obtained from ergot, by first extracting the seed with

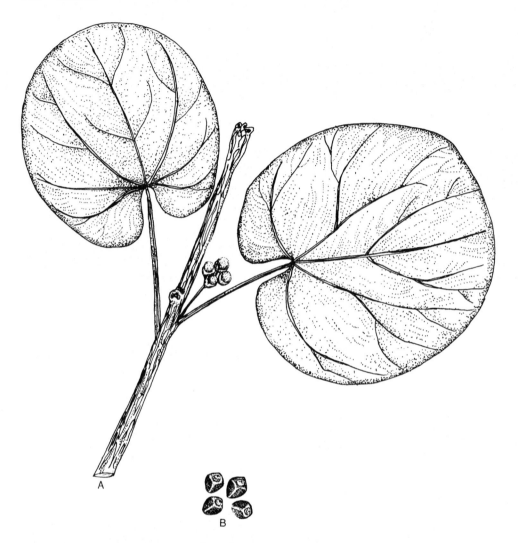

Figure 50 Argyreia speciosa **A** twig, **B** seed.

petroleum ether and then with alcohol. A paste of 8–10 seeds, after removal of seed coat, is said to have a good hallucinogenic effect. The results are more tranquil than those induced by LSD. In some people it has a depressant effect whilst in others it acts as an invigorating agent (from the internet, on the basis of some people's experience).

Chemical studies

It contains ergoline-type alkaloids, some of which are hallucinogenic. A seed contains 3 mg of ergoline and ergometrine (Chao and Dermarderosian, 1973, Agarwal and Rastogi (1974), Wealth of India, 1985).

References

Agarwal, S.K., Rastogi, R.P. (1974) Ergometrine and other constituents of *Argyreia speciosa* Sweet. *Indian Journal of Pharmacy*, 36, 118–119.

Chao, J., Dermarderosian, A.H. (1973) Identification of ergoline alkaloids in the genus *Argyreia* and related genera and their chemotaxonoimc implication in Convolvulacae. *Phytochemistry*, 12, 2435–2440

Ratsch, Christian *Plants of Love. The History of Aphrodisiacs and a Guide to their Identification and Use.* Ten Speed Press, Berkley, CA USA 1997.

Wealth of India Publication and Information Directorate, CSIR, New Delhi, India 1985.

58 Some *Rasayana* formulations

Since ancient times, classical Ayurvedic texts have mentioned *Rasayana* formulations. These have been manufactured all over the Indian subcontinent for several centuries by learned *vaidyas* (physicians). The number of these formulations is so large that it is not possible to list all of them. In recent times, many Ayurvedic physicians, using their experience and keeping the need of the society in view, have developed more *Rasayana* products which are sold under trade names. Today, Ayurvedic pharmacies manufacture both classical preparations and trade name preparations. A selection of these products is given here. The first part consists of classical formulations, which are manufactured under their Ayurvedic name, and the second part lists preparations where trade names are used.

CLASSICAL FORMULATIONS

These have been selected from the Ayurvedic literature on the basis of their uniqueness and popularity. In each formulation, the name of the ingredients and parts used have been identified from the Sanskrit name and are listed in a table. The quantity of each and the dose of the products have been converted into grams (approximately). On the basis of information in the Sanskrit texts, a summary of the method of preparation and uses of each product is given. As will be seen from these tables, quite a number of minerals/gems/poisonous substances are included in these formulations. This was probably done to potentiate the slow action of the herbs on the human system, or to provide rare minerals to the body, or may have been a result of the feudal system of society in mediaeval India, which had become so sophisticated that complex compounds with precious and rare ingredients were the need of the hour. Most of these compounds contained ambergris, saffron and musk, which are hard to find even now. Stress was laid on incorporation of inorganic compounds in organic forms. These compounds, in formulations, are actually complex organo-metallic compounds prepared by various tedious processes of treating minerals, etc. with many herbs, and subjecting them to high temperatures, so that they turn ash-like (*bhasama*) and become partly soluble in water for bioavailablity to the human system. In earlier English translations, the term calcination was used for this process of treating minerals, etc., but, as later discovered, it is not a simple process of heating raw materials but consists of subjecting them to various herbal treatments so the term, *processed* has been used in the present text. Special mention may be made of red sulphide of mercury, which is used extensively in *Rasayana* preparations. In Ayurveda there are two different processes for its manufacture. In one of the products, called *Makardhawaj*, gold is used as a catalyst, while the other product, *Ras Sindur*, is manufactured without gold.

Amrit *Rasayana*

Ayurvedic name	Botanical/English name	Plant part/processing	Quantity
Vatsnabh (*Shodhit*)	*Aconitum* spp.	Aconites (processed)	25 g
Lauha Kanta	Iron ore	Processed in *amalaki* juice	25 g
Abhrak Bhasam	Mica	Processed	25 g
Swarnmakshik Bhasam	Iron pyrites	Processed	25 g
Makardhawaj	Red sulphide of mercury (gold)	Processed	25 g
Rajat Bhasam	Silver	Processed	25 g
Vang Bhasam	Tin	Processed	25 g
Katha	*Acacia catechu*	Powder of wood extract	35 g
Sonth	Ginger	Powder	35 g
Ghee Kawar	*Aloe* spp.	Juice	As required

Method Heat iron ore in *amalaki* juice for a whole day. Pulverize all the other herbs and minerals to a very fine powder. Macerate iron ore and the fine powder of herbs and mineral in *Aloe* pulp until a thick paste is formed. Make pills of 250 mg each and dry.

Dose 250 mg with *ghee*, sugar or honey for one year.

Use A geriatric tonic, for slow and long term treatment. Cures almost all diseases of old age. In other cases, it imparts strength, vigour, intelligence and vitality. It cures impotence due to chronic diseases.

Braham *Rasayana*

Ayurvedic name	Botanical/English name	Plant part/process	Quantity
Amalaki	*Emblica officinalis*	Fruit, fresh	1,000 in number
		Fruit juice	1,000 fruits
Prashnaparni	*Desmodium gangeticum*	Root	As required
Punernava	*Boerhaavia diffusa*	Root	
Jivanti	*Leptadenia reticulata*	Root	
Nagbala	*Sida spinosa*	Root	
Mandukparni	*Centella asiatica*	Herb	
Shatawari	*Asparagus racemosus*	Root	
Shankhpushpi	*Convolvulus pluricaulis*	Herb	
Peepali	*Piper longum*	Fruiting spike	
Vavading	*Embelia ribes*	Seed	
Kawanch	*Mucuna pruriens*	Seed	
Gaduchi	*Tinospora* cordifolia	Stem	
Chandan. Lal	*Pterocarpus santalinus*	Wood	
Agar	*Aquilaria agallocha*	Wood	
Mulathi	*Glycyrrhiza glabra*	Root	

continued

Ayurvedic name	Botanical/English name	Plant part/process	Quantity
Aaak phul	*Calotropis* spp	Flower	
Neelkamal phul	Lotus, blue	Flower	
Kamal phul, safed	Lotus, white	Flower	
Chameli phul	Jasmine	Flower	
Malti phul	*Aganosma dichotoma*	Flower	
Nagbala Ras	*Sida spinosa*	Juice	4 litres
Suvaran Bhasam	Gold	Processed	As required
Rajat Bhasam	Silver	Processed	
Tamar Bhasam	Copper	Processed	
Parval Bhasam	Coral, red	Processed	
Lauha Bhasam	Iron	Processed	

Method   Blanch *amalaki* fruit with the steam generated from milk (use milk instead of water). When soft, remove the nut from the pulp, dry and pulverize it. Mix with *amalaki* powder, juice of 1,000 *amalaki* fruits prepared separately and dry. When the whole mass dries, weigh it, add to it one-eighth of its weight of the pulverized herbs mentioned above, taking each herb in equal quantity. Add to this powder of mixture of herbs and *amalaki*, four litres of *Sida spinosa* juice and dry the whole mass again in the shade. Pulverize this mixture once again, and add two parts of honey and one part of *ghee* until a thick paste is formed. Pour the paste in a container, seal, and subject it to mild heat in such a way that the heat is uniform all over. Let it remain undisturbed for two weeks, and note the weight of the product obtained. Take equal quantities of all inorganic compounds (*Bhasamas*) given in the formulations to form one-eighth of the total weight of the *amalaki* preparation obtained above. Mix the two to form a homogenous paste for the pills.

Use   This *Rasayana* is mainly used for *Kuti Parveshika* (indoor *Rasayana* treatment) for rejuvenation of the whole body under the guidance of a health provider, who monitors the condition of the patient, determines the dose and duration.

Jawahar Mohra

Ayurvedic name	Botanical/English name	Part/processing	Quantity
Mukta Pishti	Pearl	Paste	25 g
Lal Pishti	Ruby	Paste	25 g
Pukhraj Pishti	White or yellow sapphire	Paste	25 g
Panna Pishti	Emerald	Paste	25 g
Neelam Pishti	Blue sapphire	Paste	25 g
Parval Pishti	Coral, red	Paste	250 g
Agate	Agate	Paste	25 g
Kasturi	Musk	Resin	1.5 g
Ambergrease	Ambergris	Resin	1.5 g
Rajta vark	Silver	Foil	50 g
Suvarn vark	Gold	Foil	10 g
Zahar Mohra	Serpentine	Paste	10 g
Abe Resham	Silk cocoon	Powder, fine	500 g

Method   Make a paste of all the items mentioned above, except musk, silk cocoon and amber. Do not let the paste dry. To the wet paste, add silver and gold foil and triturate the whole mixture, than add musk, amber and silk cocoon powder until it becomes homogenous. Make pills of the size of a rice grain.

Dose   Remove the stone from a date palm fruit, and in its place put two pills of *Jawahar Mohra*, along with a pinch of saffron. Take this medicated date palm daily for two weeks.

Use   For high blood pressure, heart trouble, heart palpitations and irregular heart beat.

Kamdugdha Ras

Ayurvedic name	Scientific/English name	Part/processing	Quantity
Mukta Pishti	Pearl	Paste	10 g
Parval Pishti	Coral red	Paste	10 g
Mukta Shukti Pishti	Mother of Pearl	Paste	10 g
Cowrie Pishti	*Cypraea moneta*	Paste	10 g
Shankh Bhasam	Mollusc shells	Processed	10 g
Garu lal	Red ochre (Iron oxide)	Processed	10 g
Gaduchi satav	*Tinospora* spp.	Starch	10 g

Method   Take equal quantities of all the above ingredients and triturate to form a uniform mixture.

Dose   250 mg with cumin, sugar, twice daily.

Uses   It is said to have a cooling effect on the body, so it is used for inflammation, digestion, urinary tract infection, hyperacidity, headache, paralysis, mental problems, and haemorrhage.

Laxami Vilas Ras

Ayurvedic name	Botanical/English name	Plant part/processing	Quantity
Kuchla Shodhit	Nux vomica	Seed processed	75 g
Mirch kali	Black pepper	Powder	75 g
Tankan Shodhit	Borax (crude)	Dehydrated	75 g
Swaran Makshik Bhasam	Iron pyrite	Processed	50 g
Gandhak Shodhit	Sulphur	Processed	25 g
Parad Shodhit	Mercury	Processed	12.5 g
Bhringraja Ras	*Eclipta alba*	Plant juice	As required
Amalaki Ras	*Emblica officinalis*	Fruit juice	As required
Shatawari Ras	*Asparagus* spp.	Root juice	As required
Adrak Ras	Ginger (fresh)	Juice	As required

Method Triturate mercury and sulphur until a black mass is formed. Add fine powders of all herbs and minerals and triturate them in this black mass. Make paste by adding ginger juice to it. When dry, soak and dry again in the juices of *Asparagus, Emblica, Eclipta*, one after the other, three times each. Make pills of 125 mg.

Dose One pill.

Uses In wasting disease, lack of energy, provides nutrition to convalescent patients.

Laxman Vilas Ras

Ayurvedic name	Botanical/English name	Plant part/processing	Quantity
Abhrak Bhasam	Mica	Processed	40 g
Parad Bhasam	Mercury	Purified	20 g
Gandhak Shodhit	Sulphur	Purified	20 g
Mushkafoor	Camphor	Crystals	10 g
Jaiphal	Nutmeg	Seed powder	10 g
Javitri	Mace	Aril powder	10 g
Vidhara Beej	*Argyreia nervosa*	Seed powder	10 g
Dhatura Beej	*Datura* spp	Seed powder	10 g
Bhang Beej	*Cannabis*	Seed powder	10 g
Vidarikand	*Pueraria tubereosa*	Root powder	10 g
Shatawari	*Asparagus racemosus*	Root powder	10 g
Nagbala	*Sida spinosa.*	Herb powder	10 g
Atibala	*Abutilon indicum*	Seed powder	10 g
Gokshru	*Tribulus terrestris*	Seed powder	10 g
Pan Ras	*Piper betle*	Juice of leaves	10 g

Method Mix all the powders and minerals, followed by juice and camphor and divide into doses of 125 mg.

Dose 1–2 doses twice daily with milk, or macerate the powder honey and take with a spoon.

Use It is a supreme *Rasayana*, acts on all organs of the body, and rectifies all *doshas*, diseases. It is a geriatric tonic and prevents premature grey hairs, wrinkles, failing senses, and loss of immunity. It is a cardiotonic with beneficial effects on all parts of the heart and vascular system. It does not cause depression after stimulation as is the case with many other preparations. In this case heart and pulse rates remain normal. It helps sinking heart, cardiac palpitation, restlessness, and angina. It is effective in influenza nervousness, breathlessness, dry cough, oedema of head and feet, indigestion, diarrhoea and obesity.

Contraindications Fatty matters, sour, heavy food. Use under medical supervision; sometimes it increases the pulse rate.

Madanoday Modak

Ayurvedic name	Botanical/English name	Plant part/processing	Quantity
Javitri	Mace	Aril powder	15 g
Jaiphal	Nutmeg	Seed powder	15 g
Jatamansi	Nardostachys grandiflora	Root powder	15 g
Lavang	Clove	Buds powder	15 g
Mushkafoor	Camphor	Crystals	15 g
Keshar	Saffron	Stigma	15 g
Iliachi, choti	Cardamom	Fruit powder	15 g
Dalchini	Cinnamon	Bark powder	15 g
Sonth	Ginger (dry)	Rhizome powder	15 g
Mirch, Kali	Black pepper	Fruit powder	15 g
Vang	Tin	Processed	15 g
Abhrak	Mica	Processed	15 g
Lauha	Iron	Processed	22.5 g
Makardhawaj/Ras Sindur	Red sulphide of mercury	Processed	22.5 g
Shatawari	Asparagus racemosus	Root powder	22.5 g
Gokshru	Tribulus terrestris	Fruit powder	22.5 g
Draksha	Dry grapes	Fruit	22.5 g
Kakrasingi	Pistacia lentiscus	Gall powder	22.5 g
Bala	Sida spp.	Seed powder	22.5 g
Kawanch	Mucuna pruriens	Seed processed	22.5 g
Kushth	Saussurea lappa	Root powder	22.5 g
Vidhara	Argyreia speciosa	Seed powder	22.5 g
Bhang	Cannabis sativus	Leaves, flower tops	200 g
Shakar	Sugar		800 g

Method   Make syrup with the sugar, add powder of all the herbs and minerals, and form candy balls of 3–5 g each.

Use   It increases libido enormously when taken with boiled milk containing sugar and cardamom seed. It is an anabolic agent and, if used for three months, it gives extensive sexual and physical vigour.

Makardhwaj Vati

Ayurvedic name	Botanical/English name	Plant part/processing	Quantity
Makardhawaj	Red sulphide of mercury (with gold)	Processed	10 g
Mushkafoor	Camphor	Crystals	10 g
Jaiphal	Nutmeg	Powder	10 g
Mirch Kali	Black Pepper	Powder	10 g
Kasturi	Musk	Resin	3 g

Method   Triturate all dry powders mentioned in the formulation, first in camphor and after that in musk. Moisten the whole mass with water and make pills of 250 mg each.

Dose   One pill in the morning, one in the evening with milk, butter and sugar. Use in winter months only.

Use   As a physical and mental tonic, provides strength and energy to the heart, brain, nervous and urinogenital systems and thus cures impotence.

Manmath Ras

Ayurvedic name	Botanical/English name	Plant part/processing	Quantity
Parad Bhasam	Mercury	Processed	40 g
Gandhak Shodhit	Sulphur	Processed	40 g
Abhrak Bhasam	Mica	Processed	20 g
Mushkafur	Camphor	Crystal powder	10 g
Vanga Bhasam	Tin	Processed	10 g
Lauha Bhasam	Iron	Processed	10 g
Tamar Bhasam	Copper	Processed	10 g
Vidhara	Argyreia nervosa	Root powder	3 g
Jeera Safed	Cumin	Seed powder	3 g
Vidari kand	Pueraria tuberosa	Root powder	3 g
Shatwari	Asparagus racemosus	Root powder	3 g
Talamkhana	Hygrophila spinosa	Seed powder	3 g
Bala	Sida spp.	Seed powder	3 g
Kawanch	Mucuna pruriens	Seed processed	3 g
Ativisha	Aconitum heterophyllum	Root powder	3 g
Javitri	Mace	Aril powder	3 g
Jaiphal	Nutmeg	Seed powder	3 g
Lavang	Clove	Bud powder	3 g
Bhang	Cannabis sativus	Seed powder	3 g
Ajwain	Trachyspermum ammi	Seed powder	3 g
Ral Safed	Pinus spp.	Gum resin	3 g

Method   Triturate all the minerals in a pestle and mortar. Separately, in a grinder, make a fine powder of all the herbal ingredients. Mix the two, moisten with water to form a thick paste and make pills of 250 mg each.

Dose   Boil milk vigorously. When warm, take one pill with this milk in the morning and one in the evening.

Use   *Manmath* is another name for *Kamdeva*, the god of sex. *Manmath Ras* is used for regularizing all types of sexual inadequacies in men; it cures many sexual diseases, helps in senescence and keeps death away.

It is customary to add opium in preparations used for delaying ejaculation, but *Manmath Ras* is unique in that it does not contain opium but has the same effect as opium-containing recipes.

It is effective in diseases of women such as leucorrhoea, slackness of ovary and irregular ovulation. It aids in conception and helps proper development of the foetus and in retention of placenta.

Mukta Panchamrit *Rasayana*

Ayurvedic name	Botanical/English name	Processing	Quantity
Mukta Bhasam	Pearl	Processed	40 g
Parval Bhasam	Coral	Processed	20 g
Vang Bhasam	Tin	Processed	10 g
Shankh Bhasam	Molluscs	Processed	5 g
Mukta Shukti Bhasam	Mother of Pearl	Processed	5 g
Shatawari Ras	Asparagus racemosus	Juice	As required
Vidari kand Ras	Pueraria tuberosa	Juice	As required
Ghee kanwar Ras	Aloe spp.	Juice	As required
Ganna Ras	Sugar cane	Juice	As required

Method   Pulverize all animal and mineral ingredients to a fine powder. Triturate these pulverized materials in pestle and mortar, first with the juice of *Asparagus racemousus*, then let the juice dry and add juice of *Pueraria tuberosa*. When this dries add aloe pulp, dry again then add sugarcane juice. Repeat the process five times, and when moist enough make pills of 125 mg each.

Dose   One pill twice daily.

Use   Same as for pearl paste and ash. It is said to have a cooling effect on the body, so is used as a cerebral tonic, cardiotonic, in nervous diseases and sexual inadequacies.

Nari Kalyan Pak

Ayurvedic name	Botanical/English name	Plant part/processing	Quantity
Supari boiled in water	Areca catechu	Nuts boiled in water	100 g
Katha	Acacia catechu	Extract of catechu	
Musali Safed	Chlorophytum arundinaceum	Root	100 g
Aswagandha	Withania somnifera	Root	100 g
Sonth	Ginger (dry)	Root	10 g
Peepali	Piper longum	Fruiting spike	10 g
Peeplamul	Piper longum	Root	10 g
Jeera Safed	Cumin	Seed	10 g
Lawang	Clove	Flower buds	10 g
Dalchini	Cinnamon	Bark.	10 g
Tejpat	Cinnamomum spp.	Leaves	10 g
Nagkesar	Mesua ferrea	Flower	10 g
Kamarkas	Butea frondosa	Gum	10 g
Chava	Piper chaba	Fruit	10 g
Chitrak	Plumbago zeylanica	Root	10 g
Lajwanti	Mimosa pudica	Seed	10 g
Talamkhana	Astercantha longifolia	Seed	10 g
Nirgundi	Vitex negundo	Seed	10 g
Luha Bhasam	Iron	Processed	10 g
Parval Bhasam	Coral, red	Processed	10 g
Abhrak Bhasam	Mica	Processed	10 g
Vanga Bhasam	Tin	Processed	10 g
Ghee	Butter oil		300 g
Dudh	Milk		2 l

Method   Pulverize 100 g each of areca nut after boiling in decoction of catechu until soft and dry, along with *Chlorophytum arundinaceum* and *Withania somnifera* followed later by all other remaining herbs. Mix all the inorganic processed materials and make a separate fine powder.

Boil whole milk until it becomes condensed and forms a thick slurry. To this milk, add fine powders of the first three items, heat further until the whole mass becomes solidified, and fry in *ghee* (300 g). Add thick syrup of sugar to taste and the fine powder of the remaining herbs and processed minerals. Mix thoroughly and make candy balls of 25–50 g each.

Dose   As per digestive power, chew one candy with milk.

Use   It makes women's bodies healthy, keeps them in proper shape, and protects from all gynaecological problems.

Navjeevan Ras

Ayurvedic name	Botanical/English name	Plant part/processing	Quantity
Kuchla Shodhit	Nux vomica	Seed processed	25 g
Swarn Makshik	Iron pyrites	Processed	25 g
Ras Sindur	Red sulphide of mercury	Processed	25 g
Sonth	Ginger (dry)	Powder	50 g
Peepali	Long pepper	Powder	50 g
Mirch Kali	Black pepper	Powder	50 g
Adrak	Ginger (fresh)	Juice	As required

Method   Macerate all the ingredients in ginger juice, when wet enough and homogenous, make pills of 125 g each.

Dose   125 mg.

Use   It imparts a new lease of life to the body by increasing strength, and memory. It activates the nervous system and thus helps diseases caused by inactivation of this system.

Navratna Ras

Ayurvedic name	Botanical/English name	Plant part/processing	Quantity
Heera Bhasam	Diamond	Processed	14 g
Pukhraj Bhasam	Topaz	Processed	16 g
Neelam Bhasam	Aquamarine/sapphire	Processed	20 g
Lal Bhasam	Ruby	Processed	20 g
Vidurya Bhasam	Cat's eye	Processed	26 g
Gomed Bhasam	Hesonite	Processed	26 g
Mukta Bhasam	Pearl	Processed	30 g
Parval Bhasam	Coral	Processed	30 g
Panna Bhasam	Tourmaline/Emerald	Processed	16 g
Vikrant Bhasam	Silica	Processed	30 g
Ras Sindur	Black sulphide of mercury	Powder	250 g
Peepali	Long pepper	Powder	250 g

Method   Make pills containing 50 mg of above ingredients by adding binders to the mixture.

Dose   1 pill twice a day.

Use   For general debility, convalescence and wasting disease.

Navratnakalpa Amrit

Ayurvedic name	Botanical/English name	Plant part/processing	Quantity
Pukhraj Pishti	Topaz	Paste	10 g
Neelam Pishti	Aquamarine	Paste	10 g
Rajat Bhasam	Silver	Processed	20 g
Rajvart Pishti	Turquoise	Paste	20 g
Parval Pishti	Coral	Paste	20 g
Suvarn Bhasam	Gold	Processed	6 g
Yashad Bhasam	Zinc	Processed	6 g
Abhrak Bhasam	Mica	Processed	6 g
Guggal	Commiphora wightii	Oleo gum resin	12 g
Shilajit	Bituminous compound	Paste	12 g
Gaduchi	Tinospora spp.	Starch	12 g
Ghee	Clarified butter oil	Pure fat	As required

Method   Triturate all inorganic compounds and pastes. Add gum *guggal*, *ghee* and *Tinospora* starch to it, and triturate the whole mixture again until homogenous. Dissolve *Shilajit* in a small amount of water and mix it in the above mixture. When homogenous make pills of 250 mg each.

Dose   2 pills twice daily with milk for one year.

Use   As a geriatric tonic. It strengthens all parts of the human body, stabilizes *vata*, *pitta* and *kapha*. It is a boon for mental workers as it has beneficial effects on the brain and heart. It is an antidote to both internal and external toxins, particularly when *ama* is produced in the body due to the wrong type of food, irregular diet, lack of regularity in life style. It mitigates *ama* and brings *tridosha* into equilibrium.

Panchamrit Ras

Ayurvedic name	Botanical/English name	Plant part/processing	Quantity
Parad Bhasam	Mercury	Processed	10 g
Lauh Bhasam	Iron	Processed	10 g
Abhrak Bhasam	Mica	Processed	10 g
Tamar Bhasam	Copper	Processed	10 g
Shilajit Shodhit	Bituminous compound	Purified	10 g
Guggal Shodhit	Commiphora wightii	Oleo gum resin, purified	As required
Triphala Kadha	Emblica officinalis, Terminalia bellirica, T. chebula mixture	Decoction of fruits	As required
Gaduchi Kadha	Tinospora spp.	Decoction of stem	As required

Method Macerate *Guggal* gum in the decoction of *Tinospora* spp. and *Triphala*, and mix in the fine powder of all the remaining items. Knead all these together until homogenous, and make pills of 60 mg each.

Dose 1–2 pills with goat's milk, honey, *ghee* or water.

Use In wasting diseases, polyurea, weakness, tuberculosis, and as an antimicrobial and antipyretic agent. It helps in all the three *doshas* of the body.

Paraadi Ras

Ayurvedic name	*Botanical/English name*	*Plant part/process*	*Quantity*
Parad Bhasam	Mercury	Processed	10 g
Gandhak Shodhit	Sulphur	Purified	10 g
Vang Bhasam (Shatputi)	Tin	Processed (100 times)	10 g
Rasuant	*Berberis* spp.	Water extract (dry)	30 g
Lodhra	*Symplocos racemosa*	Bark powder	60 g
Vasaka	*Adhatoda vasica*	Juice of herb	As required

Method Triturate mercury with sulphur and add fine powders of the remaining items. Add the required quantity of the juice of *Adhatoda*, until a thick paste is formed. Homogenize the whole mixture further for 6 hours and make pills of 375 mg each.

Dose 1–2 pills twice daily with honey, or with rice gruel or water. For additional benefit take it with 2 g *Bergenia ligulata* powder.

Use It is a *Rasayana* for women, and the pill gives relief if vaginal flow increases due to excessive intercourse, wrong diet, wrong way of living, short temper, stress, etc. During this medication, use of intoxicants, narcotics, luxurious life, junk spicy food leading to laziness, backache, pains, stress, etc. should be avoided.

Ramchuramani Ras

Ayurvedic name	*Botanical/English name*	*Part used/processing*	*Quantity*
Mukta Pishti	Pearl	Paste	20 g
Swarn Makshik Bhasam	Iron pyrite	Processed	20 g
Suvarn Bhasam	Gold	Processed	20 g
Bhimseni Kapoor	Borneol	Powder	20 g
Jaiphal	Nutmeg	Fruit powder	20 g
Vanga Bhasam	Tin	Processed	20 g
Rajat Bhasam	Silver	Processed	20 g
Dalchini	Cinnamon	Bark powder	10 g
Tejpat	*Cinnamomum* spp.	Leaf powder	10 g
Ilaichi Choti	Cardamom	Fruit powder	10 g
Nag Kesar	*Mesua ferrea*	Bud powder	10 g
Shatawari Ras	*Asparagus racemosus*	Root juice	As required

Method Prepare a fine powder of all items and keep them in the juice of *Asparagus* for seven days. Make pills of 125 g each.

Dose 1–2 pills twice daily with milk.

Use A cooling, nutritive sex stimulant and aphrodisiac. It is considered suitable for those persons who consume items which are hot in nature, such as hot and spicy food, intoxicants, alcohol, meat preparations, etc. It does not have any narcotic or side effects and can be used throughout the year.

Rasayana for infants

Ayurvedic name	Botanical/Scientific name	Plant part/process	Quantity
Yashad Bhasam	Zinc	Processed	5 g
Parval Pishti	Coral, red	Paste with water	10 g
Heran Sing Bhasam	Deer/stag horn	Ash	5 g
Tankan Bhasam	Borax (dehydrated)	Powder	5 g
Mirch Safed	White pepper	Powder, outer black coat removed	10 g
Shathi	*Hedychium spicatum*	Rhizome powder	20 g
Kesar	Saffron	Style and stigma	5 g

Method Triturate fine powders of above, moisten with water, and make pills of 65 mg each.

Dose and Use Crush a pill in one teaspoon of mother's milk or cow's milk, and administer to child followed by milk or honey with *Embelia ribes* powder. It is an anabolic agent, acts on all the systems of the body, particularly when there are symptoms of fever, cold cough, vomiting, loose motions, indigestion and worm infestation.

Rattivalabh Pak

Ayurvedic name	Botanical/Scientific name	Plant part/process	Quantity
Gond Kikar	Gum acacia	Powder	500 g
Sonth	Ginger (dry)	Powder	100 g
Peepali	*Piper longum*	Fruiting spike powder	100 g
Piplamul	*Piper longum*	Root powder	25 g
Lawang	Clove	Powder	25 g
Jaiphal	Nutmeg	Powder	25 g
Javitri	Mace	Powder	25 g
Kamarkas	*Bombax malabarium*	Gum powder	25 g
Shilajit	Bituminous compound	Paste	10 g
Mirch Kali	Black pepper	Powder	10 g
Dalchini	Cinnamon	Powder	10 g
Tejpat	*Cinnamomum* spp.	Leaf powder	10 g
Nagkeshar	*Mesua ferrea*	Flower powder	10 g
Ilaichi	Cardamom	Fruit powder	10 g
Parval Bhasam	Coral, red	Processed (calcined)	10 g
Lauh Bhasam	Iron	Processed	10 g
Abhrak Bhasam	Mica	Processed	10 g
Keshar	Saffron	Stigma and style	5 g
Ghee	Clarified Butter		250 g
Mishri	Sugar candy		2 kg
Sukha Mewa	Dried fruits		as required

Method Fry gums in clarified butter. Separately powder ginger, long pepper fruiting spikes and roots. In another batch make a fine powder of saffron, spices, processed minerals, mix them and pass them through a fine cloth or a sieve. Chop almond, pistachio, dry grapes and coconut.

Make sugar syrup, and add to it all the powders of herbs and minerals except saffron and spices until the sugar syrup is of thick consistency. When the syrup starts to solidify and is still warm, add saffron and spices. Smear a flat plate with clarified butter, and spread the above semi solid mixture on it. Put chopped dry fruits as a top layer and make pieces of 25 g each.

Dose   25–50 g as per the digestive power of the patient. Chew it in the morning with an empty stomach, along with warm milk.

Use   It acts on the body in various ways. It provides the body with the energy required for delaying ejaculation during sex. It imparts beauty and health to women, gives enough strength for sex and relief in leucorrhoea. It is of immense use after giving birth.

Shukar Amritika Vati

Ayurvedic name	Botanical/English name	Plant part/processing	Quantity
Parad Bhasam	Mercury	Processed	40 g
Gandhak Bhasam	Sulphur	Processed	40 g
Abhrak Bhasam	Mica	Processed	40 g
Lauh Bhasam	Iron	Processed	40 g
Iliachi	Cardamom	Fruit powder	40 g
Gokshru	Tribulus terrestris	Fruit decoction	20 g
Vibhitaki	Terminalia bellirica	Fruit powder	20 g
Hariatki	T. chebula	Fruit powder	20 g
Amalaki	Emblica officinalis	Fruit powder	20 g
Tejpat	Cinnamomum spp.	Leaf powder	20 g
Rasaunt	Berberis spp.	Water extract, dry	20 g
Chava	Piper chaba	Fruit powder	20 g
Talispatra	Abies spp.	Leaf powder	20 g
Tankan Bhasam	Borax, crude	Dehydrated powder	20 g
Anar	Punica granatum	Sweet fruit seed	20 g
Guggal (Shodhit)	Commiphora wightii	Oleo gum resin (Processed)	10 g

Method   Triturate sulphur and mercury compounds until homogenous. Make a decoction of *gokshru*, and add mercury sulphur compound, and a fine powder of the remaining items to this decoction. Add additional decoction to such an extent that a paste wet enough for making pills is formed. Triturate this paste further for 12 hours and make pills of 250 mg each.

Dose   1–2 pills with milk, water or pomegranate juice as per the age and severity of the illness of the patients.

Use   It is used particularly for diseases of the nervous and urinogenital systems, until total recovery is achieved. In helps in the formation of blood in the body, makes the body muscular, thickens and purifies spermatic fluid, and acts as a mental stimulant. It helps impotence due to weakness of the nervous system. In involuntary nocturnal emission and/or premature ejaculation, 1 pill twice daily is used.

Precaution　The dose of the medication should not be increased. The patient should lead a simple, regulated, disciplined life without amorous activity of any type.

Smritisagar Ras

Ayurvedic name	Botanical/English name	Plant part/processing	Quantity
Parad Bhasam	Mercury	Processed	10 g
Gandhak Shodhit	Sulphur	Processed	10 g
Hartal	Arsenic compound	Prepared from 49 parts of arsenic and 24 parts of sulphur	10 g
Manshil	Arsenic compound	Prepared from 49 parts of arsenic and 16 parts of sulphur	10 g
Tamar Bhasam	Copper	Processed	10 g
Malkangani Tail	Celastrus paniculatus	Oil	As required
Mandukparni	Centela asiatica	Herb juice or decoction	As required
Vach	Acorus calamus	Rhizome juice or decoction	As required

Method　Take equal quantities of all the minerals, triturate them in a pestle mortar first with *Celastrus paniculatus* oil, enough to moisten the materials, and then soak and dry the mixture 21 times in the decoction or juice of *Calamus* and *Centella*. Make pills of 60 mg.

Dose　60–120 mg with butter and *ghee*.

Use　This mixture is mainly prescribed for loss of memory, but is used for any type of weakness in the nervous system (sedative, tranquilizer, antidepressant) and also for paralysis, hysteria, sudden spasm, sudden loss of memory, pain nausea, vomiting, and threatened abortion. It was tried by Tripathi and Singh (1995) in residual schizophrenia with good results.

Note　If during the administration of this compound, poisoning due to arsenic is evident, give juice of *Benincasa hispida*, cumin seed and sugar for three days.

Suvaran Malini Vasant

Ayurvedic name	Botanical/English name	Plant part/processing	Quantity
Suvaran Vark or Bhasam	Gold	Foil or processed	10 g
Mukta Pishti or Bhasam	Pearl	Paste or processed	20 g
Hingul	Arsenic compound	Processed	30 g
Mirch Safed	White pepper	Pepper with seed coat removed, powder	40 g
Yashad Bhasam	Zinc	Processed	80 g
Makhan	Butter		20 g
Nimbu ka ras	Lemon juice		As required

Method   Triturate gold and *hingul* in a pestle and mortar until mixed uniformly. If gold foils are to be used, do not add all at once but use a single gold foil at a time, triturate until mixed, add more, and so on. To this mixture add white pepper, pearl, zinc compound and butter; triturate further for three hours. Add the required quantity of filtered fresh lemon juice to the mixture, triturate until the butter becomes fully emulsified and no separate fatty matter is evident. Continue this treatment of the mixture with fresh lemon juice for 8–10 days until the product is no longer greasy. Make pills of 125 mg each.

Dose   1–2 pills twice daily with 250 mg of long pepper, and honey, for 40 days. In children the dose can be halved.

Use   It helps in all types of weakness and diseases in the body, particularly tuberculosis, AIDS, in low constant fever, liver and spleen enlargement. For weak eyesight, red eyes, and eye infection, use one pill twice daily with butter and sugar. In mental weakness, and in chronic fevers, use one pill twice daily with cold milk. In respiratory problems one pill twice daily with a teaspoon of honey and 250 mg of long pepper powder is used. For stimulating the neuromuscular system, one pill with cumin and sugar, or *Emblica* preserve, or with pomegranate juice sweetened with milk is given. For nocturnal emission, the dose is one pill twice daily, with half a spoon of honey and one spoon of butter, while other sexual inadequacies are treated with one pill twice daily with 1–2 spoons of honey in cold milk for 40 days. This preparation gives a permanent cure and can be used in any weather, by any person of any age. It is a general tonic for women with various gynaecological problems such as leucorrhoea, dysmenorrhoea, weakness due to pregnancy, etc. In leucorrhoea one pill twice daily with rice gruel for forty days is required. For proper nutrition of the foetus of expectant mothers, one pill twice daily with honey in milk, or butter and sugar should be taken.

Precautions   Sour things such as tamarind, unripe mango, and hot food such as spices, red pepper, non-vegetarian and fried items are prohibited.

Suvarna Vasant Malti

Ayurvedic name	English name	Processing	Quantity
Suvarn vark	Gold	Foil	10 g
Mukta pishti	Pearl	Paste	10 g
Ras Sindur	Red sulphide of mercury	Processed	10 g
Yashad Bhasam	Zinc	Processed	10 g
Tamar Bhasam	Copper	Processed	10 g
Mirch kali	Black pepper	Powder	10 g

Method   Make a fine powder of the minerals, mix black pepper powder, and triturate with gold foils and pearl paste until a homogenous mixture is formed. Make pills of 32 g each.

Use   1–2 pills for impotence due to chronic fevers.

Swapanmehntak

Ayurvedic name	Botanical/English name	Plant part/processing	Quantity
Vang Bhasam	Tin	Processed	25 g
Arishtak majja	Sapindus mukrosii	Kernel powder	50 g
Mishri	Sugar candy	Bold crystals	50 g

Method   Triturate the three ingredients, moisten and make pills of 350 mg each.

Dose   3–6 pills with water

Use   In diabetes, loss of spermatic fluid, spermatorrhoea, for increasing retention power of seminal discharge, and in wasting diseases. In involuntary nocturnal emission take two pills three times a day with water, do not eat in the evening.

Vasant Kusmakar Ras

Ayurvedic name	Botanical/English name	Plant part/processing	Quantity
Parval Pishti	Coral	Paste	40 g
Mukta Pishti	Pearl	Paste	40 g
Ras Sindur	Red sulphide of mercury	Processed	40 g
Abhrak Bhasam	Mica	Processed	40 g
Suvarn Bhasam	Gold	Processed	10 g
Rajat Bhasam	Silver	Processed	10 g
Lauha Bhasam	Iron	Processed	30 g
Vang Vark	Tin foils	Processed	30 g
Amber	Ambergris	Aromatic resin	30 g
Kasturi	Musk	Aromatic resin	20 g
Keshar	Saffron	Stigma and style	20 g
Vasaka Ras	Adhatoda vasica	Decoction, flower top	As required
Haldi Kwath	Turmeric	Decoction	As required
Gana Ras	Sugar cane	Juice	As required
Shatawari Ras	Asparagus spp.	Juice of root	As required
Kadli Ras	Banana (wild)	Juice of stem	As required
Chandan Kwath	Sandal	Decoction of wood	As required
Kamal Kwath	Lotus	Decoction of flower	As required

Method   Triturate all the inorganic materials in powder form, with juice/decoction of each of the herb, as per formulation one by one (*Adhatoda*, followed by decoction of turmeric sugar cane juice, lotus flower juice, *Asparagus* juice, banana stem juice, and finally decoction of sandalwood) for 3–6 hours in sufficient quantity for free movement of the mass in a pestle and mortar. Triturate further for 3 hours with musk and ambergris, and make pills of 125 mg each.

Dose   1/2 to 1 pill twice daily with milk fat or butter and sugar.

Use   It is a geriatric and sexual tonic used for rejuvenation. It gives energy to all the body systems, but is particularly useful for the brain, heart, lungs, alimentary canal, and the sexual organs. In diabetes, one pill twice daily is said to reduce sugar both from urine and blood. As a mental tonic, make a decoction of half a teaspoon each of cinnamon, cinnamon leaves and cardamom, and boil them in 200 ml water. Take one pill daily with this decoction. In haemorrhage or bleeding from any part of the body, take half a pill with sugar/honey. For male sexual inadequacy take one pill before sleep or early in the morning. In acute cases, one pill twice daily with milk may be taken. For gynaecological problems make a paste of coral, take 5 g of this paste, mix it in 2 g *Vasant Kusmakar Ras* and make 24 doses from this mixture. Take one dose twice daily with milk.

Visha *Rasayana*

Ayurvedic name	Botanical/English name	Plant part/processing	Quantity
Vatsnabh (shodhit)	Aconite	Mitigated	12 g
Ras Sindur	Red sulphide of mercury	Processed	25 g
Parad Bhasam	Mercury	Processed	12 g
Rajat Bhasam	Silver	Processed	12 g
Tamar Bhasam	Copper in mercury and sulphur	Compound Preparation	50 g
Sonth	Ginger (dry)	Powder	50 g
Peepali	Long pepper	Powder	50 g
Mirch Kali	Black pepper	Powder	50 g
Dalchini	Cinnamon	Powder	50 g
Tejpat	Cinnamomum spp.	Powder leaves	50 g
Nag Kesar	Mesua ferrea	Powder flower	50 g
Chitrak	Plumbago zeylanica	Powder root	50 g

Method Macerate all the items and make pills of 250 mg each by adding a binder.

Dose 1–2 pills.

Use This *Rasayana* gives strength and imparts immunity. It increases *internal fire* of the body, which activates liver, spleen and thus digestion. It is useful for the amorous person with multiple partners. For longevity, it should be used for two months.

Vrahida Vangashwar Rasa

Ayurvedic name	Botanical/English name	Plant part/processing	Quantity
Vang Bhasam	Tin	Processed	12 g
Parad Bhasam	Mercury	Processed	12 g
Abhrak Bhasam	Mica	Processed	12 g
Gandhak Shodhit	Sulphur	Purified	12 g
Suvarna Bhasam	Gold	Processed	3 g
Rajat Bhasam	Silver	Processed	12 g
Mukta Pishti	Pearl	Paste with water	3 g
Mushkafoor	Camphor	Crystals	12 g
Bhringraja	Eclipta alba	Juice	As required

Method   Mix mercury and sulphur, and other items in the juice of *Eclipta alba*, triturate and make pills of 125 mg each.

Dose   1–2 pills twice daily with goat's milk or yogurt.

Use   It helps in all types of chronic diabetes, and urinogenital problems. It compensates loss in the body from to excessive amorous activities.

PRODUCTS WITH TRADE NAMES

The trade name of the product along with the name of manufacturer in brackets, brief indications and detail about the ingredient is given in each case. In the labels/brochures of these products, some manufacturers gave Ayurvedic names, while others used botanical names, still other mentioned both names. Plant part is usually not mentioned. In many cases it was not clear whether the herb was used or a particular type of extract was incorporated in the formulations. In these cases whatever information was available has been given.

1-Top (Pentovax)

For rejuvenation and virility

Ayurvedic name	Botanical/English name	Part used	Quantity
Keshar	*Crocus sativus*	Style	15 mg
Akarkara	*Anacyclus pyrethrum*	Root	15 mg
Shankhpushpi	*Canscora decussata*	Herb	15 mg
Jatamansi	*Nardostachys jatamansi*	Root	15 mg
Malkangani	*Celastrus paniculatus*	Seed	15 mg
Jaiphal	Nutmeg	Seed	20 mg
Peepali	Long pepper	Fruiting spike	20 mg
Sonth	Ginger	Root	20 mg
Dalchini	Cinnamon	Bark	20 mg
Pan	*Piper betle*	Leaves	20 mg
Talamkhana	*Hygrophila spinosa*	Seed	40 mg
Lata kasturi	*Hibiscus abelomoschus*	Seed	40 mg
Ashwgandha	*Withania somnifera*	Root	40 mg
Satavar	*Asparagus racemosus*	Root	40 mg
Mundi	*Spharenthus indicus*	Flowers	40 mg
Kuth	*Saussurea lappa*	Root	40 mg
Jaiphal	Nutmeg	Seed	40 mg
Salam mishri	*Orchis mascula*	Root	40 mg
Khas	*Vetiveria zizanoides*	Root	40 mg
Lawang	Clove	Buds	80 mg

Ashree Forte (Aimil pharmacy)

Increases sexual activity, libido

Ayurvedic name	Botanical/English name	Part used	Quantity
Makardhawaj	Red sulphide of mercury with gold	–	20 mg
Kesar	Saffron	Style	20 mg
Jaiphal	Nutmeg	Seed	20 mg
Javitri	Mace	Aril	20 mg
Shilajit	Bituminous compound	–	20 mg
Swarn Vang	Processed tin	–	10 mg
Gaduchi satva	Tinospora cordifolia	Starch	20 mg
Trivang Bhasam	Processed lead, tin and zinc	–	10 mg
Gokshuru ghansatva	Tribulus terrestris	Seed Extract	20 mg
Kaunch (processed)	Mucuna pruriens	Seed	150 mg
Ashwgandha	Withania somnifera	Root	30 mg
Shatawar	Asparagus racemosus	Root	30 mg
Safed Musli	Chlorophytum arundinaceum	Root	20 mg
Bhilwa	Semecarpus anacardium	Seed	30 mg
Til	Sesame seed	Extract	20 mg
Varahi kand	Dioscorea bulbifera	Root	20 mg
Tejpatar	Cinnamomum iners	Leaf	15 mg
Dalchini	Cinnamon	Bark	15 mg
Dhtura beej (processed)	Datura spp.	Seed	10 mg
Kuchla (processed)	Nux vomica	Seed	10 mg
Akarkara	Anacyclus pyrethrum	Root	10 mg

Brento (Zandu)

A general nerve tonic

Ayurvedic name	Botanical/English name	Part used	Quantity
Shankhpushpi	Convolvulus microphyllus	Whole herb	100 mg
Mandukparni	Centella asiatica	Whole herb	100 mg
Ashwgandha	Withania somnifera	Root	100 mg
Mulathi	Glycyrrhiza glabra	Root	100 mg
Kuth	Saussurea lappa	Root	50 mg
Vacha	Acorus calamus	Root	25 mg
Serpgandha	Rauvolfia serpentina	Root	25 mg
Jatiphala	Myristica fragrans	Fruit	5 mg
Chanderody Ras	A preparation of red sulphide of mercury	–	5 mg

Fortege (Alarsin)

Aphrodisiac

Ayurvedic name	Botanical/English name	Part used	Quantity
Kamboji	Adenanthera pavonina	Seed	60 mg
Kawanch	Mucuna pruriens	Seed	30 mg
Kuchula	Nux vomica (processed)	Seed	30 mg
Samundra sosh	Salvia plebia	Seed	15 mg
Vardhara	Argyreia speciosa	Seed	15 mg
Vardhara	Argyreia speciosa	Root	15 mg
Asar	Calotropis gigantea	Root bark	15 mg
Lavang	Clove	Bud	7.5 mg
Piper	Long pepper	Fruit	7.5 mg
Vacha	Calamus	Root	7.5 mg
Marich	Black pepper	Fruit	7.5 mg
Sunthi	Ginger	Root	7.5 mg
Chini Kabab	Piper cubeba	Fruit	7.5 mg
Akarkara	Anacyclus pyrethrum	Root	7.5 mg
Sukhad	Santalum album	Wood	7.5 mg
Jaifal	Nutmeg	Fruit	4.5 mg
Javitri	Mace	Fruit	3.00 mg
Jeevanti	Leptadenia reticulata	Root	56.5 mg

Imminex (Hind Chemicals)

Immunomodulater

Ayurvedic name	Botanical name	Plant part/process	Quantity
Kutaj	Holarrhena antidysentrica	Bark	50 mg
Kutaki	Picrorhiza kurroa	Rhizome	50 mg
Chirayta	Swertia chirata	Herb	25 mg

Jaryan (Yogi Pharmacy)

For sexual disorders and disability

Ayurvedic name	Botanical/English name	Part used	Quantity
Salam Mishri	Orchis mascula	Root	33 mg
Safed musli	Asparagus adscendens	Root	33 mg
Kikar gond	Gum arabica	Gum	33 mg
Shital chini	Piper cubeba	Fruit	33 mg
Chobchini	Smilax glabra	Root	33 mg
Vang Bhasam	Tin processed	Root	33 mg
Jawahar Bhasam	Precious stones, processed	Root	33 mg
Luban	Styrax benzoin	Gum	33 mg
Gond Katira	Cochlospermum religiosum	Gum	66 mg

Mast (Herba Indica)

For powerful, consistent, and focused performance

Ayurvedic name	Botanical name	Part used	Quantity
Kwanch	Mucuna pruriens	Seed processed in milk	250 mg
Gokshru	Tribulus terrestris	Seed water extract	150 mg

Mentat (Himalaya Drug)

Activates the mind

Ayurvedic name	Botanical/English name	Part used	Quantity
Brahmi	Bacopa monnieri	Herb Extract	136 mg
Mandukparni	Centella asiatica	Herb Extract	70 mg
Ashwgandha	Withania somnifera	Root Extract	52 mg
Shankhpushpi	Evolvulus alsinoides	Herb Extract	52 mg
Jatamansi	Nardostachys jatamansi	Root Extract	52 mg
Tagar	Valeriana wallichii	Root Extract	50 mg
Babading	Embelia ribes	Seed Extract	50 mg
Badam	Almond	Seed	50 mg
Haritaki	Terminalia chebula	Fruit Extract	36 mg
Amalaki	Emblica officinalis	Fruit Extract	36 mg
Gaduchi	Tinospora cordifolia	Herb Extract	36 mg
Malakangni	Celastrus paniculatus	Seed Extract	32 mg
Shoyanaka	Oroxylum indicum	Bark Extract	32 mg
Brahmi	Bacopa monnieri	Herb Powder	80 mg
Kawanch	Mucuna pruriens	Seed Powder	18 mg
Ela	Elettaria cardamomum	Seed Powder	18 mg
Arjun	Terminalia arjuna	Bark Powder	18 mg
Saunf	Fennel	Seed Powder	18 mg
Salab mishri	Orchis mascula	Root Powder	18 mg
Sunth	Ginger	Root Powder	14 mg
Vibhitaki	Terminalia bellirica	Fruit Powder	14 mg
Jaiphal	Nutmeg	Fruit Powder	14 mg
Laung	Clove	Bud Powder	10 mg
Mukta pishti	Pearl	Paste	3 mg

Mucuna Forte (Deesons)

Aphrodisiac

Ayurvedic name	Botanical/English name	Part used	Quantity
Ashwgandha	Withania somnifera	Root	80 mg
Vidhara	Argyreia nervosa	Root	5 mg
Kawanch	Mucuna pruriens	Seed (processed)	30 mg
Akarkara	Anacyclus pyrethrum	Root	20 mg
Bala beej	Sida cordifolia	Seed	25 mg
Kuchla shodhit	Strychnos nux vomica	Seed (processed)	10 mg
Salab panja	Eulophia campestris	Root	10 mg
Makardhawaj	Red sulphide of mercury with gold	–	10 mg
Jaiphal	Myristica fragrans	Fruit	10 mg
Shilajit	Bituminous material	Paste	20 mg
Jund Bedaster	Castoreum	Oleo-resin	20 mg
Keshar	Saffron	Style and stigma	4 mg

Processed in the decoction of *Piper betle*, onion, *Withania* and *Asparagus*.
Precaution: Do not use in cardiac diseases, hypertension and bleeding piles.

Power Pills (Gambers Lab.)

For instant sexual vigour

Ayurvedic name	Botanical/English name	Part used	Quantity
Khurasani Ajwain	Hyoscyamus niger	Seed	45 mg
Makardhawaj	Red sulphide of mercury with gold	–	22 mg
Akrakara	Anacyclus pyrethrum	Root	15 mg
Jaiphal	Nutmeg	Fruit	15 mg
Javitri	Mace	Aril	7 mg
Lawang	Clove	Buds	7 mg
Ashwgandha	Withania somnifera	Root	7 mg
Kesar	Saffron	Styles	7 mg
Amber	Ambergris	Resin	7 mg

Ravin (Malabar Chemicals)

For retention power in sexual happiness

Ayurvedic name	Botanical/English name	Part used	Quantity
Talamkhana	Hygrophila spinosa	Seed	25 mg
Gokshru	Tribulus terrestris	Seed	25 mg
Kawanch	Mucuna pruriens	Seed (processed)	25 mg
Shatawari	Asparagus racemosus	Root	25 mg
Salam Musali	Bombax malabaricum	Young root	25 mg
Jaiphal	Myristica fragrans	Fruit	25 mg
Suvaran Bhasam	Gold (Processed)	–	25 mg

Spy (Yogi Pharmacy)

Sex tonic

Ayurvedic name	Botanical/English name	Part used	Quantity
Sarpgandha	Rauvolfia serpentina	Root	22.5 mg
Kuchla (shodhit)	Strychnos nux vomica	Seed (processed)	22.5 mg
Salam Mishri	Orchis mascula	Root	33.0 mg
Jaiphal	Nutmeg	Fruit	25.5 mg
Javitri	Mace	Aril on seed	25.5 mg
Akrakara	Anacyclus pyrethrum	Root	25.5 mg
Shilajit	Bitumen material	Paste	25.5 mg
Makardhawaj	Red sulphide of mercury with gold	–	16.5 mg
Trinkantmani gum	Azima tetracantha?	Gum	16.5 mg
Vang Bhasam	Tin	Processed	16.5 mg
Kesar	Saffron	Styles	16.5 mg
Amber	Ambergris	Oleoresin	16.5 mg
Mukta pishti	Pearl pulverized	Paste	6.6 mg
Jund Badastar	Castoreum	Oleoresin	6.6 mg
Kadali ras	Banana stem	Juice	13.2 mg

Processed in the decoction and fresh juice of *Pueraria tuberosa*, *Withania somnifera*, *Asparagus racemosus*, *Aloe barbadensis*, *Curcuma longa* and *Cannabis sativa*.

Strenex (Zandu)

Vitality aid. tones health

Ayurvedic name	Botanical/English name	Part used	Quantity
Ashwgandha	Withania somnifera	Root	100 mg
Kawanch	Mucuna pruriens	Seed (processed)	150 mg
Chandrodya Ras	Red sulphide of mercury	–	100 mg
Manikya Bhasam	Ruby	Processed	100 mg
Mukta Pishti	Pearl	Paste	100 mg
Abhrak Bhasam	Mica	Processed	50 mg
Shilajit	Bituminous compound	Paste	50 mg
Kuchla (mitigated)	Strychnos nux-vomica	Seed (processed)	25 mg
Kantloha	Wrought iron	Processed	20 mg
Jaiphal	Nutmeg	Seed Powder	20 mg
Mankiya Ras	Arsenic	Processed	10 mg
Bhimseni kapoor	Borneol	Crystals	5 mg
Amber	Ambergris	Resin	5 mg

Tentex forte (Himalaya Drug)

Sex stimulant for men

Ayurvedic name	Botanical/English name	Part used	Quantity
Lata Kasturi	Ablemoschus moschatus	Seed Extract	10 mg
Ashwgandha	Withania somnifera	Root	65 mg
Vidhara	Argyreia nervosa	Seed	32 mg
Kawanch	Mucuna pruriens	Seed (processed)	32 mg
Trivanga bhasam	Processed lead, tin and zinc	–	32 mg
Shilajit	Bituminous compound	–	32 mg
Kesar	Saffron	Styles and Stigma	25 mg
Kuchla Shodhit	Nux vomica	Seed (processed)	16 mg
Makardhawaj	Red sulphide of mercury (gold)	–	16 mg
Salam mishri	Orchis mascula	Root	16 mg
Akrakara	Anacyclus pyrethrum	Root	16 mg
Bala	Sida cordifolia	Seed	16 mg
Semal Musli	Salmalia malabarica	Root	16 mg
Kali Mirch	Black pepper	Seed	5 mg

Processed in the juice of *Sida, Asparagus, Ipomoea digitata, Piper betle, Withania, Tribulus, Tinospora, Argyreia, Acacia arabica* and *Dashmool* (ten roots).

Trasina (Dey's Medical Stores)

Antistress immunomodulater

Ayurvedic name	Botanical/English name	Part used	Quantity
Ashwgandha	Withania somnifera	Root Extract	90 mg
Tulsi	Ocimum sanctum	Leaf Extract	190 mg
Shilajit	Bituminous mineral	Paste	20 mg
Gaduchi	Tinospora cordifolia	Herb Extract	10 mg
Kutaki	Picrorhiza kurroa	Root Extract	10 mg
Bhringraja	Eclipta alba	Root Extract	10 mg

Vitox (Maxo Lab.)

General sex tonic

Ayurvedic name	Botanical name	Part used	Quantity
Vidarikand	Ipomaea paniculata	Root	60 mg
Safed musli	Asparagus adscendens	Root	60 mg
Shatawari	A. racemosus	Root	60 mg
Gokshru	Tribulus terrestris	Fruit	60 mg
Ashwgandha	Withania somnifera	Root	60 mg
Kawanch	Mucuna pruriens	Seed (processed)	25 mg
Salam Panja	Orchis latifolia	Root	25 mg
Nakchikni	Centipeda orbicularis	Seed	25 mg
Akrakara	Anacyclus pyrethrum	Root	15 mg
Agar	Aquilaria agallocha	Heart wood	15 mg
Jaiphal	Myristica fragrans	Fruit	15 mg
Lata Kasturi	Abelomoschus moschatus	Seed	5 mg

Vysex (Ban Pharm)

Rejuvenator, increases virility

Ayurvedic name	Botanical/English name	Part used	Quantity
Ashwgandha	Withania somnifera	Root	80 mg extract
Kavanch	Mucuna pruriens	Seed (processed)	80 mg extract
Silajit	Bituminous matter	Paste	10 mg
Bala beej	Sida cordifolia	Seed	40 mg extract
Kesar	Saffron	Styles and stigma	0.5 mg
Vishtinduk	Nux vomica	Seed (processed)	15 mg
Akarakara	Anacyclus pyrethrum	Root	40 mg
Makardhawaj	Red sulphide of mercury with gold	–	10 mg
Jundebastoor	Castoreum	Resin	4.5 mg
Rasa Sindur	Red sulphide of mercury	–	10 mg

Reference

Tripathi, J.S., Singh, R.H. (1995) Clinical evaluation of Smritisagar Rasa in cases of residual schizophrenia. *Seminar on Research in Ayurveda and Siddha, CCRAS*, New Delhi. P.35, 20–22 March 1995.

Index

1-Top 329
2.12-dimethylbenz anthracene (DMBA) 278
3-o-alpha-L-rhamnoside 293
5-hydroxytryptamine 253
5-lipoxygenase 239

α-amyrin 178
aachar 2
aak 16–18
aak phul 314
abdominal sepsis 111
Abe Resham 314
Abelomoschus moschatus 335
aberrant cells 278
abhrak 317, 321, 323, 334
Abhrak Bhasam 313, 316, 318, 319, 321, 324
abhya 37, 135
Abies 265, 324
abortion 31, 80, 325
Abroma augusta 248
Abrus precatorius 159, 177, 213
Abutilon 64
Abutilon indicum 64, 66, 68, 69
Acacia 29, 173
Acacia arabica 170, 335
Acacia auriculiformis 205
Acacia catechu 107, 313, 319
Acacia nilotica 107, 109, 170, 275
Acacia senegal 174
Acanthaceae 151, 270
acetaminophen 82, 153
acetic acid 14
acetylated oil 77
acetylcholine 37, 50, 95, 178, 203, 252, 253
acharasayana 23
achene 190
acidic *ras* 10
acidic urination 36
acne vulgaris 27, 131
aconite 295–298, 313, 328
aconitine 30, 298
Aconitum balfourii 295
Aconitum deinorrhizum 295
Aconitum falconeri 295
Aconitum ferox 295

Aconitum heterophyllum 30, 100, 109, 128, 221, 318
Aconitum laciniatum 295
Aconitum napellus 295, 298
Aconitum spicatum 295
Aconitum spp. 295, 313
Acorus calamus 31, 202, 252, 253, 257, 281–287, 330, 331
adaptogen 48, 53
adaptogenic 37, 53, 205, 214, 277
Adenanthera pavoniana 331
adenomas 52
adenosine triphosphatase 230
Adhatoda 126, 257, 266
Adhatoda vasica 30, 37, 109, 322
adjuvant-induced arthritis 78
adrak 265, 320
adrak Ras 315
adrenal gland 52, 187, 235, 277, 307
adrenaline 145, 191, 193, 234
adrenergic 88, 121
adrenergic beta blocking 233
adrenocortical 37, 51, 53
Adriamycin 77
adusa 37
Aegle marmelos 34, 38
AFB1 toxicity 224
Afghanistan 59, 135, 136, 141
aflatoxin 167
Aganimantha 37
Aganosma dichotoma 314
agar 14, 313, 335
agaru 37
agate 314
aggressiveness 285
agni 4, 99
ahara 1, 3
AIDS 3, 326
Aimil Pharm 330
ajwain 318
akrakara 20, 21, 329–331, 333–335
Akrakaradi Vati 21
alantolactone 235
Alarsin 331
albumin 37, 229, 330
alcoholism 3, 307

aldose reductase 90
Algeria 20
Allium macleani 242
allopathic tonic 260
almond 75, 173, 245, 274, 305, 332; nut cream 60; oil 60
Aloe 127, 222, 313, 319
Aloe barbadensis 334
Aloe extract 127
alpha galactosidase activity 253
alpha-2-macroglobulin 54
Alpinia 161
Alpinia galanga 31, 180–182
Alpinia officinarum 180
Alstonia scholaris 109
alterative 46
Alternaria alternata 90
alui 151
alum 29, 149
Alzheimer's disease 53, 72
ama 4, 99, 126, 272, 321
amalaki 6, 10, 22–39, 67, 86, 107, 258, 301, 313, 324, 332
amalaki ras 315
Amalaki Rasayana 25, 32
Amanita 263
Amanita muscaria 262
Amanitaceae 262
Amaranthus polygamous 75
Amaryllidaceae 212
amavata 126
amber 333, 334
ambergris 312, 314, 333, 334
amenorrhoea 275
America 262
American Sarsaparilla 43
amla 23–39
amla juice 32
Amomum subulatum 38, 151, 259
amphetamine 34, 144, 203
Amrit Rasayana 313
Amrita 37, 107, 135
Amrita Bhallatak 77
Amritadi kwath 109
Amritarishat 109
Amrutadiguggulu 111
amygdalin 60
amygdaloid kindling 51

Amygdalus communis L. var. *dulce* 59
amyrin 178
anabolic 120, 182, 224, 268, 317;
    activity 53, 161; agent 25, 48,
    51, 173, 230; effect 204; steroids
    37
Anacamptis 242
Anacardiaceae 74
Anacyclus 245, 167
Anacyclus officinarum 20
Anacyclus pyrethrum 16, 20, 159,
    265, 329–331, 333–335
anaesthesia 52
analeptic 224
analgesia 52, 53
analgesic 31, 48, 60, 69, 111, 161,
    200, 203, 222, 239, 276, 299
anantmul 43
anaphrodisiac 278
anar 324
Andamans islands 196
androgenic activity 160
Andrographis paniculata 151, 186
andrographolide 152–154, 186
angina 2, 192, 316
angina pectoris 121, 234, 305,
    306
angioplasty 154
angiotensin 89
ankylosing spondylitis 239
ankylostomiasis 77, 216
anodyne 165, 297
anorexia 162
anorexia nervosa 160
anthelmintic 31, 131, 151, 160,
    170, 216, 221, 233, 267, 282,
    286
anthraquinones 306
anthropometric 7
anti-*ama* 265
anti-*vata* 265, 144
antiageing effect 54, 161
antiallergic 152, 233
antiamoebic 224
antianginal 131
antianxiety 52, 96, 253
antiarterosclerotic 198
antiarthritic 77
antiasthmatic 235, 301
antiatherogenic 27
antiatherosclerotic 28, 100
antibacterial 69, 72, 294
antibiotics 8
antibody 26
anticancerous 18, 51, 111, 167,
    187, 205, 223, 278
anticancerous activity 96
anticancerous property 223
anticarcinogens 181
anticholestatic activity 186
anticomplementary 186, 239
anticonvulsant 198, 224, 252
antidepolarizing agent 306
antidepressant 161, 253, 325

antidiabetic 31, 89, 193, 217, 293,
    300
antidiarrhoeal 26, 146, 293
antidipsotropic 307
antidote 166, 272
antidysentric 237
antiemetic 25, 268
antiendotoxic 112
antiepileptic 51, 253, 285
antifertility 101
antifever 184
antifilarial 205, 216, 267
antifungal 26, 90, 267, 299
antigastric 178
antigastroduodenal ulcer effect 293
antigiardial 224
antihemorrhagic 82, 278
antihepatotoxic 4, 60, 69, 80, 82,
    84, 153, 182, 224, 230
antihypertensive activity 83
antiinflammatory 29, 31, 54, 60,
    66, 77, 105, 110, 111, 127, 146,
    153, 186, 192, 205, 209, 212,
    214, 217, 267
antiinflammatory agent 8, 53, 80,
    83, 130
anti-*kaph* 144, 219
antileprotic 170, 215
antimalarial 299
antimicrobial 26, 83, 139, 180,
    187, 192, 217, 224, 235, 267,
    322
antimutagenic 26, 106, 139
antineoplastic 52, 278
antinociceptive 90
antioxidant 26, 30, 54, 90, 96,
    112, 167, 187, 267, 278, 293,
    307
antioxytocin 259
anti-PCA 152
antiperiodic 274, 297
antiplatelet 154, 267
antiprogestational 101
antipyretic 31, 111, 161, 198, 237,
    277, 297, 299, 322
antiscretagogue 286
antisecretory 181
antiserotonergic 51
antispasmodic 16, 51, 90, 138,
    143, 235, 285, 301, 306
antistress 52, 54, 112, 274, 277,
    335
antithrombogenic 154
anti-*tridosha* 125
antitubercular 37
antitumour 45, 77, 168, 181, 192,
    211, 217, 259, 268, 271, 294
antitussive 301
antiulcer 153, 178, 181, 187, 193,
    210, 224, 267
antiulcerogenic effect 53, 110, 153,
    217, 253, 277
antiurolithic 120
antivenomous effect 83

antiviral 83, 89, 186, 267
anxiety 52, 53
anxiety neurosis 52, 96, 203, 250,
    252
anxiolytic 96, 204
aphrodisiac 14, 16, 36, 46, 60, 66,
    82, 103, 116, 122, 126, 143,
    147, 148, 158, 159, 161, 166,
    180, 182, 193, 196, 212, 242,
    244, 247, 258, 265, 270, 274,
    297–299, 309, 322, 323
apigenin 153
Aplotaxis auriculata 190
Apomorphine 276
apoptosis 205
appetite suppressant 193
appetizer 184
apricot oil 60
aqua 13
Aqua Mundi 210
aquamarine 320
Aquillaria agallocha 14, 37, 67,
    313, 335
Araceae 281
Areca catechu 319
areca nut 222
arginine 60
Argyreia 48, 159, 167, 317, 318,
    335
Argyreia nervosa 309–310, 333, 335
Argyreia speciosa 309, 49, 50, 331
Arishta 13, 14, 105, 215
arishtak majja 327
arjun 332
aromatic lichens 67
Arq Mundi 210
arrhythmia 298
arrow root 177
arsenic 325, 328, 334
arterial stenosis 154
arterial thrombotic diseases 154
arterial wall 72
arthritis 29, 50, 53, 54, 60, 74, 80,
    110, 127, 167, 217, 267
arthropathies 48
Aryans 1, 2, 262
asafoetida 31, 128, 141–143, 283,
    291
asar 331
asarledehyde 286
asarone 281, 285–287
asav 13, 14, 105
ascites 181, 229
Asclepiadaceae 16, 43, 262
ascorbic acid 52
asgand see asgandh
Asgandh 47, 50, 51
Asgandh Nagori 46, 48
Asgandh pak 50
Ashree Forte 330
Ashtavarga 33, 34, 37, 67
ashwa 46
ashwagandha 8, 23, 50, 60, 309,
    319, 329, 330, 332–335

Ashwagandha Rasayana 54
Ashwagandhadi Churn 49, 309
Ashwagandhadi Ghrit 49
Ashwini Kumars 33
asiaticoside 205, 206
asiatic acid 205
asparagines 60, 69
Asparagus 49, 67, 98, 159, 178, 244, 245, 248, 252, 265, 307, 309, 315–319, 323, 335
Asparagus adscendens 33, 214, 255, 331, 335
Asparagus falcats 259
Asparagus filicinus 214, 255
Asparagus gonoclados 214, 255
Asparagus officinalis 255
Asparagus racemosus 29, 33, 38, 50, 119, 139, 213, 255–260, 313, 315, 322, 330, 333–335
Asparagus sarmentosus 255
aspartate transminase 307
aspartic acid 60
aspirin 34, 53, 153, 267
Asteraceae 190, 209, 233
Astercantha 259
Astercantha longifolia 119, 270, 319
asthma 221, 274, 301
asthmatic cigarette 191
astringent 10, 170, 237, 299
astringent ras 10
astverga 258
atherogenesis 198
atheroma 77
atheromatous plaques 198
atherosclerosis 71, 72, 182
Atherveda 125
atibala 64–66, 316
ativisha 318
ATPase 230
augmentative 270
aushidhis 1
avleh 14, 33
axillary raceme 237
ayuh 1
Ayurvedic materia medica 1
Ayurvedic Pharmacopoeia 35
Azadirachta 109, 125
Azadirachta indica 29, 94, 107, 109, 215–218
Azima tetracantha? 334
azoospermia 48

β-adrenergic receptors 96
babading 332
Baby Rosewood 309
Bacopa 94–96, 204, 252, 283
Bacopa monnieri 94, 332
bacosides 96
bacosine 96
bactereolytic enzyme 18
Bacteriosides fusobacteria 193
badam 59–62, 332
badshah 242
bahera 299

bal haritaki 135
bal vacha 281
bala 38, 64–70, 204, 317, 318, 335
bala 4
bala beej 333
Bala oil 67
Bala Phanjivika 65
Balachaturya 66
Baladighrit 68
Baladivya 66
Balapanchak 66
Balatriya 66
Balayadighrit 66
Baliospermum montanum 31, 229
Balsamodendron roxburghii 124
Baluchistan 59
balyi 135
bamboo concretion 38
bamboo manna 31, 33, 50, 67, 106, 117, 149, 159, 245, 266
Bambusa arundinacea 71
banana stem 334
Banar 159
Banar gutika 159
Bandhani Hing 143
Banslochan 38, 71, 72
Banya 289
banyan tree 289
barbiturate 276
barbiturate hypnosis 50, 95, 203, 252
barbiturate potentiation 50, 96
hari peepal 219
barley 67
basil leaves 202
basil, holy or sacred 272
Basra (Iraq) 102
Basti 5
baya 11
bee pollen 309
Beejband 66
Belladonna 297
Bengal 151
Benincasa hispida 325
benzodiazepine 96, 306
benzoin 196
berberine 109, 110, 113
Berberis 31, 109, 322, 324
Berberis extract 127
Bergenia ligulata 120, 322
beta-endorphin 223
betain 72
bhalatak 74–78
Bhalatak Rasayana 76, 77
Bhaltakadi Modka 77
bhang 317, 318
bhang beej 316
bhangra 80
bharati 94
bhasam 14, 312, 320–323, 325, 327, 328
Bhavamisra 33
Bhavaprakasa Nighantu 33
Bhavprakasha 1

Bhela ka mela 74
bhilwa 330
Bhimseni kapoor 322, 334
Bhisk priya 135
bhringraja 80, 315, 335
bhuiamalaki 38, 86
bhuiamla 86–90
bhumibala 66
bidhara beej asli 309
bifidobacteria 193
Biju 22
bikh 295
bikhaconitine 298
bile 267, 268; acids 130, 187, 293
bilva 38
biochemical 7
bios 11
bipinnate 170
bishaconitine 298
bishatisine 298
bitter almonds 59
bitter glucosides 186
bitter gourd 24
bitter ras 10
bituminous: compound 321, 323, 330, 333–335; material 333, 334; mineral 335
black bean 60
black grape 30, 67, 106, 221
Black oil 196
black salt 15, 30, 275
black sulphide of mercury 320
Blepharis edulis 159
blood cell, total count 52
blood: cleansers 4; coagulation 167; glucose levels 193; pressure 2, 214; purifier 29, 109, 170, 209, 215; urea 204, 293
blue flag 281
blue sapphire 314
Boerhaavia 67, 229
Boerhaavia diffusa 39, 227, 313
Boerhaavia repanda 227, 230
Boerhaavia verticillata 277
Bombacaceae 247
Bombax 213
Bombax ceiba L. 247
Bombax malabaricum 173, 247, 323, 333
bone marrow 26, 112, 186; cellularity 7, 52, 204; radio protection 278; radio sensitivity 278
borax 178, 315, 323, 324
Borneo 147
borneol 322, 334
Boswellia 54, 237–240
Boswellia carteri 237
Boswellia erecta 227, 237
boswellic acid 239
bradycardia 51
Brahma Rasayana 7, 204, 313
brahmi 94–96, 332
Brahmi ghrit 200, 202

Brahmi rasayana 96, 205
brahmic acid 206
brahmine 95, 96
brahminoside 205
brahmoside 205
brain stroke 3
brain tonic 274
branchiospasm 112, 235
Brazil 144
breathlessness 316
Brento 330
Brhati 38
Bright's disease 116
bromelain 18
bronchial asthma 18, 224, 274, 286
bronchial problems 171, 191, 219, 229, 265
bronchodilator 105, 192, 233, 301
bronchiospasm 223
bronchitis 126, 147, 149, 274
brucine 178
Brufen 53
Buchanania latifolia 245
buchu 116
budhi 2
Budhism 135
burning micturition 18, 44
burning urination 177
Burseraceae 124, 130, 237
Butea 29, 32, 224, 266
Butea frondosa 118, 172, 213, 319
buttressed trunk 247

cadmium 54
cadmium chloride 54
caecal amoebiasis 224
caecal ligation 111
calactin 18
Calamus 18, 128, 159, 201, 203, 229, 266, 281–287
calcium magnesium imbalance 72
calculus affection 116
Calendula 164
California (USA) 59
Callicarpa macrophylla 31, 159, 168, 222
calotoxin 18
calotrop fruit 116
calotropin 18
Calotropis 16, 134
Calotropis gigantea 16, 18, 331
Calotropis procera 16, 18
camphor 159, 166, 182, 284, 316–318
camphoraceous 233
cancer 3, 273; therapy 52
Candida albicans 217, 299
cannabinomimetic 285
Cannabis 1, 60, 262, 285, 316–318
Cannabis sativa 334
carbon tetrachloride 17, 54, 82, 84, 88, 153, 185, 186, 307
carboxylated tryptamine 69
carcinogen 52, 111, 187, 260

carcinogenesis 7
cardamom 35, 49, 50, 71, 60, 105, 106, 149, 159, 173, 222, 224, 265, 274, 275, 276, 317, 322, 323, 324
cardiac failure 234
cardiac glycogen 27
cardiac glycoside 139, 301
cardiac palpitation 316
cardiac problems 277
cardiac stimulant 210, 192
cardiodepressant 83
cardiomyopathy 3
cardioprotective 131, 234
cardiotonic 139, 147, 229, 230, 276, 297, 298, 316, 317
cardiotoxic 297
cardiovascular 83, 162
carminative 28, 143, 201
carotene 167
carotenoids 165, 168
Carthamus 164
cartilage 71
Carum carvi 229, 259
carvacrol 278
caryophyllene 278
Cassia auriculata 88
Cassia fistula 76
Cassia tora 76, 257
castor oil 30, 128, 192, 221, 299
castoreum 333, 334
cat's eye 320
catabolic diseases 36
catalase 230
cataplasm 233, 306
catarrh 147, 274
catarrhal matter 174
catatonia 253
catechin 77
catecholamine 50, 160, 203, 253, 306
catechu 50
catechutannic acid 249
cathartic 184
cauline 141
Cedrus 67
Cedrus deodara 229, 266
Celastraceae 196
celastrine 198
Celastrus 196–198
Celastrus paniculatus 196, 325, 329, 332
celery 31, 128, 265
cellular cytotoxicity 26
cellular immune response 154
cellular transcriptase 89
Centella 94, 95, 200–207, 252, 253, 276, 281, 283, 284
Centella asiatica 24, 94, 200, 285, 313, 325, 332
Centipede orbicularis 335
Central Asia 262
central nervous system 178, 198
Centurea behen 33

cephalic tonic 210
cerebral: blood flow 306; circulation 306; edema 167; excitant 143; ischaemia 250; stimulant 20, 283
cervical: spondylitis 131; spondylosis 53
cesium chloride 26
chameli phul 314
chandan 38
chandan, lal 313
Chanderody Ras 330, 334
Charak Sanhita 1, 11, 35
chataki 135
chava 319, 324
Chavan 32, 33
Chavanprasha 25, 32–37, 258
Chavanprasha Avleh 33, 36
Chavanprasha Special 36
chebulin 139
chebulinic acid 139
chemical kindling 51
chemiluminescence 218
chemokines 192
chemopreventive 278
chemoprotector 51
chemotactic 52, 111, 187, 290
chemotherapy 7
chemotype 46, 55
Chenopodium ambrosiodes 176
chicken pox 109
childbirth 275
chilka harar 135
china berry 218
Chinese medicine 165, 201
chini kabab 331
chiryata 151, 331
chitrak 98–101, 319, 328
Chlamydia trachomatis 217
chloestasis 186
chloretic 186; activity 186
chloroform 297
Chlorophytum tuberosum 214
Chlorophytum 159, 244, 245, 248, 265, 274
Chlorophytum arundinaceum 34, 118, 159, 214, 319, 330
chloropromazine 193, 203
chobchini 331
cholagogue 82, 151, 193
cholera 109
choleretic 151
cholesterol 27, 53, 77, 89, 100, 120, 129, 130, 138, 167, 187, 198, 235, 268, 286, 293, 306; oxygenated 130
cholesterolemia 174
choline 69, 72, 113
cholinergic 53, 83
cholinesterase 95
chromosomal aberrations 26, 96
chromosome 186; breakage 51
chronic bronchitis 24
chronic dysentery 24
chronic fever 28

chronic headache 29
chronic syphilis 149
chuara 102–104
Chupchap 102
churn 13
Chyavanprasha 32
cimetidine 178
cineole 182
cinnamic acid 186
Cinnamomum 39, 50, 67, 105, 106, 117, 222, 265, 275, 319, 322–324, 328
Cinnamomum iners 330
Cinnamomum tamala 235, 275
Cinnamomum zeylanicum 39
cinnamon 36, 50, 71, 173, 177, 222, 245, 265, 275, 276, 317, 319, 322, 323, 328–330; leaves 35
Cipla 129
cirrhosis 3, 106–108, 229
cisplatin 167, 168
Cissampelos pariera 39, 128, 222
citric acid 252
Citrullus colocynthis 31, 45
clacined ruby 334
clastigenic activity 186
clastogenic effect 26
Clerodendrum phlomoides 34, 37
Clerodendrum serratum 128
Clitoria ternatea L. 250
Clonazepam 51
Clostridia 193
clove 16, 50, 196, 221, 245, 317–319, 323, 329, 331–333
CNS 178, 276
CNS depressant 52, 145
CNS excitation 121
Cochlospermum religiosum 331
cognition facilitating 54
Colchicum 166
colic 253, 283
collagen 72, 205
colon cleanser 30
Combretaceae 135, 299
Commiphora 28, 107, 109, 111, 234
Commiphora mukul 124
Commiphora wightii 29, 45, 124, 321, 324
common cold 153
common salt 15
Compositae 190, 209, 233
conception 67
condensed tannins 301
conjunctivitis 221
Conscorea decusata 250, 329
constipation 24, 178
consumption 46
convalescence 29, 178
Convolvulaceae 309, 250
Convolvulus 283, 284
Convolvulus arvensis 202, 250, 285
Convolvulus microphyllus 250, 330
Convolvulus pluricaulis 313, 250

convulsion 52, 53, 77, 143, 237, 252
copper 314, 318, 324, 325, 328
coral 173, 319–321; red 314, 319, 323
coronary: artery 121; artery diseases 131, 234; circulation 121; heart problems 72
corticosteroids 25
cortisone 217
costunolide 192, 193
Costus 190
cotyledons 175
cough 316
coumarins 45
coumestans 82
Cowrie Pishti 315
Crateva religiosa 120
creatine 36
crocetin 165
crocin 165, 167, 168
Crocus longiflorus 168
Crocus sativus 38, 164, 329
cromoglycate 152
crotalid venoms 83
cryptolerin 69
cubebin 149
cubebol 149
cubic acid 149
culumbin 83
cumin 107, 128, 259, 275, 307, 318, 319
Curculigo 211, 244, 259
Curculigo orchioides 33, 39, 159, 212
Curcuma 54
Curcuma longa 334
Curcuma zedoaria 39
cutaneous anaphylaxis 223
Cyanaprasa 32
cyanide 60
Cycas 303
cyclic AMP 88
cyclophosphamide 7, 51, 182
Cydonia vulgaris 118, 245
Cymbidium aloifolium 242
Cyperus 59
Cyperus rotundus 38, 109
Cyperus scariosus 29, 30, 31, 45, 50, 100, 128, 159, 222, 229, 266
Cyprea monata 315
cyprohepatidine 51
Cyptolepis bruchani 31
cystitis 82, 147
cytochrome P-450 224
cytocidal 217
cytodestructive 286
cytokines 268
cytoprotectant 26, 139, 181, 286
cytotoxic 18, 139, 193, 239
cytotoxicity 26, 88, 223

d-galactosamine 186
d-isolysergic acid amide 309
d-lysergic acid amide 309

d-lysergic acid diethylamide 309
d-pinene 182
Dactylorhiza hatagirea 242
daidzein 306, 307
daidzin 307
dalchini 39, 317, 319, 322, 323, 328–330
Dalton's lymphoma 167
Darjeeling 295
Dashmula 33, 34, 38, 67, 109, 116, 335
date palm 102–104, 309
Datura 147, 316, 330
debility 46
deer 323
Deesons 333
degenerative diseases 72
dehydrocostus lactone 192
delirium 78, 274
demulcent 143, 212, 213
deobstruent 46
depressant 143, 203, 285
depression 50, 52, 53, 252
depressive illness 52, 161
dermatophytes 180
Desmodium gangeticum 34, 39, 258, 313
development of breast 209
Dey's Medical Stores 335
Dhanwantri 1
Dhara 69
Dhatri 22
Dhatriyadi yoga 260
Dhatu 4
Dhatu parivartan 290
Dhatu Paushtik Churn 119, 149
dhatura beej 316, 330
DHBV 89
Dhup 237
diabetes 3, 24, 28, 110, 235, 244, 278, 327
diabetes mellitus 107, 109, 131, 180, 193, 234
diamond 320
diaphoretic 274, 297
diarrhoea 17, 24, 110, 173, 316
diarylhepatanoids 182
diastase 271
diastolic blood pressure 7
diazepam 51, 204
dietary supplement 158
digestive 28, 147
digestive agent 267
digestive problem 80, 177
Digitalis 16, 227
di-hydroxycatechol 77
dill 67
Dioscorea bulbifera 33, 39, 330
diosgenin 121
Dirofilaria immitis 205
disability 331
diterpenoids alkaloids 298
diuretic 24, 43, 113, 120, 126, 170, 229, 270, 303

divy 94, 135
Divyadhara 22
DLA 167
DNA 239
DNA polymerase 88
Dolichos biflorus 67
dopamine (DA) 198, 204
dopaminergic: receptors 160;
    system 52
dosha 2, 11, 23, 165, 316
Draksha 38, 105, 106, 317
Draksharishta 14, 106
Drakshasav 106
Drakshavleh 106
dropsy 24, 299
duck hepatitis B virus 89, 139
dudh 319
duodenal: lesion 217; tumour 287;
    ulcer 28, 83, 187, 193, 205,
    258, 293
duodenitis 187
dysentery 17, 24, 110, 127, 151,
    173
dysfunctional uterine bleeding 306
dysmenorrhoea 177, 166, 202, 258,
    306, 326
dyspepsia 24, 28, 152, 184, 283
dysphonia 234, 286
dysuria 212

ECG 121
Echinops latifolia 193
Eclipta 30, 178, 210, 252
Eclipta alba 24, 30, 202, 315, 335
Eclipta prostrata 80
ecstasy 144
eczema 16, 173, 202, 277
egg shell ash 49
Ehrlich: ascites carcinoma 271;
    ascites tumour 205
ela 332; (big) 38; (small) 38
electrical kindling 51
electrocardiogram 286
electrographic activity 51
elephantiasis 202
Elettaria cardamomum 38, 67, 332
ellagic acid 26, 28, 37, 90, 139,
    301
ellagitannins 89
Embelia ribes 27, 29, 31, 76, 100,
    128, 203, 222, 229, 266, 286,
    313, 323, 332
Emblica 109, 159
Emblica officinalis 10, 22, 50, 86,
    110, 119, 202, 221, 229, 260,
    275, 313, 315, 321, 324, 332
emerald 314, 320
emetic 16
emmenagogue 165, 306
endocrine 7, 162
endosperm 178
endothelial antagonist 89
endothelial integrity 205
endotoxaemia 112

enlarged liver 24
Entamoeba histolytica 224, 267
enuresis 143
eosinophilia 301
Ephedra vulgaris 362
ephedrine 69
epicatechin 77, 106
epidermoid carcinoma 77
epigallates 301
epigastric pain 83
epilepsy 20, 94, 96, 250, 252, 285
epistaxis 82
Epstein-Barr virus 167
erectile dysfunction 212
ergoline 309
ergometrine 309
ergot 309
erogenous zone 165
erythrocyte 51, 239
erythrocyte sedimentation 53, 54,
    239
erythrocyte, norchromatic 52
erythrocyte, polychromatic 52
Escherichia coli 69, 121, 146, 259
essential oils 131
oestrogen 129
oestrogenic 306
eugenol 278, 286
Eulophia campestris 333, 242
Eulophia hormusjii 242, 244
Eulophia nuda 242
Euphorbiaceae 22, 86
Evolvulus alsinoides 250, 332
Evolvulus emarginatus 207
Exogonium purga 136
expectorant 16, 24, 274
eye: diseases 24; infection 326

Fabaceae 303
Fabry's disease 253
facial paralysis 74
fatty degeneration 198
febrifuge 151
fennel 31, 265, 307, 332
fenugreek 76, 266
ferrous sulphate 127
Ferula asafoetida 141
Ferula foetida 141
Ferula rubricaulis 141
fibrinogen 112
fibrinolysis 167
fibromyalgia 20, 244
Fibronytic activity 131
fibrositis 239
Ficus 289–294
Ficus bengalensis 289
Ficus benghalensis 289–294
Ficus racemosa 293
Ficus religiosa 289, 291–294
flatulence 30, 36, 177, 221, 229,
    289
flavones 306
flavonoid 69, 89, 90, 306
fly-agaric 262, 263

foetal abnormality 231
formalin 90
Fortege 331
Fo-Ti tieng 206
fractures 131
France 164
frankincense 237
free fatty acid 27, 293
free radical scavenging 54, 186
free radicals 26, 139
Fritellaria oxypetala 34
fructsopeptide 69
Fumaria indica 30, 109
fungi 83
furostanoic 121

GABA 205, 230
gaduchi 48, 107–113, 313, 321,
    332, 335
gaduchi satva 110, 315, 330
gaj 219
gaj peepal 219
galactagogue 49, 66, 257, 259,
    303, 307
galactosamine 121, 153
Galanga 180
galangin 182, 286
galangol 180
Galgumn-tang 306
gallic acid 37, 69, 90, 139, 161,
    174, 217, 301
Gamber's Lab. 333
Gambhari 38
gamma radiation 52, 204, 278
gandha 46
gandhak 328
Gandhak Bhasam 324
Gandhak Shodhit 315, 316, 318,
    322, 325
gangeran 64
ganna ras 319
Gardnerella vaginalis 217
gaseous distension 152
gastric: juices 153, 178; lesion 28;
    motility 139; mucosa 224;
    mucosal damage 187; secretion
    267; ulcer 52, 53, 193, 205,
    267, 293; ulceration 205; volume
    187
gastro-duodenal mucosa 286
gastro-enteritis 43, 100, 103, 110,
    127, 173, 212, 221, 222, 299
gastro-intestinal canal 245
gastro-intestinal motility 193, 293
gastropathy 286
geeldikkop 122
Gemlina arborea 38
Gemology 2
Gentamycin 112, 120
Gentiana kurroo 187
Gentianaceae 187
geraniin 89, 90
geratric tonic 53, 313, 212
ghansatva 13

ghee 13, 14, 23, 25, 30, 32, 38, 48, 50, 60, 76, 119, 125, 138, 159, 160, 170, 172, 174, 176, 191, 196, 202, 203, 210, 213, 220, 245, 255, 257, 258, 265, 267, 275, 291, 319, 321, 322, 325, 332
ghee kanwar 313
ghee kanwar ras 319
ghor vacha 281
ghrita 14
ghritam 14
Giardia duodenalis 224
Giardia lamblia 224
Giardia spp. 267
giloe 107
ginger 20, 21, 29, 30, 45, 50, 109, 111, 119, 120, 159, 173, 177, 221, 224, 227, 229, 265–268, 274, 275, 313, 315, 317, 319, 320, 323, 328, 329, 332; fresh 315
gingerol 182, 267, 268
ginseng 53, 309; Indian 46
gitogenin 121
glangin 182
glaucoma 162
globulin 37
glomerular filtration 230
glucine 69
glucose metabolism 193
glutamic acid 60
glutamic purvic transaminase 307
glutamino oxaloacetic transaminase 307
glutathione 100, 161, 186
glycaemia 174
glycaemic levels 111
glycerol 14
glycogen 153, 235, 306
glycogenolysis 198
glycolate dehydrogenase 120
glycolate oxidase 120
glycosidase inhibitor 253
glycosides 293
glycowithanolide 53, 54
Glycyrrhiza 48, 67, 69, 209, 211, 252, 253, 257–259, 266, 307, 313, 330
Glycyrrhiza glabra 29, 313, 330
Gmelina arborea 34
go 116
goat milk 30
gokhru 116
gokhru kalan 122
gokshru 116–122, 149, 270, 316, 317, 324, 332, 333, 335
gokshru (big) 38
gokshru (small) 38
Gokshru ghansatva 330
Gokshuradi churn 118, 119
Gokshuradi guggal 131
gold 36, 313, 321, 322, 325, 326, 330, 333–335

gold foil 325
gomed 320
gond katira 331
gond kikar 323
gonorrhoea 103, 127, 147, 212
gossypol 249
GOT 307
gotu kola 200, 309
gout 20, 34, 196
GPT 307
Grahwal 295
Granada 144
Greater *galanga* 180
Greco-Arabian system of medicine 165, 242
Greek and Roman mythology 242
Grewia asiatica 103
Grewia hirsuta 64
Grewia populifolia 64
Grewia tenax 64
guggal 28, 124–131, 237, 321, 322, 324
guggalsterone 130, 130
Guggulu 8
Guglip 129
gugulipid 130, 131
Guitika 159
gum acacia 170, 323
gum arabica 170, 172, 331
gum guggal 128
gum kino 172
gum tragacanth 118, 119, 172
Guru Padamsambhav 135
gustatory nerve 153
gyantantu 60
Gymnadenia 242
Gymnema 211
gynaecological problems 80, 172, 177, 319, 326
gypsies 242

H4IIEC3 rat hepatoma cells 223
Habenaria 242
Habenaria commelinifolia 242
Habenaria intermedia 34, 38
haematuria 82
haemoglobin 53, 204, 260
haemolytic antibody response 51
haemorrhages 82, 177
haemorrhagic lesions 83; ulcer 230
haemorrhoidas 67, 221
hair: care 160; darkener 192; growth 81; melanin 53; tonic 24
Haleileh e Jung 135
hallucinogenic 144, 262, 263, 281, 285
Halwa 76
Halwa Mundi 210
hara chirayta 151
harar 135
harar jangi 135
harar kabuli 136, 138
haritaki 77, 135–139, 221, 324, 332

harmine 120
hartal 325
Hathjori 243
Hawaiian Baby Rosewood 309
HbsAg 88
HBV 88, 89
HDL 198
headache 17, 81, 192
heart: attack 2; diseases 131, 233, 274; palpitation 315; problems 27
Hedychium spicatum 182, 266, 323
Hedyotis auriculata 45
heera 320
Helleborus niger 187
Helminthosporium sativum 90
hemidesmine 45
hemidesmol 45
Hemidesmus indicus 31, 67, 107, 127
hemidsterol 45
hemiplegia 20, 198, 244
henna 118
hepatectomised 88
hepatic: amoebiasis 138; congestion 83; damage 186; lactate dehydrogenase 120; lipid peroxidation 82; tenderness 88
hepatitis 60, 82, 88, 212, 153
hepatitis B surface antigen (HbsAg) 192
hepatitis B virus 186, 214
hepatocarcinogen 287
hepatocellular carcinoma 77
hepatocyte 88, 121, 153
hepatoma 88, 223
hepatoprotective 17, 26, 82, 84, 111, 121, 153, 186, 214, 217, 224, 235, 270, 300
hepatotoxic lesions 167
hepatotoxicity 54, 151, 217, 268, 307
heran singhhasam 323
Herba Indica 332
herpastine 96
herpes 286
Herpestis monniera 94
hessonite 320
hexabarbitol 145, 277, 285
Hibiscus abelomoschus 329
hicogenin 121
high blood pressure 252, 273, 315
high density lipoprotein 138
Himachal Pradesh 201
Himalaya Drug 332, 335
Himalayan 201, 269
Himalayas 190, 196, 233, 243, 262; foothill 157
Hind Chemicals 331
Hindu mythology 135
hing 141–143
hingul 325, 326, 328
Hingvastika churn 143
Hippocrates 1

histamine 37, 51, 83, 161, 203, 235, 253, 285
histaminergic 83
histidine 69
histopathological aberrations 51
HIV 69, 153, 217, 299
HIV-protease 139
Holarrhena antidysenterica 109, 229, 331
Holarrhena pubescens 27
homeostasis 186
homeostatic action 82
Homoeopathic 202
homosexual mounting 246
hook worm 286
hormonal imbalance 72
horn 323
human hepotoma Hep 3B cells 192
human papilloma 16 virus 217
human polymorphonuclear leucocyte 218
humoral activity 186
humoral components 239
humoral immune response 154, 274
humoral imuunity 186
humours 11
hydrocortisone 54, 285
Hydrocotyle asiatic minor 206
Hydrocotyle asiatica 200
Hydrocotyle javanica 207
Hydrocotyle rotundifolia 207
hydrocyanic acid 60
hydrolyzable tannins 26, 88, 301
hydroxyl 37
hydroxyl radicals 130
hydroxyproline 37
Hygrophila 48, 159, 245, 318
Hygrophila auriculata 270
Hygrophila spinosa 270, 309, 329, 333
hygrophytic 209
Hyocyamus 116
Hyoscyamus niger 333
hypaphorin 69
hyperacidity 27, 106, 177, 259, 315
hyperactivity 178, 285
hyperchlorhydria 27, 83, 259
hypercholesterolaemia 27, 129
hyperglycaemia 111, 234, 278
hyperhidrosis 27
hyperlipidaemia 129, 130, 240
hyperoxalurea 120
hyperseborrhic 160
hypertension 48, 52, 131, 167, 234, 274, 277, 305
hyperthermia 52, 100
hyperthyroidism 129, 130
hypertriglyceridaemia 129
hypnosis 276; potentiation 253
hypnotic activity 83
hypocholesterolemic 77
hypocholesterolic effect 77, 293
hypochondria 143

hypochondriasis 143, 201
hypoglycaemia 293, 305
hypoglycaemic 31, 89, 174, 217
hypoglycaemic effect 111, 193
hypolipidaemic 27, 100, 138, 146, 168, 182, 187, 198, 235, 293
hypolipidaemic agent 129–131
hypotensive 51, 162, 252, 306
hypotensive: activity 238; effect 121, 277; palpitation 162
hypothalamus 160
hypothermia 203
hypothyroidism 130
hypo-uricaemic effects 268
hysteria 143, 198, 252, 325

Ibn-Al-Baytar 180
ibotenic acid 263
Icnocarpus 45
Icnocarpus frutesecence 67
illiachi 323, 324
illiachi choti 317, 322
Imminex 331
immune system 268
immunity 2
immunity booster 60
immunoactive 82, 88
immunobuilder 118
immunodepression 51
immunoelectrophoresis 53
immunoglobulin 68, 230
immunohaemolysis 239
immunomodulator 26, 51, 54, 68, 88, 111, 112, 139, 167, 204, 218, 239, 268, 276, 277, 331, 335
immunomodulating effect 186, 259, 277
immunopotentiating effect 204
immunoresponse 186
immunostimulant 7, 72, 112, 154, 186, 211, 305
immunostimulating 224, 277
immunosuppression 112
immunosuppression effect 239, 276
immunosuppressive 51, 110, 111, 277
immunotherapeutic 111
immunotoxicological potential 239
imparipinnate 141, 237
impotence 48, 116–118, 149, 166, 265, 318
improvement of eyesight 210
incontinence of urine 177
indaconitine 298
Indian ginseng 46
Indian olibanum 237
Indian Pharmacopoeia 151
Indian sarsaparilla 43
Indian thyme 82, 265, 275
indigestion 30, 316, 323
Indo-gangetic plains 206
indomethacin 96, 267, 286
Indonesia 107, 144, 147, 200, 219

infectious hepatitis 82, 109
inflammation 18, 34, 43, 47, 48, 83, 54, 110, 229, 306, 315
inflammatory diseases 180
inflammatory pains 130
influenza 274, 316
inotropic 267
insanity 48, 94
insomnia 96, 204, 252, 255
insulin 24, 89, 111, 233, 235, 293
intelligence quotient 96
interferon 25
interlukin 52, 111, 260, 298
intestinal worms 109
intraocular tension 24
Inula 234
Inula racemosus 39, 131, 190, 193, 233, 265
inulin 21, 193
involuntary muscles 192
ipecacuanha 16
Ipomoea digitata 38, 303, 335
Ipomoea jalap 136
Ipomoea paniculata 335
Ipomoea reniform 207
Ipomoea turpethum 203
Iran 59, 141, 164, 242
Iraq 102
Iridaceae 164
iridoid glycosides 185
Iris 190
Iris florentina 233
Iris germanica 233, 281
iron 128, 167, 173, 178, 317–319, 321, 323, 324; ore 313; oxide 315; pyrite 313, 315, 320, 322
ischaemia 112, 214
ischaemic aorta 192
ischemic heart diseases 286, 233, 234
isobrahmic acid 206
isoflavins 306
isoflavone 307
isoflavonoids 307
Italy 164

Jadwar khatai 295
jaifal 331
Jain monks 60
jaiphal 144, 316–318, 322, 323, 329, 330, 332–335
jal brahmi 94
jal neem 94
jalap 136
jalap harar 136
Jamaican Sarsaparilla 43
Jammu 164
Jamu 182
Jaryan 331
jasmine 31, 314; flower 203; oil 210
jatamansi 329, 332
jatiphal 329
jattorhizine 113

jaundice 80, 82, 88, 89, 107, 108, 110, 112, 151, 217, 229
Java 144, 147
javitri 144, 316, 318, 323, 330, 331, 333, 334
Jawahar Bhasam 331
Jawahar Mohra 314, 315
jeera safed 318, 319
jeevak 33
jeevanti 331
Jiva 135
Jiva priya 135
jivak 33, 38
jivanika 135
jivanti 38, 135, 313
junde bedaster 333–334

kabab chini 147–149
Kabul 135, 136
Kabuli harar 136
kachula 331
kadali ras 334
Kaempferia galangal 182
kajjali 30
kaknasa 38
kakoli 33, 34, 38
kakra singhi 38, 317
kala azar 224
Kalami Amla 25
kali mirch 323, 328, 335
kalmegh 151–154
Kalmi 22
kamal phul. safed 314
kamarkas 319, 323
kamboji 331
Kamdeva 318
Kamdugdha Ras 315
kanghi 64, 66
kantkari 38
kantloha 334
kapha 11, 12, 28, 170, 297, 303, 321
kapur kachari 182
Karengro 242
Karnataka 60, 147
Kashmir 59, 164, 190, 281, 295
kasmiri 38
kasturi 314, 317
katha 313, 319
kawanch 157–162, 305, 313, 317, 318, 330–335
kaya kalp 5, 200, 202
Kayastha 135
KB human carcinoma cells 52
Kerala 74, 88
keratitis 54
kesar 38, 323, 330, 333–335
keshar 164–168, 317, 323, 333
khajur 102
kharanti 66
khas 329
Khulanjan 180
Khurasan 187
khurasani ajwain 333

khurasani kutaki 187
Khursani vacha 281
kikar 170–174
kikar gond 323, 331
kindling: amygloid 51; chemical 51; electrical 51
Kishtwar 164
Ko for 305
Krimighan 215
Krishna 272
Krishna tailam 196
ksheer kakoli 33, 34
Ksheer pak 167
Ksheerbala tailam 204
Kshir 69
Kshirdhara 69
kshru 116
kuchla 175–178, 330, 333, 334
kuchla oil 176, 177
kuchla shodhit 315, 316, 320, 335
kudzu 305
kulanjan 180–182
kundru 237
kushtha 317
kutaj 331
kutaki 184–187, 331, 335
kuth 190, 192, 329, 330
Kuti Parveshika 6, 200, 314
kuti prevesh 6
kutkin 186
kutkoside 186

L 3, 4 dihydroxyphenylalanine 160
L-dopa 160
Labiate 272
lac 131
Laccha zafran 164
lactate dehydrogenase 120
lactation 275
lactic acid 14, 306
laghu 34
Laghu raahmriga 275
Lahaul 190
Lahore 242
lajwanti 319
lal 320
Lal Pishti 314
Lamiaceae 272
lanceolate 151
laryngo-pharyngitis 277
lata kasturi 329, 335
lauha 317
Lauha bhasam 314, 318, 319, 321, 324
Lauha Kanta 313
lawang 317–319, 323, 329, 331–333
laxative 24, 28, 30, 139, 184, 186, 282, 299
Laxman Vilas Ras 316
Laxmi Vilas Ras 178, 315
LDH 5, 27, 120
LDL 28, 130, 198
Lea aquata 38

lead 26, 128, 176, 330, 335
lecithin 161
Leguminosae 157, 170, 303
lehya 14
Leishmania donovani 224
lemon juice 325
leprosy 16, 28, 100, 107, 196, 202, 277, 299
Leptadenia 259, 307
Leptadenia reticulata 38, 67, 313, 331
lesser *galanga* 180
leucocyte 7, 192
leucocyte count 239
leucocytosis 8, 52, 112, 120
leucodelphins 90
leucoderma 43
leucorrhoea 18, 28, 32, 43, 48, 49, 66, 106, 127, 131, 159, 172, 177, 202, 212, 217, 231, 244, 257, 275, 293, 318, 323, 326
leukaemia 77, 154, 259, 273
leukaemia HL–60 239
leukaemia L12120, P388 77
leukopelargonidin 293, 294
leukopenia 7, 52
leukotriene 267
levodopa 161
Li She Chin 305
liana 157
libido 48, 60, 68, 143, 161, 317
lignan 88, 90
Liliaceae 214
Lilium polyphyllum 34, 38
limonoids 217
lipase 271
lipid peroxidation 31, 54, 96, 153, 307, 278
lipid peroxide 37, 77, 90
lipoma 32
lipopolysaccharide 192
liquorice 20, 30, 31, 49, 204, 224
lithium-pilocarpine model 51
live vaccine virus 186
liver damage 82; DNA 186; glycogen 51, 193, 198; problems 229; stimulant 151; tonic 184; torpidity 152; toxicity 52
Loban 237
Lodhra 322
Loganiaceae 175
long pepper 21, 30, 35, 48, 50, 54, 71, 99, 106, 108, 109, 119, 126, 128, 149, 159, 167, 173, 177, 209, 224, 229, 245, 255, 275, 319, 320, 328, 329, 331
loose motion 30, 323
Lorazepam 96
loss of libido 10
loss of memory 325
lotus 31, 314; blue 314; flower 30; white 314
love amulet 242
love drug 144

low density lipoprotein 130, 138
LSD 309
luban 331
lumbago 82
Luminal 96
lymphocytes 52, 205
lymphoid organ 277
lysergic acid 309
lysosomal 96
lysosomal enzyme 77
lysosomal membrane 77, 78

mace 16, 21, 144–146, 159, 166, 167, 196, 245, 257, 266, 316, 318, 323, 330, 331, 333, 334
Macrohyporia extensa 285
macrophage 8, 52, 111, 112, 187, 193, 239
macrophage function 7
macrophage migration index 186, 224
Madanody Modak 317
madecassic acid 205
madecosside 205
Madagascar 200
madhu 38
magnesium carbonate 141
mahabala 64–66
mahameda 33, 34
Maharasayana yoga 305
mahashatawari 255
Mahatriphaladi Ghrit 30
Mahayograj guggulu 126, 128
Makardhawaj 36, 167, 313, 330, 333–335
Makardhawaj Ras 317
Makardhawaj Vati 317
makhan 325
Malabar Chemicals 333
malaria 197, 151, 217
Malaysia 144, 200, 219
male infertility 259
malkangani 196–198, 329, 332
Malkangani tail 325
Mallotus philippinensis 286
malti phul 314
Malva rotundifolia 207
Malvaceae 64
malvidin 3 glucosides 106
mammary tumour 211
Mandi 201
mandukparni 200, 313, 325, 330, 332
mango 326
Mankiya Ras 334
Mankya bhasam 334
Manmath 318
Manmath Ras 318
manshil 325
Maranta arundinacea 177
marich 331
marihuana 67
marking nut 74
marn 14

Marytenia diandra 38
mashparni 38
Mast 332
mast cell 152
Mastagi roomi 172
Mastomys 186
Mastomys natalensis 153, 186
masturbation 48
materia medica 126, 166
mating behaviour 161
Maxo Lab. 335
MDA 144
Meda 33, 34, 38
Medha Rasayana 7, 200, 250
medhya 82, 94
Medohar Guggal 128
medulla 192
meetha 190
meetha kuth 190
melancholia 166
Melaphis chinensis 39
melatonin 130
Melia azedarach 218
Meliaceae 215
Melocanna bambusoides 71
melon seed 60
memory enhancer 96, 97
Menispermaceae 107
menopausal syndrome 306
menorrhagia 212
menstruation 109, 159, 166, 202, 258; delayed 177; excessive 305
mental confusion 292
mental diseases 7
mental illness 196
mental retardation 60, 204, 285
mental tonic 250, 283
Mentat 332
mercury 2, 30, 178, 315, 318, 321, 322, 324, 325, 328
Merremia emerginata 207
mescaline 285
Mesua ferrea 35, 39, 50, 105, 106, 109, 117, 118, 159, 168, 173, 222, 266, 275, 319, 322, 323, 328
metallurgy 2
metaphase block 51
metastic pain 161
methicillin resistant 139
methyl cinnamate 182
methyl eugenol 278
metrinidazole 112
Mexico 67, 262
mica 36, 67, 128, 167, 173, 313, 316–319, 321, 323, 324, 334
Michelia champaca 168
Micostyllis wallichi 39
micronuclei 223
Microstylis spp. 34
Microstylis wallichii 34
migraine 17, 161, 177, 209, 268, 283, 305, 306
Mimosa pudica 319

Mimusops elengi 159
mint 275
mirch kali 315, 317, 320, 323, 325, 326, 328
mirch safed 323, 325
miscarriage 80
mishri 15, 323, 327
mitigation 178
mitochondria 30, 31, 106
mitotic abnormality 51
mochrus 247
mollusc 319; shell 315
molluscicidal 267
Moluccas Island 144
Momordica charantia 24
monamines 198
Mongra zafran 164
Moniera cuneifolia 94
monocyte 112
monoecious 141
mononuclear 268, 298
Moraceae 289
morning stiffness 54
Morocco 20
morphine 51, 111, 238, 277
mother of pearl 315, 319
Mucuna 147–149, 167, 213, 245, 248, 270, 274, 317, 318
Mucuna Forte 333
Mucuna pruriens 119, 157–162, 313, 330–333, 335
Mucuna prurita 157
Mucuna utilis 161
mucus 30
mukta 320, 322, 325
Mukta Bhasam 319
Mukta Panchamrit Rasayana 319
Mukta Pishti 314, 315, 322, 325, 326, 332, 334
Mukta Shukti Bhasam 319
Mukta Shukti Pishti 315
Mul 233
mulathi 313, 330
mundi 209–210, 329
Mundi Resinoid 210
munjatak 242
Muraba Harar 138
murine macrophage 52, 187
Musalyadi Churn 213
muscarine 69, 263
muscarinic receptors 161
Muscat 102
muscimol 263
muscle relaxant 198
muscular weakness 224
mushkafoor 316–318
musk 36, 312, 314, 317
musli 34, 212
musli, black 212
musli safed 319
musli, white 214
musta 38
mustard 128
mutagenesis 26

mutation 106
mycobacterial 186
Mycobacterium tuberculosis 286
mycotoxins 224
myeloid 154
myelosuppression 7, 51, 205
myocardial: contractility 298; infraction 154; ischemia 121; necrosis 27, 301
myotoxic effect 83
Myrica nagi 229
Myristica 253
Myristica fragrans 144, 333, 335
Myristica malabarica 146
myristicin 144, 146, 286

nag kesar 322, 328
nagbala 64–66, 313, 314, 316
nagkesar 39, 168
nagkeshar 319, 323
nakchikni 335
naphthalene derivatives 249
naphthaquinones 101
narcosis 51, 198, 276, 277
narcotic 1, 49, 101, 193, 194, 206, 299, 322
Nardostachys 204
Nardostachys grandiflora 67, 69, 222, 260, 266, 292
Nardostachys jatamansi 112, 221, 253, 292, 329, 332
Nari Kalyan Pak 319
Narmada 242
Narsimah churn 119
natural killer cell 26, 204
nausea 83, 162, 259, 265, 268, 325
Navjeevan Ras 320
Navjovan Ras 177
Navratna Ras 320
Navratnakalpa Amrit 321
Navsari peepal 219
Naysay 5
neck stiffness 305
necrosis factor 298
necrospermia 259
neelam 320, 321
Neelam Pishti 314
neelkamal phul 314
neem 6, 107, 215–218
Neem giloe 107
Neem oil 217
Neem tawagadi kashyam 217
nematodes 83, 216
nembutal hypnosis 96
neoandrographolide 152, 153
neogetogenin 121
neoplasms 77
neotigogenin 121
Nepal 255
Nepeta elliptica 253
Nepeta hindostana 253
nephroprotective 120
nephrotic 116, 229
nephrotic syndrome 230

nervine tonic 46, 82, 158, 196, 330
nervous: apoplexy 143; breakdown 201, 283; debility 47, 180, 201, 244, 292; irritability 143; tension 50
nervousness 316
Neta 215
neuralgia 166, 297
neuralgic affections 20
neurasthenia 94
neuritis 201
neurohumors 37, 252
neuroleptic effect 193, 203
neuromuscular blocking agent 306
neuromuscular system 177
neuropsychopharmaceutical 96
neuroticism 252
neurotransmitter 112
neutrophil 8, 112
nicotenolytic 51
nicotine 84
nicotinic acid 37, 83
Nigella 259
Nimba 215
nimbidin 217
nimbin 217
nimbnin 217
nimbu ka ras 325
nirgundi 319
niter 15
nitro-o-phenylenediamine 26
nitrogen balance 32, 120
Niwa Institute of Immunology 26
nocturnal emission 118, 122, 245, 290, 326, 327
non-steroidal 239
non-ulcer dyspepsia 82, 83
nootropic 96
norchromatic erythrocyte 52
norepinephrine (NE) 198, 204
normoglycaemic 217
North America 281
nortropane alkaloids 253
nutmeg 16, 21, 50, 60, 117, 144–146, 159, 166–168, 173, 196, 245, 257, 275, 286, 290, 316, 317, 322, 323, 329–334
nutritive tonic 27
nux vomica 175–178, 315, 320, 330, 331, 335
Nyctagenaceae 227
Nyctanthes arbor-tristis 277
Nymphea stellata 39

obesity 3, 29, 31, 129, 180, 221, 316
ochratoxin A 52, 111, 187, 260
Ochrocarpus longifolius 168
Ocimum sanctum 202, 272, 335
Ocimum tenuiflorum 272–278
oedema 34, 227, 239, 316
ojas 66
oligosaccharide 69
oligospermia 259

Onosma bracteatum 253
Operculina turpethum 149, 229
ophthalmology 1
opiate binding 223
opiodergic 96
opium 1, 21, 116, 176, 197, 290, 318
Orchidaceae 242
orchids 242
Orchis 33, 147, 148, 161, 167, 214, 242, 244, 245, 274
Orchis latifolia 34, 242–244, 335
Orchis laxiflora 242
Orchis maculata 242, 246
Orchis mario 242
Orchis mascula 33, 242, 329, 331, 332, 334
Orchis militaris 242
Orchis pyramidalis 242
Orchis sambucina 242
Orchis simia 242
organo-metallic compounds 312
organo-phosphate pesticides 197
Oroxylum indicum 34, 39, 332
orris 233
osteoarthritis 8, 130, 239
osteoporosis 71, 72
otorhinolaryngology 1
overiectomised 306
ovulation 318
oxalate 120
oxalic acid 69
oxygenated cholesterol 130

P388 lymphocytic leukemia 77
p-methoxy salicylic aldehyde 45
Pachak Peepali 221
Pachoni 135
Paederia foetida 33
paediatrics 1
pak 14
Pakistan 59, 242
Palmae 102
palmatine 113
pan 329
Pan ki Jar 180
pan ras 316
Panchamrit Ras 321
panchang 292
panchbala 64
panchkarma 5, 6, 32
pancreas 24
pancreatic islet 54, 111
panicle 151
paniculatine 198
panna 320
Panna pishti 314
papain 18, 267
papaverine 51, 121, 138, 285
papilloma 167
papillomagenesis 278
Paraadi Ras 322
paracetamol 26, 153
parad 315, 325, 328

Parad Bhasam 316, 318, 321, 322, 324
Parad shodhit 315
paralysis 20, 177, 196, 315, 325
paralytic attack 143
Paris polyphylla 281
parkinsonianism 160
Parsik vacha 281
parturition 66
parval 320, 321, 323
Parval bhasam 314, 319
passive cutaneous anaphylaxis 152
patala 39
patha 39
patra 39
Pavonia odorata 45, 50
peach oil 60
pearl 314, 315, 319, 320, 322, 324, 325, 332, 334
pearl paste 334
Pedalium 245
Pedalium murex 38, 110, 116, 122
peepal 291, 292
Peepal avleh 292
peepali 219–225, 303, 313, 319, 320, 323, 328, 329
Peepali asav 221
Peepali churn 221
Peepali pak 221
Peepali quath 221
Peepla mul 219
Peganum harmala 262
Penicillium expansum 299
penile erection 193
pentabarbitone 223, 276, 285
pentabarbitone hypnosis 34
pentabarbitone sodium 83
Pentatrapsis microphylla 38
Pentovax 329
pentylene tetrazole (PTZ) 51, 276
pepper: black 29, 50, 80, 109, 119, 159, 173, 177, 202, 221, 229, 274–276, 315, 317, 320, 323, 324, 328, 331, 335; white 323, 325
peppermint 147
pepsin 28
pepsin hydrolysis 60
peptic ulcer 28, 82, 273; dyspepsia 83
peptide 89
Periploca aphylla 262
petiolate 151
phagocytic activity 224
phagocytic function 239
phagocytic index 112
phagocytosis 8
pharyngo-tonsilitis 153
Phaseolus aconitifolius 39
Phaseolus mungo 60, 159, 170
Phaseolus trilobus 39
phenolic acid 69
phenylbutazone 54, 285
phenylethylamine 69

phenytoin 223, 253
Philippines 197
Phoenix dactylifera L. 102
Phoenix sylvestris 102
phosphaturia 116
phospholipid 28, 89, 100, 130, 293
photochemotherapy 187
photosensitivity 122
phototoxic 83
phyllanthin 88, 90
Phyllanthus 86–90
Phyllanthus amarus 38, 86–89
Phyllanthus debile 86, 88
Phyllanthus emblica 22, 28, 30, 31, 37, 131
Phyllanthus fraternus 86–89
Phyllanthus maderaspatensis 86
Phyllanthus niruri 178, 86, 89, 90
Phyllanthus simplex Retz. 86
Phyllanthus urinaria 86, 87, 89
Phyllanthus virgatus 86, 87
phyllembin 301
physiotherapy 2, 8
Pichumarda 215
picrocrocin 167, 168
Picroliv 185, 186
Picrorhiza 227
Picrorhiza kurroa 31, 45, 100, 109, 128, 187, 331, 335
Picrorhiza kurrooa 184
picroside I 185
piles 24, 147, 149, 212, 221
pillasterol 225
Pind khajur 102
pine kernel 60
Pinus 67, 318
Piper 331
Piper betle 18, 147, 166, 210, 222, 316, 329, 333, 335
Piper chaba 105, 128, 319, 324
Piper cubeba 21, 105, 118, 147, 159, 221, 222, 229, 249, 265, 275, 284, 331
Piper longum 18, 31, 39, 50, 105, 177, 219–225, 229, 313, 319, 323
Piper nigrum 18
Piper peepuloides 219
Piper retrofractum 219
Piperaceae 147, 219
piperine 223, 224, 225
piperlonguamine 225
piplamul 225, 319, 323
piplartine 225
pippali 39, 60
Pippali Rasayana 224
pishti 322, 325
pistachio 174, 245
Pistacia galls 67
Pistacia lentiscus 172, 221, 229, 245, 248, 317
Pit shamak Rasayana Churn 110
pitta 11, 12, 28, 33, 59, 170, 255, 321

Pitta jawar virodhi 184
plasma 233; cortisol 7; insulin 193; lecithin 187
Plasmodium 217
Plasmodium berghei 153, 186
Plasmodium falciparum 299
Platanthera 242
platelet aggregation 131, 167
Pluchea lanceolata 265
plumbagin 100, 101
Plumbaginaceae 98
Plumbago 98–101
Plumbago capensis 98
Plumbago indica 98
Plumbago rosea 98
Plumbago zeylanica 50, 98, 105, 128, 222, 229, 319, 328
Pohkarmul 233
poliomyelitis 69
polyacetylenes 83
polychromatic erythrocyte 52
polycyclic alkaloids 259
Polygala 285
Polygonatum verticillatum Moench. 34, 38
Polygonum aviculare 149
polyhydroxy tropane 253
polymorphonuclear neutrophils 239
polypeptide 83
polyphenolic flavonoids 293
polyphenols 301
polysaccharides 193, 217
polysomnographic 112
polyurea 36, 109, 209, 212, 322
pomegranate 103, 326
poppy seed 60, 159
potassium nitrate 118, 193, 229
power pills 333
Prananda 135
prasha 33
prashnaparni 313
Pratpathya 135
precious stones 331
pre-convulsive dyspnoea 277
pregnancy 49
premature ejaculation 48, 60, 119, 149, 161, 245, 290
premature graying of hair 30, 81
Premna integrifolia 37
preulcerogenic 187
primordial tissue 4
prishanparni 39
procyanidins 106
progestrogenic 306
prolactin 161
propranol 111
prostaglandin 96, 182, 239, 267, 268, 277
prostaglandin E-2 192, 234
prostate gland 77, 110, 147
prostate problem 44
protease 271
protein kinase catalytic subunit 88

proteolytic enzyme 267
protoberberine 113
protolytic enzyme 18
protozoal 217
Prunus amygdalus 59
Prunus paddam 67
pseudoaconitine 298
pseudoephedrine 69
pseudotannin 69
pseudotropane 253
psoriasis 160, 192, 202
psychedelic 182, 309
psychiatric disturbances 162
psychiatry 1
psychic anxiety 204
psychoactive 94
psychological 7
psychomotor performance 53, 204
psychosomatic 7
psychotropic 50, 95, 252, 277
Pterocarpus santalinus 38, 258, 266, 276, 313
Ptychotis 229
Ptychotis ajwain 82
Pueraria 245, 259, 265, 303, 316, 318, 319
Pueraria hirsuata 306
Pueraria lobata 305
Pueraria thomsonii 305, 306
Pueraria thunbergiana 307
Pueraria tuberosa 33, 39, 49, 258, 303, 334
puerarin 306, 307
pukhraj 320
Pukhraj Pishti 314, 321
pulmonary 162
puncture vine 116
punernava 39, 227–231, 313
Punernava Mundur 229
pungent *ras*
Punica granatum 324
Punjab 242
purgative 80
Purvakarma 5
Pushkar 233
Pushkar guggal 131, 234, 235
pushkarmul 39, 126, 190, 233–235
Putana 135
putranjivain A 26
pyknotic nuclei 167
pyrethrin 21
Pyrethrum germanicum 20
pyrexia 34
pyro-type alkaloids 298
pyrogallol 139
pyrrolidine 253

quarternary alkaloids 113
quercetin 26, 90, 106, 293
Quercus 29

radiation 100
radiation induced toxicity 26
radical 141

radioprotective effect 278
radiosensitizing 52, 100
Radix puerarie 306
rajat 322, 328
rajat bhasam 313, 321
rajat vark 314
Rajvari Pishati 321
rakt pitta 59, 66
rakta soksha 5
ral safed 318
Ram 272
Ramchuramani Ras 322
ramdzan 102
Randia dumetorum 266
Ranunculaceae 295
ras 10
Ras sindur 177, 245, 313, 320, 326, 328
rasa 4
Rasaunt 322, 324
Rasayana chikitsa 200
Rasayana therapy 5
rasna 180, 233
Rativallabh churn 245
Rativallabh Pak 173, 245, 323
Rauvolfia 253
Rauvolfia serpentina 112, 330, 334
Ravin 333
Ravisamha 215
red coral 323
red eyes 326
red ochre 315
red sulphide of mercury 36, 167, 245, 317, 320, 324, 328, 330, 333–335
refrigerant 24
relapse of anus and vagina 172
relaxant 51
renal disease 229
reserpine 203, 286
respiratory stimulation 51
restonsis 154
restorative 242
reverse transcriptase 26
Rheum palmatum 118
rheumatic pain 166, 127, 233
rheumatism 20, 46, 111, 126, 196, 201, 217, 237, 239, 283, 306
rheumatoid arthritis 111, 130, 192, 239, 267
Rhus succedanea 38
riddhi 33, 34, 39
rifampicin 186
Rigveda 32, 262
ringworm 233
rishbhak 33, 34, 39
RNA 186, 239
rock salt 67
Roghan badam 60
rohini 135
Roscoea purpurea 214
round worm 286
Rubia cordifolia 67
ruby 314, 320

ruscogenin 121
Russia 193

Sacharomyces cerevisiae 106
sacred basil 202
safed musli 255, 330, 331, 335
saffron 36, 60, 103, 173, 174, 292, 312, 317, 323, 330, 333–335
safranal 167, 168
sahastr 14
sahastra puti 14
Sahlep 242
Sakariya 102
salab mishri 332
salab panja 333
salai guggal 124, 237
salam badshah 242
salam lahori 242
salam lahsunia 242
salam mishri 329, 331, 333, 334, 335, 242, 244
Salam pak 245
Salam pak forte 245
salam panja 242
Salem 242
Salep 242–246
Salmalia 159
Salmalia malabarica 247, 335
Salmonella typhi 68, 187, 217
Salmonella typhimurium 26, 139, 301
saltpeter 15
salty *ras* 10
Salvia plebia 331
samshodhna 5
samunderphul 309
sandal 50
sandalwood 21
Santalum album 31, 149, 222, 266, 331
Sapindus mukorosii 24, 327
saponins 259, 301
sapphire 314, 320; blue 314
sapt dhatu 10
Sarangdhara 103
Saraswat ghrit 203
Saraswati 94
sarcoma 180 52, 181, 271
sarcoma 180 solid tumour 167
sarcoma180 ascites tumour 217
Sarcostemma brevistigma 262
Sardai 60
sariva 43
sarpagandha 334
Sarsaparilla: American 43; Indian 43; Jamaican 43
Sarswat churn 284
satavari 305, 329
sathi 39
Satyrion 242
Satyrium nepalensis 242
Saussurea 201, 222, 253
Saussurea costus 190

Saussurea lappa 31, 39, 190, 202, 203, 229, 233, 234, 317, 329, 330
Saussureae Radix 190
saussureamine A 193
saussurine 192, 193
Sayastha 22
schizonticidal 217
schizophrenia 198, 253, 325
sciatica 20, 74, 77, 130, 221
Scindapsus officinalis 128, 159, 219
Scitamineae 180, 214
scorpion sting 66
scrofula 202
Scrophulariaceae 94, 184
sedative 46, 51, 145, 165, 203, 285, 325
semal musli 247, 335
Semecarpus anacardium 74, 119, 176, 330
Semecarpus oil 286
seminal vesicles 160
seminal weakness 110
senescence 71
senna 166
sennoside 139
Senseveria roxburghiana 128
septicaemia 112, 187, 217
Serankottai Nei 77
seratonin 51, 161, 198
Serpentine 314
Serpgandha 330
serum alkaline phosphate 84
serum cholesterol 234, 293
serum glutamic oxaloacetic transminase 27
serum glutamic pyuruvate transminase 27
serum insulin 293
serum lactic dehydrogenase 27
serum lipid 235
serum proteins 53, 54, 260
sesame 77, 119, 330; oil 24, 39, 177
sesamin 225
Sesamum indicum 76
sesquiterpene 193
sesquiterpene glycosides 211
sex stimulant 20, 322, 335; tonic 246, 334, 335
sexual: behaviour 160, 161; debility 50, 117, 122, 248, 305, 331; inadequacies 67, 110, 119, 149, 231, 244, 245, 290, 291; vigour 333
sexually transmitted diseases 108, 127
SGOT 27
SGPT 27
Shaddharna yoga 100
Shahi zafran 164
shakar 39, 317
Shakla shreshta 135
shalparni 39

Shankh bhasam 315, 319
shankh pushpi 250–253, 313, 329, 330, 332
Shankhpushpi pills 252
Shankhpushpi syrup 252
Sharad 94
Sharma 94
shat 14
shatawari 60, 149, 255–260, 270, 313, 316–318, 330, 333–335
Shatawari ghrit 258
Shatawari pak
Shatawari ras 315, 319, 322
shathi 323
shatputi 14, 322
Shay rat 153
Shay ulceration 217
sheetal 147, 215
sherbet 24
shilajit 127, 173, 321, 323, 330, 333–335
shital chini 147, 331
Shitavirya 290
Shitphal 22
Shiva 22
shodhit 313, 328
shogaols 268
shoynka 39, 322
Shreephala 22
Shreyasi 135
Shukar Amritika Vati 324
shukra 6
Siberia 262
Sida 34, 265, 317, 318, 335
Sida acuta 64, 65, 67
Sida alba 64, 65
Sida alnifolia 64, 65
Sida althaefolia 64, 65
Sida caprinifolia 64, 65
Sida cordifolia 38, 64, 65, 68, 119, 149, 159, 257, 333, 335
Sida grewioides 64
Sida herbacea 64, 65
Sida humilis 64, 65
Sida lanceolata 64, 65
Sida orientalis 64, 65
Sida ovata 64
Sida retusa 64, 65
Sida rhombifolia 64, 65, 67–69, 119
Sida rhomboidea 34, 64, 65, 69
Sida rhomboidea var. *rhomboidea* 65
Sida rotundifolia 64, 65
Sida spinosa 64, 65, 68, 119, 313, 314, 316
Sida veronicaefolia 64–66, 68, 69
Siddha 77
silicic acid 50, 72, 106
Silent Valley 88
silica 31, 71, 72
silicious concretion 71
silk cocoon 314
silver 128, 313, 314, 328; foil 36
Silybium marianum 153
silymarin 69, 153, 186

Simhanda guggal 126
sindur 317
Singalila range 295
sinusitis 283
sitoindosides VII-X 54
sitosterol 83
skeletal muscle depressant 145
skin eruption 160
sleep inducer 48
sleeplessness 49, 50
sluggish liver 151
small pox 109
Smilax aristolochaefolia 43
Smilax chinensis 53, 149
Smilax glabra 331
Smilax ornate 43
Smritisagar Ras 325
smundra sosh 331
snake venom 83
soap nut 24
soap stone 118
sodhna 14
sodium bicarbonate 147, 149
sodium phenobarbitone 203
Solanum indicum 34, 38
Solanum surattensis 30, 38
Solanum xanthocarpum 30, 34
Som ras 262
soma 289
somnifera 48
sonth 265, 267, 268, 313, 317, 319, 320, 323, 328, 329, 332
Sooksham Triphala 30, 31
South Africa 200
South India 144
Spain 20, 59, 164
spasmolytic 285
spermatic fluid 327
spermatogenesis 160, 178
spermatogenic 210, 258, 303
spermatorrhoea 116, 119, 122, 149, 184, 231, 245, 290, 327
spermatozoa 160
spermotoxic 182
Sphaeranthus africanus 209
Sphaeranthus amaranthoides 211
Sphaeranthus indicus 209, 213, 329
spinescent 270
Spiti 190
spleen 277
spleen enlargement 80, 326
spondylitis 239
Spy 334
Sri Lanka 144, 147, 200, 201
sringi 39
stag 323
stag horn 36
stalactite tears 237
Staphylococcus 192
Staphylococcus aureus 68, 69, 121, 139
status epilepticus 51
Stephania hernandifolia 100
Stereospermum suvalens 34, 39

Stereospermum tetragonum 39
sterility 48, 49
steroidal 51, 306; glycosides 260;
    lactone 54; sapogenin 121, 260;
    saponin 121
stigmasterol 83
stomach: ache 109; diseases 219;
    troubles 24, 30
Strenex 334
Streptococcus 192
strychnine 18, 95, 178
Strychnos nux vomica 175, 316, 333,
    334
Strychnos potatorum 118
style and stigma 335
Styrax benzoin 331
Subhagya Shunthi Pak 265
sudden deafness 305
sudorific 43, 209, 282
Sukha Mewa 323
Sukhad 331
sulphide of mercury 177, 312
sulphonyl urea 217
sulphur 178, 315, 316, 318, 322,
    324, 325, 328
Sumatra 144, 147
Sunder Vati 27
sunth 331
supari 319
superoxide 31, 37, 90
superoxide dismutase 111, 153
Sureshta 94
surface antigen expression 88
Sushrut Samhita 1, 129
suvaran bhasam 314, 333
Suvaran Malini Vasant 325
suvaran vark 314, 315, 326
suvarn 321, 322
Suvarna Vasant Malti 326
Swapan mehtank 327
swarn makshik 315, 320
swarn makshik bhasam 313, 322
swarn vang 330
sweet *ras* 10
Swertia 29, 151, 227
Swertia chirata 331
swimming stress 53
Symplocos racemosus 222, 322
syphilis 16, 43, 44, 100, 107, 127,
    149, 172, 202, 209, 292
Syrian golden hamster 307
Syzygium cumini 24

T-lymphocyte 112, 193
tabashir 71, 72
Tacca aspera 33
tagar 332
tagets 164
tajpatr 330
talamkhana 270–271, 318, 319,
    329, 333
talisman 242
talispatra 324
tamar 325, 328

Tamar Bhasam 314, 318, 321, 326
tamarind 326
tankan 323
Tankan Bhasam 316, 324
Tankan shodhit 315
tannins: condensed 301;
    hydrolyzable 301
tejpat 39, 319, 322, 323, 324, 328
tenesmus 17
Tentex Forte 335
Teramnus labialis 38
Terminalia arjuna 68, 117, 234,
    332
Terminalia bellirica 28, 30, 31, 75,
    119, 229, 299–301, 321, 324,
    332
Terminalia chebula 15, 28, 30, 31,
    37, 75, 76, 99, 100, 119, 135,
    203, 229, 258, 321, 324, 332
terpenoids 240
terrestronis A-E 121
terrestroside F 121
testosterone 37, 120
tetanic convulsion 178
thankuni 206
thermic changes 52, 53
Thespesia populanea 224
thioacetamide 186
thiophene 83, 84
thirst quencher 103
threadworm 286
throat problem 257
thrombi 154
thrombogenic 154
thymecotomy 285
thymocyte 112
thymus 187, 277
thyrogenic 224
thyroid 129, 193
thyroid peroxidase activity 224
thyroid stimulation 131
Tibet 190, 295
tigogenin 121
til 330
til oil 39
tin 36, 49, 128, 173, 313,
    317–319, 321, 322, 327, 330,
    331, 334, 335
Tincture asafoetida 143
Tinospora 29, 30, 33, 44, 48, 67,
    125, 127, 159, 213, 252, 321,
    322, 335
Tinospora cordifolia 37, 43, 107,
    205, 313, 332, 335
Tinospora crispa 107, 109, 111
Tinospora malabarica 107
tissue culture 51
tocopherol 186
tolbutamide 111
tonic 242
topaz 320, 321
tourmaline 320
toxicology 1
Trachyspermum ammi 318

tranquillizer 83, 197, 238, 285,
    325
Trapa bispinosa 60
Trasina 335
triacylglycerols 293
Trianthema monogyna L. 227
Tribestan 121
tribulin activity 53
Tribulus 53, 116–122, 159, 172,
    213, 265, 274, 316, 317
Tribulus alatus 112
Tribulus terrestris 34, 38, 116, 131,
    324, 330–333, 335
Trichodesma indicum 202
tridosha 2, 43, 297, 321
trifacial neuralgia 297
trifoliate 157
triglyceride 28, 32, 89, 100, 129,
    130, 138, 198, 235, 240, 293
Trigonella 257
Trikatu 221, 225
Trinkantmani 334
Triphala 25, 28–30, 32, 124, 125,
    128, 130, 138, 159, 229, 284,
    299, 321, 322
Triphala guggul 31
triterpenic acid 240
triterpenoid 84
triterpenoid sapoinins 204
Triumfetta rotundifolia 64, 69
Trivang Bhasam 330, 335
tropane alkaloids 253, 263
tropinone 253
Trypanosoma 217
tubercular meningitis 96
tuberculosis 103, 112, 126, 322,
    326
tubular damage 198
tulsi 272–278, 335
Tulsi arshta 275
tumour 26, 51, 52, 100, 167, 205
tumour necrosis 121
tumour necrosis factor 52, 111,
    260
Turkey 59, 141, 164, 242
turmeric 29, 31, 107, 109, 203,
    222, 229, 239, 321
twak 39
tyrosine 69

ulcer 28, 53, 192, 202, 205, 286
ulceration 267
ulcerogenic effect 239
Umbelliferae 141, 200
Unani medicine 165
Unani-Tibb 242
uraemia 139, 301
Uraria lagopoides 39
Uraria picta 34, 39, 258
urethane 52
urethra 177, 193, 209
urethritis 147, 149
uric acid 268
urikinase 167

urinary: inflammation 209; nitrogen 36; problems 275; tract infection 131, 315
urinogenital 127, 209, 324; diseases 108, 172
urolithiasis 120
Urtica 66
uscharidin 18
uterine haemorrhage 80
Utopian Bliss Balls 309
utpala 39
Uttar Pradesh 74
uva-ursi 116

vacha 281–287, 325, 330, 331
Vacha, Bal 281
Vacha, Ghor 281
Vacha, Khurasani 281
Vacha, Parsik 281
Vagbhatta 250
vagus nerves 192
vaidyas 312
vajikarna 1, 6
valerian 50, 222
Valeriana wallichii 332
valeric acid 193
vamna 5
van mung 39
Vanda 211
vang 317, 327, 332
vang bhasam 313, 318, 319, 322, 331, 334
vanillic acid 186
varahi kand 330
vardhara 331
Vardhman Peepali 224
Varunadi kwath 120
vasaka 322
Vasant Kusmakar Ras 327
vascine 69
vascular sclerosis 253
vasicinone 69
vasoconstrictor 89, 170
vasodilater 180, 223
vasodilation 178, 206
vasopressin 198
vata 11, 33, 49, 50, 59, 67, 68, 255, 297, 321

vata vriksh 289–294
vatsnabh 295, 297, 313, 328
vavading 313
vayastha 94
vayu 11
veda 1
vedic 262
Veerya Shodhna Churn 173
vegetable mercury 16
venereal diseases 147, 172, 297
venous enlargement 83
venous hypertension 205
vermifuge 107, 109
Verpamil 120
vesical irritability 147
vesicant 74, 78
Vetiveria 45, 222, 266
Vetiveria zizanoides 329
vibhitaki 299–301, 324, 332
vichar 2
vidari kand 39, 149, 303–307, 316, 318, 319, 335
vidhara 49, 309–310, 317, 318, 333, 335
vidhara beej 316
Vidharaiadi churn 245
vidurya 320
vijaya 135
vincristine 77
Viola bicolor 276
Viotex 335
viral hepatitis 153, 186
virechna 5
virility 66
virya 33, 290
vish 295
Visha Rasayana 328
Vitaceae 105
vital fluid 33
vitamin A 167
vitamin C 27, 35, 37
Vitex agnus-castus 128
Vitex negundo 105, 319
vitiligo 187
Vitis vinifera 38, 105
vomiting 325
Vrhida Vangeshwar Rasa 328
Vridhi 33, 34

Vrihata 34
Vrishya 22
vyahar 3

wadelolactone 83, 84
walnut 60, 245
wasting disease 176, 321, 322, 327
Wedelia calendulacea 80, 84
weight loss 31
white pepper 323, 325
whooping cough 143
withaferin A 51–55
Withania 67, 147–149, 159, 190, 239, 245, 253, 257, 275
Withania ashwagandha 46
Withania somnifera 29, 30, 31, 33, 38, 46–55, 319, 329, 330, 332–335
withanolide D 51, 54
withanolide E & F 55
withanolide G & H 55
withanolides 52, 54, 55
withanone 55
woodchuck hepatitis virus 88
Woodfordia 221, 222
Woodfordia floribunda 14
Woodfordia fruticosa 105, 106, 120
worm infestation 323
Wrightia tinctoria 100, 128
wrought iron 334

yamogenin 121
yashad 321, 322, 323, 325
Yashad Bhasam 326
yeast 83, 180
Yogi Pharmacy 331, 334
Yograj Guggal 128
yukti 2

zafran 164
Zahar mohra 314
Zandu 330, 334
zero glycemic index 193
Zharkhalati 102
zinc 239, 321–325, 330, 335
Zingiber officinale 27, 265–268
Zingiberaceae 265
Zizyphus 67

CPSIA information can be obtained at www.ICGtesting.com
Printed in the USA
BVOW09*0939300916

463785BV00022B/24/P